Family-Oriented Primary Care

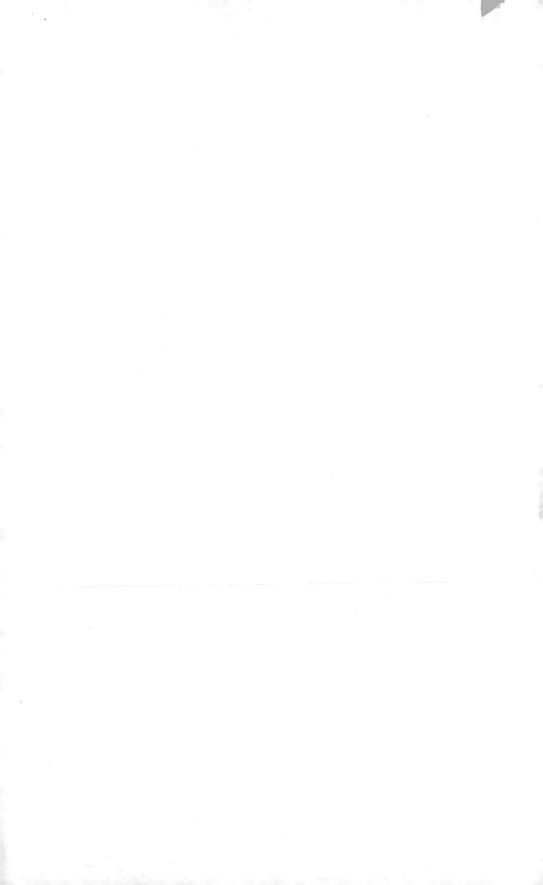

Susan H. McDaniel   Thomas L. Campbell
David B. Seaburn

Family-Oriented Primary Care

A Manual for Medical Providers

With a Foreword by Jack H. Medalie

With 11 Illustrations

Springer-Verlag

New York Berlin Heidelberg London Paris
Tokyo Hong Kong Barcelona Budapest

Susan H. McDaniel
Thomas L. Campbell
David B. Seaburn
University of Rochester
School of Medicine and Highland Hospital
Jacob B. Holler Family Medicine Center
Rochester, NY 14620
USA

Library of Congress Cataloging-in-Publication Data
McDaniel, Susan H.
  Family-oriented primary care : a manual for medical providers /
Susan H. McDaniel, Thomas L. Campbell, David B. Seaburn.
    p.   cm.
  Includes bibliographical references.
  ISBN 0-387-97056-8 (alk. paper)
  1. Family medicine. 2. Family. I. Campbell, Thomas L. (Thomas
Lothrop) II. Seaburn, David B. III. Title.
  [DNLM: 1. Family. 2. Family Practice—methods. 3. Primary Health
Care—methods.   WB 110 M478f]
R729.5.G4M3735   1989
610—dc20
DNLM/DLC
                                                              89-21890

Printed on acid-free paper.

Typeset by Caliber Design Planning, Inc.
Printed and bound by Braun-Brumfield, Inc., Ann Arbor, Michigan.
Printed in the United States of America.

9 8 7 6 5 4 3 2

ISBN 0-387-97056-8 Springer-Verlag New York Berlin Heidelberg
ISBN 3-540-97056-8 Springer-Verlag Berlin Heidelberg New York

This book is dedicated to our children:
Hanna, Marisa, Megan, Rachel, & Emily

Foreword

Integrating the family into Family Medicine has been recognized to be vital for the continued existence and development of the discipline. However, inserting a family orientation into primary care is somewhat revolutionary but seems logical if we accept Richardson's simple dictum, that the "family is the unit of living so it must be the unit of illness"(1). In this context, this book is a timely and important addition. The authors review the theory and centrality of the family orientation in primary care practice, discuss the different levels of practice, and then skillfully illustrate the principles of a family-oriented practice using examples of patients and their families. They emphasize biopsychosocial and family system concepts, a family orientation toward patients with chronic disease, specific health problems, health care during life-cycle transitions, and finally detail the organization of a family-oriented clinical practice.

It is interesting to reflect on the historical context of this orientation and to see how society and medicine interacted to produce a family orientation. Following World War I (1914–18) there were interrelated changes in many areas of human endeavor. Industrialization, urbanization, labor mobility, unemployment, and depression in the 1920s and 1930s led to many social changes and to the conflagration of World War II (1939–45) with its associated depravity and unimaginable horrors of the concentration camps and holocaust.

In reaction to all this there was, on the one hand, a rise in idealism and enthusiasm for a better, equal-opportunity world with rethinking, rebuilding, and new construction in almost every field of activity. On the other hand, a few governments were involved in a "no holds barred" race to harness atomic energy and power for space exploration and defense purposes, despite the potential for destruction of our planet.

These societal forces and changes influenced ideas, innovations, experiments, and publications pertaining to the family in three interrelated areas. These were: society in general, in medicine in the generic sense, and in the emergence of primary care as an important factor in medical care and education.

In society in general, numerous publications appeared which reflected these changes. These included: *Families in Trouble* by Koos (2), *Families Under Stress* by Reuben Hill (3), *La Vida* and other stories by Oscar Lewis (4), and the writings of Margaret Mead, the Gillins (5), Ben Paul (6), and Carol Stack (7). These publications highlighted the cultural, emotional, and socioeconomic aspects of societal changes, emphasizing both the upheavals and the strengths of families. They strengthened the theory that whatever changes society undergoes, the family will adjust to these and remain a "haven in the storm." The period from 1920 to 1950 (under the influence of Burgess and colleagues) has been referred to by Adams (8) as the period of scientific study of the family. From 1950 to the present has been the period of systematic attention to family theory building. These theories include structure-functionalism, developmentalism, symbolic interactionism, exchange and equity theory, and the systems approach. This book relates to various aspects of a number of these theories but it is the systems approach and the biopsychosocial model that they use as a basis for their work.

An experiment to combine the best in society and medicine was formulated in the late 1920s and with the building of the Pioneer Health Center in 1935, the Peckham Experiment reached fruition. They attempted to build a healthy and functioning community centered around the family as the unit of social structure. This venture, so well described in a number of publications by Williamson, Pearse, and Crocker (9,10) and succinctly analyzed by Ransom (11), inspired generations of physicians despite its own premature demise. Among these inspired physicians who built modified versions of family and community health centers was Kark (12), who in addition to building prototypes, influenced and helped others like Cassel (13), Medalie (14), and Geiger to build health centers in Africa, Israel, and the United States. Although some of the basic family lessons of the Peckham Experiment seem to have disappeared with time, many excellent centers are still functioning and have been the nucleus around which the Community-Oriented Primary Care (C.O.P.C.) movement has developed (12,15,16). An interesting American development has been a Cleveland neighborhood health center which was developed by two Family Practice graduates (Drs. Barbara Toeppen-Sprigg and Ann Reichsman) in which the community operates the practice and the physicians and staff are their employees.

Parallel to this the more traditional fields of medicine, aided by technological development spawned by the world wars, exploded in a rash of exciting biological discoveries. This was part of the rise in specialization and sub-specialization in the 1950s to 1970s with a re-

ductionistic approach to medical problems and a consequent decrease
in the status and numbers of the general practitioner. This was also a
period of greater social awareness and responsibility with increased
interest and activities in public health, community psychiatry, Office
of Economic Opportunity health centers, open wards, free clinics, less-
restricted visiting hours in hospitals, maternal and child health care
programs, and patient education and rights.

During this same period, a number of good publications were produced by various medical disciplines. These influenced the understanding of psychosocial and familial aspects of health and disease.
Notable from Psychiatry were publications on maternal care and
mental health by Bowlby (17), childhood and society by Erikson (18),
psychodynamics of family life by Ackerman (19), the patient, doctor,
and the illness by Balint (20), and works by Spiegel, Kluckhohns,
Bell, Waller, and Gerald Caplan. In addition to Ackerman, a group of
psychiatrists began concentrating more on the interrelationships and
interactions between the identified patients and their families. These
family psychiatrists and therapists like Howell in the United King-
dom and Americans like Don Jackson, Haley, Whitaker, Satir, Minuchin, Bowen, and Epstein have given our understanding of families
a quantum leap forward and in many instances have directly influenced primary care physicians as well as psychologists and social
workers who work in areas of primary care. Pediatrics produced
Spence's landmark study of 1,000 families in Newcastle-on-Tyne as
well as important studies by Hagerty, Alpert, and their colleagues,
and by Klaus and Kennel on maternal–infant bonding. Social Medicine produced Ryle of Oxford, Kark of South Africa and Israel, and
George Reeder in the United States. Epidemiology extended its field
of operation to social and family problems through some excellent
people: Frost (familial aggregation of infectious diseases) (21), Fox
(family-based epidemiological studies), Dingle (illness in families)
(22), Cassel and co-workers (applications of epidemiological methods
to psychosocial problems, the integration of biopsychosocial factors in
epidemiology, and studies in primary care) (13), and the classic work
of a rural family doctor, Pickles (epidemiology in country practice)
(23).

This leads us to the 1960s where the social upheavals in the
United States set the stage for three national health reports all published in 1966—the Willard, Millis, and Folsom Reports. By 1969,
Family Practice, which had been rejected in 1919 and 1944, was recognized as the 20th medical specialty in the United States. The subsequent increase in numbers of Family Practice departments and residency training programs was phenomenal and unprecedented in
medical history. Within Family Practice a small group of people emphasized and laid the foundation for the incorporation of the family

into Family Medicine and Practice. This group rallied around a task force of the Society of Teachers of Family Medicine and the chief proponents of the family in Family Medicine have been meeting annually for the past nine years at Amelia Island.

By the early 1980s the spiraling costs of medical care, the aging of the population, the increase of chronic diseases, and the predicted oversupply of physicians led to the rise in importance of primary care as a way of decreasing costs while giving a good service. Additionally, a large amount of funding became available for primary care educational and other programs. These funds plus pressure from health insurance companies "convinced" many Medicine and Pediatric departments to seriously enter the primary care field.

The major attributes of primary care were defined by a National Academy Task Force, chaired by Dr. Harvey Estes, as being: accessibility, comprehensiveness, coordination, continuity, and accountability (24). They did not include a family orientation! Despite some pioneers from Medicine and Pediatrics like Richardson, Engel, Silver, Hagerty, Kennel, and so on, and the emphasis on the medical encounter by the Task Force on the Medical Interview and Related Skills of the Society of General Internal Medicine (among their leaders are Putnam, M. Lipkin, Jr., Novack, Suchman, and Cohen-Cole), the emphasis on the family in primary care has virtually been confined to a group in Family Medicine. This group consists of behavioral scientists (Ransom, Doherty, Worby, Kosch, Thrower, Cole-Kelly, & Zyzanski), family physicians with family therapy training (Glenn, Christie-Seely, Talbot, Baird, Comley, Crouch, & Sawa), and family physicians without special family therapy who emphasize the family in their daily activities (Huygen, Medalie, Smilkstein, Gerard, Blake, Mullins, Widmer, Reeb, & Ramsey). As could be expected, some of the best results are achieved when there has been close collaboration between a family physician and a behavioral scientist, namely Doherty and Baird, McDaniel and Campbell.

We have reached the stage in our history where the authors of this book believe that the time is ripe for a family orientation in primary care. Contributing to this optimistic view, I believe, is the point they emphasize about family orientation. They define it as an approach or way of thinking that a physician can bring to any patient encounter, with or without accompanying family members. They say their approach applies to levels 2–4 of Doherty and Baird and it also applies to Medalie's third and fourth levels of practice, that is, family orientation and family as unit of practice (25,26). The ability to have a family orientation even when seeing an individual patient is vital if a family orientation is to infiltrate primary care. The fact remains that the majority of contacts with patients in primary care are with individual patients. Although I accept the fact that the most valid family assessment and intervention takes place when the whole family is observed and interacted with, this will only occur in perhaps 1 percent of our patients at any one time. Thus, to deal with the majority of our patients we must learn to have a family orientation even if we do not meet the rest of the family in the practice setting, in the home, or in the hospital. This family orientation with and without the rest of the family is the core of this book. It fills an important void in our education and therefore is highly recommended. I wish it every success because if it succeeds, we all win.

JACK H. MEDALIE, M.D., M.P.H., F.A.A.F.P.
Dorothy Jones Weatherhead Professor of Family Medicine
Case Western Reserve University

Selected References

1. Richardson, HB: *Patients Have Families*. New York, Commonwealth, 1945.
2. Koos, EL: *Families in Trouble*. New York, King Crown Press, 1946.
3. Hill, R: *Families Under Stress*. New York, Harper, 1949.
4. Lewis, O: *La Vida*. New York, Penguin, 1950.
5. Gillin, JL, Gillin JP: *Cultural Sociology*. New York, MacMillan, 1948.
6. Paul BD (ed.): *Health, Culture and Community*. New York, Russell Sage, 1955.
7. Stack, C: *All Our Kin: Strategies for Survival in a Black Community*. New York, Harper and Row, 1974.
8. Adams, BN: *The Family: A Sociological Interpretation* (4th ed.). Orlando, FL, Harcourt-Brace-Jovanovich, 1986.
9. Pearse IH, Williamson GS: *The Case for Action*. London, Faber and Faber, 1931.
10. Pearse IH, Crocker L: *The Peckham Experiment*. London, Allen and Unwin, 1943.
11. Ransom, DC: The evolution from an individual to a family approach. In *Principles of Family Systems in Family Medicine* (eds. Henao, S and Grose, N). New York, Brunner/Mazel, 1985, pp. 5–23.
12. Kark, SL: *The Health Center in Social Medicine* (ed. Clover, EH). Johannesburg, Central News Agency, 1948. Kark, SL: *The Practice of Community-oriented primary care*. New York, Appleton-Century-Crofts, 1981.
13. Cassel, JC: *Comprehensive Health Program Among South African Zulus in Health Centers and Community* (ed. Paul, BD). New York, Russell Sage, 1955. Cassel, JC, Hulka, BS, Ibrahim, MA: Evolution of primary care. In *Family Medicine: Principles and Applications* (ed. Medalie, JH). Baltimore, Williams and Wilkins, 1978, pp. 255–268.
14. Mann, KJ, Medalie, JH, Lieber, E, et al: *Visitors to Doctors: A Medical Social Study of a Family Health Center in a Developing Community*. Jerusalem, Academy Press, 1970.

15. Mullan, F: *Community-oriented primary care. New Engl J Med* 1982; **307**:1076–1078.
16. Mettee, TM: Urban community diagnosis. In *Urban Family Medicine* (ed. Birrer, RB). New York, Springer-Verlag, 1987, pp. 163–170.
17. Bowlby J: *Maternal care and Mental Health.* Geneva, World Health Organization, 1952.
18. Erikson, E: *Childhood and Society.* New York, Norton, 1968.
19. Ackerman, NW: *Psychodynamics of Family Life.* New York, Basic Books, 1959.
20. Balint, M: *The Doctor, the Patient and Illness.* New York, International University Press, 1964.
21. Frost, WH: *Papers of Wade Hampton Frost.* New York, Commonwealth Fund, 1941.
22. Dingle, JH, Badger, GF, Jordan, Jr., WS: *Illness in the Home.* Cleveland, Case Western Reserve University Press, 1964.
23. Pickles WN: *Epidemiology in Country Practice.* Devon (UK), Devonshire Press, first publsihed 1939 and reissued 1972.
24. Estes, HE (chairman): *primary care in Medicine: Report of a Task Force.* Washington, D.C., National Academy of Sciences, 1977.
25. Medalie, JH: *Family Medicine: Principles and Applications.* Baltimore, Williams and Wilkins, 1978, pp. 3–20.
26. Medalie, JH: Family diagnosis in family practice. In *Family Medicine and Supportive Interventions* (eds. Kaplan BH, Ibrahim MA). Chapel Hill, University of North Carolina Press, 1981, pp. 24–40.

Preface

This book is a manual for physicians who want to enhance their skills in working with patients in the context of their families. It has evolved out of our work with physicians, patients, and families in a primary care medical setting, as well as our teaching within the Department of Family Medicine at the University of Rochester School of Medicine and Dentistry. Respected colleagues, such as Medalie, Doherty and Baird, and Christie-Seely, have made contributions to the theory of family systems medicine, but little has yet been written about the practicalities and skills involved in day-to-day family-oriented primary care. Building on this theoretical work, we are taking the step of integrating theory into the daily practice of primary care physicians.

Family-oriented primary care offers the practitioner a useful perspective that will help in caring for both the individual patient and the family. The skills that operationalize this approach enable the physician to utilize the support inherent in most families to the benefit of the patient. The National Heart, Lung, and Blood Institute has recognized the importance of the family in increasing compliance and promoting continuity of care. Based upon research studies and clinical experience with hypertension, they recommend the physician:

> Enhance support from family members—identifying and involving one influential person, preferably someone living with the patient, who can provide encouragement, help support the behavior change, and, if necessary, remind the patient about specifics of the regimen (1).

In this book, we have extended this basic strategy to apply to all of primary care.

While family-oriented primary care can result in more effective care of a patient, we also feel it is important to note that this perspective can be useful to the physician. Primary care can be a stressful and taxing, albeit rewarding, career. Recognizing the importance of the family and utilizing its resources allows the physician to share the responsibility of care and decision-making with those who care most about the patient. This approach can help to prevent physician burn-out so that energy can be conserved for the physician's own personal and family life.

We begin the manual with a section that spells out our theory of family systems medicine, reviews the relevant research, and provides a guide for assessing and interviewing families in primary care. This section is called "The Biopsychosocial Assessment of the Family." We then turn to a section entitled "Health Care of the Family in Transition," and discuss how to treat specific health care issues that arise when the patient and his or her family are facing normal developmental challenges. These issues range from the concerns of new couples, pregnancy, and adolescent difficulties, to sexual issues, aging, and death. In the next section, "A Family-Oriented Approach to Specific Medical Problems," we provide guidelines for a family-oriented approach to substance abuse, anxiety and depression, chronic illness, somatic fixation, and sexual and physical abuse. The final section, "Implementing Family-Oriented Primary Care," addresses general issues: the implementation of a family-oriented practice; hospitalization; collaborating and making referrals with family therapists; and managing personal and professional boundaries.

Throughout the book we will use case material to illustrate how to approach specific treatment problems in a family-oriented way. The case examples are actual primary care cases, or composites of cases; however, identifying data have been changed and pseudonyms added to protect the confidentiality of our patients. Protocols appear at the end of each chapter to be used as a quick guide in daily practice.

Many people have helped us in the completion of this project. Our patients have provided us with invaluable opportunities to learn about family-oriented primary care. The residents who we teach and the faculty with whom we work at the University of Rochester Department of Family Medicine have provided important feedback on our ideas and our clinical practice. Our colleagues in the Division of Family Programs in the Department of Psychiatry have also stimulated and informed our work. Particularly, the thinking and teaching of M. Duncan Stanton, the Director of the Division, and Judith Landau-Stanton have influenced and broadened our perspectives. The administration of the Department of Family Medicine, and Highland Hospital, have provided us with the financial support to work on this project. We would like to especially thank Jay Dickinson, the Chairman of the Department of Family Medicine, for his guidance and support.

We would also like to acknowledge the many people who read and reviewed these chapters before publication. Their responses helped us to clarify our theories and sharpen our techniques. We are most grateful to three people who read the entire book in process and provided us with constructive feedback: Kathy Cole-Kelly, Eugene Farley, and Thomas Schwenk. Numerous colleagues read specific chapters along the way and responded from their areas of expertise. Thank you to: Marvin Amstey, Macaran Baird, Richard Botelho, T. Berry Brazelton, Christine Charbonneau, Frank deGruy, Steve Eisinger, Barbara Elliott, Annmarie Groth-Junker, Jeff Harp, Allison Kempe, Judith Landau-Stanton, Pieter le Roux, Grover McDaniel, Beth Maher, Carol Maskiell, Cathy Morrow, Steve Munson, Elizabeth Naumburg, Paul Rapoza, Deborah Richter, Eric Schaff, Joseph Scherger, Cleveland Shields, Bernard Shore, David Siegel, Earl Siegel, Lucy Siegel, David Stoller, Sarah Trafton, Donald Treat, Michael Weidner, and Lyman Wynne.

Finally, thank you to our families for their understanding and support during a project of this size. Thank you to our editor, Shelley Reinhardt, for her helpful support and guidance. Thank you to our colleague, Peter Franks, for his technical assistance. Our thanks to Sally Rousseau for her endless and creative efforts in producing and refining the tables and figures. And many thanks to our secretary, Jeanne Klee, who helped us with her typing, her editing, and her always present smile.

Reference

1. Working Group on Health Education and High Blood Pressure Control (1988). *The physician's guide—improving adherence among hypertensive patients*. Bethesda, MD, U.S. DHHS, PHS, NIH.

Contents

A Family-Oriented Approach to Specific Medical Problems

Implementing Family-Oriented Primary Care

The Biopsychosocial
Assessment of the Family

CHAPTER 1

Basic Premises of Family-Oriented Primary Care

Utilizing the Family as a Resource

There is a tendency for all living things to join up,
establish linkages, live inside each other,
return to earlier arrangements, get along whenever possible.
This is the way of the world.

LEWIS THOMAS
The Lives of a Cell (1)

Who Is the "Family" in Family-Oriented Primary Care?

Physicians are involved daily in managing and treating the illnesses of patients who are linked with, joined to, and living within a larger context—the family. In fact, despite the popular attention given recently to singles living alone or with a nonfamily roommate, still a majority of the American population make their home with other family members (2). The family remains the most basic relational unit in society.

When we speak of the family, each of us develops a picture in our minds of what that means. For some, it is Mom and Dad, brother and sister, as well as the family dog. For others, it may be Mom and Dad, Grandma and Grandpa, and a few aunts and uncles. For still others, the arrangements are less "traditional": single-parent families, gay relationships, adoptive families, remarried families. Beyond that, there are those who feel their truest family is found in a religious community or among a set of friends. All of us have a personal sense of what the family is, but when it comes to defining the "average American family," the task becomes more difficult.

The television stereotype of the American family in the 1950s, which was comprised of a working dad, a mother at home, and one or more children, constitutes only 13% of American households (3). What have emerged in the 1970s and 1980s are more single-parent families and "nonfamily households," which are composed of single persons or persons living with nonrelatives (4). The American family is a mix of couples (30%), two parents and children (28%), single-parent households

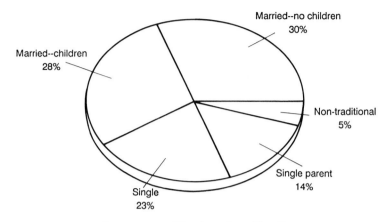

FIGURE 1.1.   The American Family

(14%), and nonfamily households (28%). (See Figure 1.1.) Even with these societal changes, it is the family, however constituted, that addresses the individual's need for physical and emotional safety, health, and well-being. Research supports the view that the family plays a vital role in the health and illness of its members. (See Chapter 2.) Since the nature of the American family is evolving, our understanding of it also needs to evolve in order to capture its rich diversity.

We define *family* as *any group of people related either biologically, emotionally, or legally.* The family-oriented physician gathers information about family relationships, patterns of health and illness across generations, emotional connections with the extended family, and life cycle transitions in order to understand the patient within his or her larger context. In daily family practice, though, the family physician is most often involved with family members who live within the same household. Even though involvement of nonhousehold family members can be important to a patient's medical care, the household is most often the primary focus of the family-oriented physician's care (6). It is important for the physician to encourage the whole household to register with him or her. In this way the physician has direct access to the people who may influence each other's illness and health most.

Without considering the patient in his or her family context, the physician may inadvertently eliminate not only a wider understanding of illness, but a broader range of solutions as well. "Family-oriented primary care" does not mean the physician always sees entire households together. Rather, by "family-oriented" we mean an approach or way of thinking that a physician can bring to any patient encounter, even without accompanying family members. We will address both treating a patient with family members involved and treating the individual patient from a family perspective. This approach involves thinking about a symptom or problem in the context of the whole person and the person's significant others. At times this way of thinking may mean the inclusion of other important persons in the assessment and treatment process, at other times it may not.

We do not advocate family-oriented primary care because we believe that the family alone can cure disease. Instead, we believe – and research is beginning to support – that planned and purposeful family participation in health care improves health care for the patient, family, and, also, the physician. Not including family members can at times run the risk of incurring roadblocks or, at least, detours on the road to effective and efficient primary care. Including family members can mean the physician has enlisted his or her most potent ally in the treatment of his or her patients. We now turn to the basic premises that underpin this manual, illustrate them with case examples, and then describe the level of skills presented in subsequent chapters.

Basic Premises of Family-Oriented Medical Care

A family-oriented approach to medical care incorporates, expands upon, and, at times, differs from a biomedical approach. Some of the basic premises of a family-oriented approach include:

Premise #1: Family-oriented medical care is based on the biopsychosocial model. The biomedical model, based primarily on molecular biology, assumes that disease can be reduced to "measurable biological variables" (7). The task of the physician operating from a biomedical approach is to analyze and eliminate all factors in the development of illness until the simplest biological elements are identified. The disease-producing factors are isolated and treated as the primary causes of the problem. The central problem with the biomedical approach is that it focuses on biological factors to the exclusion of social and psychological factors, a focus based on the belief that complex situations can be explained entirely by biology. Physicians educated in a narrow biomedical model are more likely to be overly reductionistic and will conceptualize illness from one vantage point. For example, from a biomedical perspective, the cause of tuberculosis is the tubercule bacillus, yet the dramatic decline in the incidence of the disease has resulted from public health measures and improvements in social environment, not from the introduction of antitubercular drugs (8). The physician who defines disease within somatic boundaries alone will miss the impact of other factors, such as the person, the provider–patient interaction, the family, and the social setting, and how these factors may be connected in the creation of symptoms. The biomedical approach is a paradigm that fosters the view that "the body is sum of its parts, separate from mind and impervious to the influences of external forces" (9). A biopsychosocial approach recognizes that psychosocial factors can play as important a role in health and illness as biological factors.

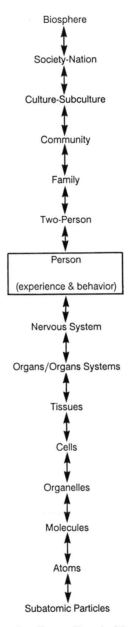

FIGURE 1.2 Systems hierarchy. From: Engel, GL: The clinical application of the biopsychosocial model. *Am J Psychiatry.* Copyright May 1980. The American Psychiatric Association. Reprinted by permission.

The biopsychosocial model, as presented by Engel (7), places illness within a larger framework involving multiple systems. To understand a disease the physician must not only attend to the biological contributors (molecules, cells, organs), but also to the person, the family, the patient–physician relationship, and the social context. (See Figure 1.2.) Rather than being discrete unrelated factors, these various elements are interrelated in such a way that changes in any one level can have an effect on the others. The relationship among these various levels involves continuous and reciprocal feedback.

Medalie describes and illustrates how the various levels in the patient's experience interact (10,11). Each level responds and adjusts to changes in other levels. In that way, stability is maintained through a process of change, much the same as a tightrope walker keeps his or her balance by making frequent shifts and adjustments (12). Dym (13) illustrates this process with a simple case of childhood asthma.

> In John and Mary's relationship, John drinks frequently. When he drinks Mary criticizes him. Their son, Harry, 14, unable to deal with the stress leaves the field. As the fight continues, George, 11, becomes more anxious and has an asthma attack. Mary shifts her focus to George and gives him an inhaler. She then blames John who feels guilty. He leaves and the fight stops. The next day he drinks again and the cycle continues.

From a biomedical perspective, the illness is the asthma. From a biopsychosocial perspective the illness is the problem-maintaining relational pattern that fosters a biopsychosocial symptom: wheezing. For a family-oriented physician the primary focus of diagnosis is the multilevel cycle in which the symptom plays an integral part. One of the most important issues in settling on a treatment plan is deciding at which level or levels to intervene (14).

Premise #2: The primary focus of medical care is the patient in the context of the family. The physician who operates from a biopsychosocial perspective focuses on the patient in the context of the family. While this is the starting point of medical care, it does not eliminate consideration of the other multiple levels included in a biopsychosocial approach, levels ranging from molecules, cells, organs, and organ systems to community, culture, society, and biosphere (7). Rather this focus highlights the patient's family context as the primary arena in which medical care issues typically are addressed.

Leaders in the field of family medicine have disagreed on the efficacy of considering the family as the "unit of care" (15–20). There are those who feel the individual is the primary "unit of care," while others argue for the family. We feel this argument is not useful because in a reductionistic way it pits two levels of the biopsychosocial model against each other, that of the "individual" vs the "family," and forces a choice of what will be the "unit of care." While a physician might choose to intervene primarily at only one of these levels in a given case, to argue for only one of them to be the sacred "unit of care" results in conceptual confusion. (What does it mean for the family to be the "unit of care"?) It is also antithetical to the interrelationships among levels that are fundamental to the original meaning of the biopsychosocial model. For that reason we have chosen to think of the patient in the context of the family as the "focus" rather than the "unit" of medical care. From this perspective, the physician is reminded of the importance of the person as a biological and emotional entity as well as the significance of the family's influence on illness and health. For example,

> Billy Smith's diabetes was first diagnosed at the age of 13 when he was admitted to the hospital with diabetic ketoacidosis. He adjusted well while in the hospital and shortly thereafter began to manage his own insulin and diet. An only child, Billy received support from his parents, especially his mother who did not work outside the home. Billy's diabetes was stable until his senior year in high school, when he began to spill large amounts of glucose in his urine. His blood sugars were often in the 300's. Billy claimed to be taking his insulin and sticking to his diet. But his situation worsened until he was finally admitted to the hospital to get his diabetes under control.

In cases such as this, the family-oriented physician explores family issues to see how they may influence or be a resource in a crisis. As part of this process, four considerations influence family-oriented primary care:

a) **The family is the primary source of many health beliefs and behaviors.** The initial appraisal of physical symptoms is usually made within the family and is based upon family beliefs about health. Many families have a health expert, often the oldest female. The family health expert often makes an initial health assessment and treatment plan and decides whether a physician should be consulted. In our case, for example, it was Mrs. Smith who typically made the first contact with Dr. B.

Many health behaviors and risk factors are shared by members of a family. Children are more likely to smoke if their parents smoke (21). Most families share the same diet, which along with genetic influences result in elevated cholesterol levels occurring within certain families (22). A family approach to health promotion and risk reduction is therefore likely to be more efficient and cost effective (23).

b) **The stress that a family feels when going through developmental transitions can become manifest in physical symptoms.** The family-oriented physician is sensitive to the impact of life-cycle changes on the health of family members. Marriage, birth of the first child, adolescence, leaving home, midlife, death of a parent, retirement are all normal developmental transitions in the life of a family (9,24). Due to the stress that can occur during these periods, the health of family members may be more vulnerable to illness.

The Smiths were going through three significant transitions simultaneously. Mr. Smith has made a career shift at midlife. Mrs. Smith has experienced the death of her mother. And Billy, soon to graduate from high school, was facing the issue of leaving home. Each family member was under tremendous strain. The family as a whole was being transformed by the demands these changes are placing upon it.

c) Somatic symptoms can serve an adaptive function within the family and be maintained by family patterns (25). Dr. B. learned that Billy had a very close relationship with his mother. Mrs. Smith was protective of her son, and Bill depended on his mother's support during his illness. Mr. Smith supported the family primarily through his role as breadwinner and provider. While Mr. and Mrs. Smith were not very close, Billy and his father were able to maintain a good relationship. In the year prior to the acceleration of his illness, Mrs. Smith's mother died, and Mr. Smith had been traveling more since receiving a promotion. Billy was also making plans to leave home for college. Mrs. Smith's needs for closeness increased because of the loss of her mother. Her neediness coincided with her husband's frequent absence. Billy found himself in the position of having to meet his mother's needs while feeling angry and frustrated over his father's absence. It was during this time that Billy developed symptoms. As his symptoms worsened, Mr. Smith began to curtail his traveling. Mr. and Mrs. Smith also began to pull together to try to help their son.

Billy's symptoms can be understood as a barometer of the pressure felt within the family. In a sense, the symptoms were both a problem and a solution. They were obviously a problem in that they presented a challenge to his health and well-being and they created great concern for his parents who loved him. But Billy's symptoms may also be seen as a solution in that they brought Billy's parents together to care for him, thus stabilizing their marital difficulties. The symptoms kept Billy from leaving home too quickly at a time when he was clearly concerned about his parents; and they sounded an alarm for the alert physician that the whole family was in need.

Studies by Salvador Minuchin, a leader in the family therapy field, have shown that increased family stress can adversely affect the management of chronic childhood illnesses (26–28). In particular, he demonstrated that when diabetic children are involved in their parents' conflicts, the stress resulted in an acute rise in free fatty acids and worsening of the diabetic control (see Chapter 2).

d) Families are a valuable resource and source of support for the management of illness. Physicians do not treat illness: they recommend treatment that is usually carried out in the home by the patient and family members. Physicians must rely upon the assistance of the family in management of most chronic illness.

In Billy's case, he had taken responsibility for his insulin and diet with the support and supervision of his parents. As Dr. B. addressed this recent crisis, he once again engaged the parents in planning for the management of their son's illness. Despite their differences, Mr. and Mrs. Smith's commitment to their son made planning for and carrying out his treatment possible.

Dr. B's approach to Billy's diabetes takes not only his symptoms into account but the family context as well. It highlights how the family is a factor in both illness and health and sets the stage for utilizing the family as a resource in developing and carrying out a treatment plan.

Premise #3: The patient, family, and physician are partners in medical care. In a biomedical approach the physician uses a process in which various factors are eliminated or ruled out until the most critical biological factors emerge (29). Unfortunately, what also may get eliminated is the person as well as other supraperson levels that may contribute to the illness (29). Since family-oriented physicians consider multiple systems when diagnosing and treating illness, the patient and family are very important resources. It is through these people that the physician gains the most significant information for understanding symptoms and planning treatment. In this way, the family is a natural partner in medical care.

The perspective of partnership destroys what Doherty and Baird have called "the illusion of the dyad in medical care" (3, p. 12). The illusion is that medical care only involves a one-to-one relationship between physician and individual patient. Doherty and Baird point out that except in the most rare situation the family is involved in what takes place between physician and patient. Even when the family is not physically in the room, the patient's role within the family, the family's expectations of medical care, and the family's relational patterns as they pertain to health and illness play a part in what transpires.

In place of a dyadic approach, Doherty and Baird propose a "triangular perspective" (3, p. 13). This triangle involves the physician, patient, and family working in a medical-care partnership. Together they define what needs to be done. This includes identifying symptoms, establishing a treatment plan, and clarifying responsibilities. When this partnership is not in place, medical treatment can go awry.

> Dr. L prescribed medication and a low-salt diet for Mr. Samuel's hypertension. Mr. Samuel's parents, with whom he lived, had doubts about the efficacy of medical treatment in general. They questioned the medication and also felt the diet would mean their lifestyle would have to change as well. Mr. Samuel was caught between opposing expectations from his physician and his parents. He resolved the dilemma by complying with the treatment plan only in part. He took his medication irregularly and followed his diet for a few days. Ironically, partial compliance convinced both Dr. L and the family that each was right. Dr. L saw it as confirmation that the patient must try harder. The family was convinced that the treatment wasn't working. Both sides escalated

their positions and Mr. Samuel continued his compromise. In the meantime, his blood pressure remained elevated.

Dr. L soon recognized the situation and invited the patient's parents to come in with their son. Dr. L explained their son's hypertension and the rationale for the treatment plan. He enlisted their help, clearly indicating that they could bring about some change for their son. Mother was utilized as an expert on diet. The parents gave their "permission" for their son to take the medication.

The role of the family in a patient's compliance with medical treatment is well documented. (See Chapter 2.) The family-oriented physician engages the patient and the family as an ally and a resource not only around compliance issues but for medical care in general.

Premise #4: The physician is seen as "a part of" rather than "apart from" the treatment system. A traditional biomedical approach supports physicians being objective outsiders who assess, diagnose, and treat their patients' illnesses. One important factor in medical care that can be missed by this approach is how physicians may influence and be influenced by their patients' behavior. For example, when treatment does not go well, physicians may see their patients as "difficult" or "noncompliant." How the interaction between physicians and patients influences the course of treatment is not considered adequately.

Physicians who operate from a systems or biopsychosocial perspective believe that "the observer constantly alters what he observes by the obtrusive act of observation"(12, p. 129). Biopsychosocially oriented physicians observe the interaction between themselves and their patients. In that sense they understand themselves as part of a circular process in which their behavior contributes as much to what transpires as their patients'. Consequently, when treatment does not proceed well despite biomedical interventions, these physicians will consider the interaction of additional parts of the overall treatment system. This includes how their interaction with the patient and family system may unwittingly contribute to rather than relieve the problem.

Mrs. Jackson brought Mary, age 11, to the doctor's office for the third time in three months with symptoms of a sore throat. Dr. K, alert to larger, systemic issues, invited Mr. and Mrs. Jackson in to discuss their daughter's recurring symptoms. In the course of the interview, she learned that Mr. Jackson had been working very long hours and some weekends for the past six months. Mrs. Jackson was very upset that her husband did not spend more time with her and with Mary. Mrs. Jackson complained that she was always the one to leave work if Mary was in need of care and that her husband did not help out much at all. Mr. Jackson said he could not control his work schedule and did not feel he needed to be more available. Mary said she just didn't feel well and things weren't the way they used to be at home.

Dr. K quickly realized that her exclusive focus on Mary's symptoms in the past two months may have become part of an ongoing argument between Mr.

and Mrs. Jackson over Mr. Jackson's work and involvement in the family. If Dr. K continued to focus only on the biomedical problem, more fuel would have been added to the fire of Mr. and Mrs. Jackson's disagreement and Mary's resultant stress. By including the family, Dr. K saw the larger picture and recognized how she fit into it. She then treated not only Mary's sore throats, but encouraged Mr. and Mrs. Jackson to resolve their differences regarding her work. This was successfully done in several primary care counseling sessions.

It is important for physicians to be aware that they are a part of the larger treatment system. When treatment is faltering, it is useful for the physician to raise questions about how his or her own involvement with patients and families may contribute to patterns that maintain rather than eliminate the problem. A change in the physician's behavior may help facilitate change throughout the system. In the case of the Jackson family, calling a family meeting began to shift the focus from a narrow biomedical perspective to one that respected multiple factors. Dr. K changed her behavior, i.e., she called a family meeting, and involved the family in treatment in a qualitatively different way.

Developing Skills for Family-Oriented Medical Care

Given our basic premises about the family and primary care, our goal is to develop the skills necessary to implement family-oriented medical care. Doherty and Baird describe five levels of physician involvement with families (30). Level One involves minimal emphasis on the family. The family is included only when necessary for practical and medical/legal reasons. At Level Two, the physician is primarily biomedically focused and communicates regularly with the family about medical issues. The physician functioning at Level Three not only gathers information but addresses family stress and feelings by actively eliciting family feelings in a supportive way. At Level Four the physician not only gathers information and deals with family affect but intervenes in ways that may alter the family's interactional patterns. The physician at this level has an understanding of family systems theory and a grasp of the skills to counsel the families to make constructive changes. Level Five is family therapy, which addresses more deeply rooted family patterns of dysfunction. Most physicians (except those who received postresidency training in family therapy) will refer families who need this level of intervention to trained family therapists.

This manual focuses primarily on developing skills at Levels Two through Four. We will mention the importance of Level Two—basic communication with the family. We will encourage physicians to use the skills involved at Level Three when it is important to elicit family feelings and deal with them in a supportive manner. Many physicians already operate at Levels Two and Three. The goal of this book is to increase skills and comfort with Level Four—where the physician is able to assess family interaction, utilize family resources and when necessary engage the family in primary care counseling in order to treat illness in the most effective, efficient way. In so doing, we hope to move family-oriented primary care farther along the continuum (31) from an exclusively biomedical approach to a biopsychosocial approach.

References

1. Thomas L: *The Lives of a Cell: Notes of a Biology Watcher*. New York, Bantam Books, Inc., 1974, p. 147.
2. U.S. Bureau of the Census: *Population Characteristics*. Washington, DC, U.S. Government Printing Office, 1980.
3. Doherty W, Baird M: *Family Therapy and Family Medicine*. New York, Guilford Press, 1983.
4. U.S. Bureau of the Census: *Families, Marital Status, and Living Arrangements*. Washington, DC, U.S. Government Printing Office, March 1984.
5. U.S. Bureau of the Census: *Statistical Abstract of the United States: 1987*, 107th edition. Washington, DC, U.S. Government Printing Office, 1986.
6. Report of the North American Primary Care Research Group (NAPCRG) Committee on Standard Terminology: *A Glossary for Primary Care*. Presented at the Annual Meeting of NAPCRG, Williamsburg, VA, March 1977.
7. Engel GL: The need for a new medical model: A challenge for biomedicine. *Science* 1977;**196**:129–136.
8. McKeown T: *The Role of Medicine: Dream, Mirage, or Nemesis*. Princeton, NJ, Princeton University Press, 1979.
9. Saba G, Fink DL: Systems medicine and systems therapy: A call to a natural collaboration. *J Strat Sys Ther* 1985;**4**(2):15–31.
10. Medalie JH: A family-oriented approach in primary care, in Noble J (ed.): *Primary Care and the Practice of Medicine*. Boston, Little, Brown and Co., 1976, pp. 53–63.
11. Medalie JH (ed.): *Family Medicine: Principles and Applications*. Baltimore, MD, The Williams and Wilkins Co., 1978.
12. Keeney BP: *The Aesthetics of Change*. New York, Guilford Press, 1983.
13. Dym B: The cybernetics of physical illness. *Fam Proc* 1987;**26**:35–48.
14. Campbell T, McDaniel S: Applying a systems approach to common medical problems in Crouch M, and Roberts L (eds.). *The Family in Medical Practice: A Family Systems Primer*. New York, Springer-Verlag, 1987, pp. 112–139.
15. Carmichael LP: Forty families—a search for the family in family medicine. *Fam Syst Med* 1983;**1**(1):12–16.
16. Christiansen CE: Making the family the unit of care: What does it mean? *Fam Med* 1983;**15**(6):207–209.
17. Schwenk TC, Hughes CC: The family as patient in family medicine: Rhetoric or reality? *Soc Sci Med* 1983;**17**:1–16.
18. Schmidt DD: The family as the unit of medical care. *J Fam Prac* 1978;**7**(2): 303–313.

19. Ransom DC: On why it is useful to say "the family is the unit of care" in family medicine: Comment on Carmichael's essay. *Fam Syst Med* 1983; **1**(1):17–22.

20. Frank SH: The unit of care revisited. *J Fam Pract* 1985;**21**(2):145–148.

21. Bewley RB, Bland JM. Academic performance and social factors related to cigarette smoking by school children. *Br J Prev Soc Med* 1977;**31**:18–24.

22. Hartz A, Giefer E, Rimm AA. Relative importance of the effect of family environment and heredity on obesity. *Ann Hum Genet* 1977;**41**:185–193.

23. Doherty WA, Campbell TL: *Families and Health*. Beverly Hill, CA, Sage, 1988.

24. Carter EA, McGoldrick M (eds.): *The Family Life Cycle: A Framework for Family Therapy*. New York, Gardner Press, Inc., 1980.

25. Watzlawick P, Weakland J, Fisch C: *Change: Principles of Problem Formation and Problem Resolution*. New York, W.W. Norton and Company, Inc., 1974.

26. Baker L, Minuchin S, Rosman B: The use of beta adrenergic blockage in the treatment of psychosomatic aspects of juvenile diabetes mellitus, in Snart A (ed.): *Advances in Beta Adrenergic Blockage Therapy*. Princeton, NJ, Exerpta Medica, 1974, pp. 67–80.

27. Baker L, Minuchin S, Milman L, et. al.: Psychosomatic aspects of juvenile diabetes mellitus: A progress report. *Mod Prob Paediatr* 1975;**12**:332–343.

28. Minuchin S, Bosman BL, Baker L: *Psychosomatic Families*. Cambridge, MA: Harvard University Press, 1987, pp. 21–50.

29. Engel GL: The clinical application of the biopsychosocial model. *Am J Psychiatry* 1980;**137**:535–544.

30. Doherty WJ, Baird MA: Developmental levels in family-centered medical care. *Fam Med* 1986;**18**(3):153–156.

31. Doherty WA, Baird MA, Becker LA: *Family Medicine: The Maturing of a Discipline*. New York, Haworth Press, 1986.

PROTOCOL
Basic Premises of Family-Oriented Primary Care

We define "family" as any group of people related either biologically, emotionally, or legally. While involvement of nonhousehold family members can be important to a patient's medical care, the household is more often than not the primary focus of the family-oriented physician's care.

1. Family-oriented medical care is based on the biopsychosocial model.
2. The primary focus of medical care is the patient in the context of the family.
   a. The family is the primary source of many health beliefs and behaviors.
   b. The stress that a family feels when going through developmental transitions can become manifest in physical symptoms.
   c. Somatic symptoms can serve an adaptive function within the family and be maintained by family patterns.
   d. Families are a valuable resource and source of support for the management of illness.
3. The patient, family, and physician are partners in medical care.
4. The physician is seen as "a part of" rather than "apart from" the treatment system.

How Families Affect Illness
Research on the Family's Impact on Health

A basic premise of the biopsychosocial model is that various subsystems (biological, individual, family, community, etc.) impact each other in ways that affect both health and illness. Clinical experience supports the premise that families influence and are influenced by the health of their members and that family-oriented primary care can lead to better care and improved health for both the individual and the family as a whole. However, assumptions and experiences that point toward a new approach to medical care should be scientifically validated through empirical research. This chapter will examine some important lines of research on the family's impact on health. While much of the family and health research suffers from conceptual and methodological problems (1), there is now a body of well-designed studies and randomized controlled trials (see Table 2.1) which demonstrate that the family has a powerful influence on health. The clinical implications of this research are presented in the Protocol section of the chapter. This research lends support to the contention of family-oriented medical care that a partnership among physician, patient, and family may provide the most effective and efficient form of health care.

Three areas of research on the family's impact on health will be reviewed: the influence of family stress and support on overall mortality, the family's influence on cardiovascular risk factors and the prevention of heart disease, and the impact of family functioning on the course of chronic disease. Research in these areas have produced the most substantial and consistent evidence for the importance of the family and are particularly pertinent to the practicing physician. More comprehensive reviews are available (2–4) for those who are interested. This chapter does not discuss any of the excellent and voluminous research on

TABLE 2.1.   Randomized Controlled Trials of Family Interventions in Physical
Illness

Study	Illness	Intervention	Results
Lask 1979 (70)	Asthma	Family therapy	Improvement in symptoms and thoracic gas volumes
Clark 1981 (93)	Asthma	Family education	Less fear and better management of illness
Gustafsson et al. 1986 (94)	Asthma	Family therapy	Improvement in overall pediatric assessment
Baranowski 1982 (95)	Cardiovascular risk factors	Multifamily support groups	More supportive behaviors to change diet & exercise
Earp 1982 (96)	Hypertension	Family involvement in home visit	No effect
Morisky et al. 1983 (67)	Hypertension	Family support	57% reduction in overall mortality
Brownell 1978 (97)	Obesity	Spouse involvement	Maintained weight loss
Saccone 1978 (98)	Obesity	Spouse reinforcement	Increased weight loss
Wilson 1978 (99)	Obesity	Family involvement	No effect
Pearce 1981 (100)	Obesity	Spouse involvement	Greater weight loss and maintenance
Brownell 1983 (101)	Obesity	Mother involvement	Group with mother and daughter seen separately lost the most weight

families and mental health: in this area, the reader is referred to
reviews on schizophrenia (5), depression (6), alcoholism (7), drug abuse
(8), chronic pain (9), and eating disorders (10).

Family Stress

Stress has become widely accepted by patients and physicians as influencing health. Patients often explain to their physicians that they are
"under a lot of stress" and that their ulcer, back pain, or headache is "acting up." However, stress is difficult both to define and to study (11). One
successful method for studying stress and health has been to examine

the relationship of stressful life events to illness. In 1967, Holmes and Rahe (12) developed a life event scale by asking a random sample of the population to rank how stressful they perceived each of 43 common life events to be. Many retrospective and prospective studies using this scale have shown that an increase in stressful life events precedes the development of a wide range of different diseases (13).

Most of the events on the Holmes and Rahe scale occur within the family, and 10 of the 15 most stressful events are family events. Since children are likely to be affected by this stress, a number of studies have looked at the relationship of family life events and child health. Meyer and Haggerty (14) found that chronic stress was associated with higher rates of streptococcal pharyngitis, and that 30% of the strep infections were preceded by a stressful family event. In a study conducted in a day care center, children who experience more stressful life events had longer but not more frequent respiratory illnesses (15). A prospective study of over 1000 preschoolers found that family life events were strongly correlated with subsequent visits to the physician and hospital admissions for a wide range of conditions. Children from families with more than 12 life events during the four-year study period were six times more likely to be hospitalized (16).

The death of a spouse is the most stressful common life event, and the health consequences of bereavement have been extensively studied (17,18). From examining U.S. census data, Kraus and Lillienfeld (19) found that young widowers had 10 times the normal death rate for many illnesses. In a classic prospective study, Parkes et al. (20) followed London widowers for nine years after the death of their spouses. The men had a forty percent higher mortality rate during the first six months of bereavement when compared to the general population. A population study of 4032 widowed persons (21) found that when potential confounding variables (especially smoking and socioeconomic status) were controlled for, widowers, but not widows, had increased mortality rates, which persisted throughout the 10 years of the study. However, widowers who remarried had a lower death rate than the control, nonwidowed group, suggesting that marriage had a protective effect on health. In a study of 95,647 widowed persons in Finland, death rates were highest and twice the expected rate during the first week of bereavement (22).

Divorce or marital separation is also an extremely stressful event, and is ranked second on the Holmes and Rahe scale. Several cross-sectional studies (23–25) have demonstrated that divorcees have a higher death rate from all diseases than single, widowed, or married persons. However, research has also shown that chronic physical illness has an adverse affect on marital satisfaction (26,27) and may eventually lead to divorce. Prospective studies of divorce and health are needed to determine which is cause or effect.

Recent research in psychoimmunology has suggested one of several possible biological mechanisms for the adverse health effects of bereavement and divorce. Studies in animals and humans reveal that stress can lead to immunosuppression and an increase in illness (28,29). Two well-controlled studies demonstrated a decrease in cellular immunity (T-lymphocyte stimulation) during bereavement (30,31). However in a third study, T-cell function was reduced only in those bereaved subjects who were clinically depressed (32). Divorced or separated women have significantly poorer immune function than sociodemographically matched married women (33). Among the married women in the same study, poor marital quality correlated with both depression and decreased immunity. Immune function is also impaired in major depression, and researchers have suggested that changes occurring in the central nervous system during depression may be a final common pathway (29).

Family Support

Although family stress can have harmful effects on health, family support can be beneficial. Social support can be defined as "the emotional, instrumental and financial aid that is obtained from one's social network" (34). An extensive body of research has demonstrated that social networks and supports can directly improve health, as well as buffer the adverse effects of stress (35,36). Furthermore, the family has been found to be the most important source of social support.

In a seminal study of over 6000 adults, Berkman and Syme (37) showed that social networks were a major predictor of mortality over a nine-year period, independent of socioeconomic status, previous health status, or health practices. The most socially isolated adults had more than twice the death rate of the least-isolated group. Marital status and contacts with relatives and friends were the most powerful predictors of health. A similar study (38) confirmed the strong association between social isolation and mortality, but for men only. Again, the family components of social support were the most predictive. In a six-year follow-up study of 17,433 Swedish men and women, those with the fewest available social contacts had over three times the death rate of those with the most social contacts (39).

Studies of social supports in the elderly have shown that the relative importance of different aspects of family support may change over the life span. Two studies found that older persons with impaired social supports have two to three times the death rate of those with good supports (40,41). Unlike studies of younger populations, marital status was not associated with mortality. The presence and number of living children were the most powerful predictor of survival. This finding suggests that adult children become the most important source of social support in the elderly.

Family supports play a particularly important role in the outcome of pregnancy. Highly stressed women with low family and social supports have higher rates of obstetrical complications (42,43). Women who live apart from their families deliver smaller babies than those who live with their partners or families of origin (44). However, those women who are excessively close or enmeshed with their extended families also tend to deliver smaller babies, suggesting that the quality as well as the quantity of family support influences health. Ramsey and colleagues have hypothesized that the extended family's overinvolvement during pregnancy may be detrimental by not allowing enough autonomy or psychological space for a new family member (44).

These lines of research clearly demonstrate that family support and family stress, especially bereavement, can have a powerful influence on overall mortality. An understanding of the family and their potential sources of stress and support can provide the physician with ways to reduce family stress, bolster family supports, and improve health.

Cardiovascular Risk Factors in Families

Heart disease remains the leading cause of death in the U.S., and a major target of preventive medicine (45). Changes in lifestyle can substantially reduce the risk of heart disease, but are difficult to accomplish. Several studies have shown that there is a high concordance of the cardiovascular risk factor within families (46); that is, family members are more likely to share the same risk factors including smoking, obesity, hypercholesterolemia, and hypertension, than would be expected by chance. This sharing of risk factors occurs both between spouses and among parents and their children. For example, the Framingham Heart Study found a higher than expected concordance between spouses for blood pressure, cholesterol, triglyceride, blood sugar, smoking, and lung function (47).

The sharing of cardiac risk factors within families can be explained by several different mechanisms. Family members can influence each other's lifestyle and health habits. Adolescents are much more likely to smoke if either of their parents smoke (48). Families usually eat a similar diet, and therefore similar amounts of salt, saturated fats, cholesterol, and even calories. An emphasis on physical fitness and maintaining ideal body weight is often a shared family value.

Since genetics can influence some of these risk factors, similarities between parents and children may be inherited. While a recent study of adopted children concluded that obesity in children is largely determined by genetics (49), other studies have demonstrated a significant effect of the familial environment (50,51). One study of twins demonstrated that most of the concordance of cholesterol levels is due to similar diets (52).

Spouses may share cardiovascular risk factors because they married someone with similar habits. This tendency to marry someone with the same traits or behaviors is quite common and is called assortative mating. Smokers tend to marry other smokers (53), and couples tend to smoke the same number of cigarettes per day (54). Obese men tend to marry obese women. Marital partners may even choose each other (consciously or unconsciously) based upon their dietary or exercise habits. In the Framingham study, the concordance of risk factors between spouses did not increase over time, suggesting that these similarities existed at the time of marriage (47).

Whatever the cause of this phenomenon, it has major implications for health care providers. If one member of a family has a particular cardiovascular risk factor, other family members are likely to be more difficult to change if it is shared by other members of the family. Smokers are more likely to stop smoking if no one else in the family is a smoker (55) and remain abstinent longer if their spouse or friends do not smoke (56,57). Changing one member's risk factor may have a ripple effect and influence the entire family. For example, if one family member starts an exericse program, other family members may want to join in. Smoking couples tend to quit smoking at the same time (54). An intervention designed to change the risk factors within the family rather than in only one individual may be more successful, time efficient, and cost effective.

The ability of an individual to make lifestyle changes and reduce the risk of cardiovascular disease is strongly influenced by the support of family members. Several studies have demonstrated that support from the spouse is associated with successful smoking cessation (55,56). In one smoking cessation program (57), smokers who had the cooperation and reinforcement of their partners had lower relapse rate, while "nagging" and "policing" by the partners had the opposite effect. In a study of an exercise program for men with multiple cardiac risk factors (58), those men whose wives had positive attitudes about the program were twice as likely to complete the program than those men whose wives were neutral or negative.

The family's health beliefs about prevention will influence their support for changing risk factors. As part of a cholesterol-reduction study, Doherty and colleagues (59) examined the relationship of spouses' support and health beliefs to compliance with medication. The wife's beliefs regarding how susceptible she thought her husband was to elevated cholesterol were correlated with both her support and her husband's compliance with a cholesterol-lowering drug. In addition, the wife's interest in the program and reminding her husband about medicine or diet correlated with compliance, while nagging about medicine was negatively correlated with compliance.

An unhealthy behavior sometimes plays a role within a family that can hinder attempts to change the behavior. For example, studies suggest that eating behavior and obesity itself play an important homeostatic function within many families (60). In a survey of eating behavior within families, 25 percent of mothers reported that they used food as a reward for their children and 10 percent used it as punishment (61). In one weight-reduction program, 91 percent of the spouses of obese women reported that they wished their wives would lose weight, but only 49 percent were willing to help (62). Fifty-three percent of the men anticipated that weight loss would have an adverse effect on the marriage due to loss of eating as a shared activity, loss of power in marital conflicts, and concern over marital commitment and sexual fidelity. During recorded mealtime conversations, these husbands were seven times more likely to talk about food than their dieting wives, and four times more likely to offer food to the other. The men criticized their dieting wives 12 times more often than they praised them. When health-related behaviors, such as eating, serve important functions in the family, these behaviors may be resistant to change unless attention is paid to how changing the behavior will affect the family.

The family can have a significant effect on the treatment of obesity. Several randomized controlled trials of weight reduction have demonstrated that spouse or partner involvement in weight reduction programs can significantly improve results (63–65). These studies have used a behavioral paradigm in which family members provide immediate and long-term reinforcement for weight loss or dieting. When the partner participates in the weight reduction program, the obese individual is not only able to reduce more weight, but is able to maintain the weight loss.

Despite the fact that hypertension is relatively easy to identify and treat and that adequate treatment significantly lowers the risk of heart attacks and strokes, only one-fourth of all hypertensive individuals are under treatment and only one-half of those under treatment have their blood pressure adequately controlled (66). Compliance with medication is a major problem in the treatment of hypertension and reduction of cardiovascular disease. In a randomized controlled study, Morisky and colleagues (67) demonstrated a dramatic effect of family involvement on hypertension compliance and overall mortality. They studied the impact of three different educational interventions (brief individual counseling, instructing the spouse or significant other during a home visit, and small patient group sessions) on appointment keeping, weight control, and medication compliance. Involving the spouse not only improved overall compliance, but resulted in a significant reduction in blood pressure and overall mortality. Overall the experimental groups had a 57 percent overall reduction in mortality compared to the controls, and those groups that received family education tended to do the best. The family intervention was included in this study after a survey indicated that 70 percent of the clinic's hypertensive patients wished that family members knew more about hypertension (68). Based upon this and other studies of the role of social supports in improving compliance, the National Heart, Lung, and Blood Institute has stressed the importance of "the help that patients receive from their family and friends to carry on with their treatments" (69).

This body of research demonstrates that there is strong evidence for both the healthy and unhealthy influences by families on cardiovascular risk factors. Numerous randomized controlled trials have demonstrated that family involvement improves the results of weight reduction and one study shows a similar result for hypertension control. Similar studies are needed for exercise programs, smoking cessation, and dietary changes (low salt and cholesterol). Despite the proven efficacy of a family aproach to prevention, health-care providers remain focused on the individual. A major challenge to the health profession is to become more effective in health promotion and to incorporate a family approach to prevention.

Families and Chronic Illness

In the past decade there has been an increasing number of studies on the influence of the family on chronic illnesses, including research on asthma (70,71), chronic renal failure (72,73), heart disease (74,75), and cancer (76,77). Amongst this research, work on diabetes has shown the most consistent relationship between family functioning and disease outcomes (78–80). Adequate control of blood sugars in diabetes can prevent many of the long-term complications of disease, but is difficult to achieve and maintain. Diabetic control is related both to intrinsic metabolic factors (as in the "brittle diabetic") and compliance with insulin and diet. Several studies have shown that overall family dysfunction is strongly correlated with poor diabetic control (81–83). Most of the families of 30 poorly controlled diabetic children studied by White et al. (84) had numerous dysfunctional psychosocial factors, including absent fathers, poor living conditions, inadequate parental function, chronic family conflict, and lack of family involvement with the diabetes. On the other hand, clear organization in the family has been associated with good metabolic control (85). High parental self-esteem is also associated with good control and is an important mediating factor between family functioning and diabetes (81).

How emotionally close or cohesive a family is seems to be particularly important for the care of diabetes. Both low cohesion or disengagement and high cohesion or enmeshment have been associated with poor blood sugar control. (See Chapter 3 for discussion of these family systems concepts.) Fischer and Dolger (86) identified two common maternal reactions to diabetes: overprotection and rejection. The overprotective parent had either a submissive or rebellious adolescent diabetic, while the rejcting parent had a resentful and belligerent child. In a carefully controlled study, Anderson and colleagues (87) found that low cohesion and high conflict were associated with poor diabetic control. Parental indifference can result in the worst diabetic control and lead to depression in the diabetic child (88). Thus in emotionally distant or disengaged families, inadequate supervision and parental support results in noncompliance with insulin and diet and poor diabetic control.

Minuchin and his colleagues at the Philadelphia Child Guidance Clinic (89,90) have studied poorly controlled diabetic children from families with high cohesion. These children had recurrent episodes of diabetic ketoacidosis, despite adherence to diet and insulin. When hospitalized and removed from the family environment, their diabetes were easily managed. It appeared that stress and emotional arousal within the family directly affected the child's blood sugar. In studying these families and the families of children with severe asthma and anorexia nervosa, Minuchin discovered a specific pattern of interaction, characterized by enmeshment (high cohesion), overprotectiveness, rigidity, and conflict avoidance. He called these families "psychosomatic families."

To determine how these family interactions can affect diabetes, Baker, Minuchin, and colleagues (91) studied the physiologic responses of diabetic children to a stressful family interview. During the family interview, the children from psychosomatic families had a rapid rise in free fatty acids (a precursor to diabetic ketoacidosis), which persisted beyond the interview. The parents of these children exhibited an initial rise in FFA levels, which fell to normal when the diabetic child entered the room. Minuchin hypothesized that in psychosomatic families, parental conflict is detoured or defused through the chronically ill child, and the resulting stress leads to exacerbations of the illness. In a larger sample of diabetic families, Cederblad and colleagues (92) demonstrated that high cohesion in the mother, rigidity in the father, and anxiety in the diabetic child were all associated with poor metabolic control. Minuchin and his colleagues (89) have also reported the successful treatment of these diabetics and their psychosomatic families using structural family therapy to help disengage the diabetic and establish more appropriate family boundaries. In all 15 cases, the pattern of recurrent ketoacidosis ceased and insulin doses were reduced.

These studies suggest that the mechanisms by which the family influences diabetic control depends upon the style of family functioning, especially its cohesion. Both high and low cohesion are associated with poor diabetic control. In enmeshed families, diabetic control is physiologically linked to emotional processes within the family. In disengaged families, inadequate family structure and support results in noncompliance. Optimal management of diabetes requires the support and supervision of the family along with respect for individuality and age-appropriate autonomy. While these results suggest specific clinical interventions with each type of families, no controlled studies have been conducted yet.

Conclusion

Research on families and health demonstrates the powerful influence of the family on health and illness. Family stress and support have an effect on overall mortality. Bereavement is associated with an increased risk of death. Spousal support has a direct protective effect on health and buffers the impact of stress. Cardiovascular risk factors are often shared by family members, and a family approach is an effective way to change unhealthy lifestyles. Studies of chronic disease indicate that family dysfunction is associated with poor health outcomes. We are just beginning to understand the relationship of families and health, and much more research is needed. This research should have a sound theoretical base and develop from clinical observations. In addition to research on the impact of families on health, there needs to be studies of the process of family-oriented medical care, including studies on the reliability, validity, and efficiency of different methods of family assessments and the impact of family conferences on patient and family satisfaction and health outcomes.

References

1. Litman TJ: The family as a basic unit in health and medical care: A sociobehavioral overview. *Soc Sci Med* 1974;**8**:495–519.
2. Campbell TL: Family's impact on health: A critical review and annotated bibliography. *Fam Syst Med* 1986;**4**(2&3):135–328.
3. Doherty WJ, Campbell TL: *Families and Health*. Families studies text series. Beverly Hills, CA, Sage Publishing, 1988.
4. Turk, DC, Kerns RD (eds.): *Health, Illness, and Families: A Life-Span Perspective.* New York: Wiley, 1985.
5. Goldstein M: Psychosocial issues. *Schizophr Bull* 1987;**13**(1):157–171.
6. Keitner GI, Baldwin LM, Epstein NB, Bishop DS: Family functioning patients with affective disorders: A review. *Inter J Fam Psychiatry* 1985; **6**:405–437.

7. Steinglass P, Robertson A: "The alcoholic family," The biology of alcoholism. *Psychosocial Factors* 1983;**VI**:243–307.
8. Stanton MD: Drugs and the family: A review of the recent literature. *Marr Fam Rev* 1979;**2**:1–10.
9. Hepworth J: "Families and chronic pain." In Rosenthal D (ed.), *Families in Stress*. Family Therapy Collection. Rockville, MD, Aspen, 1987.
10. Yager J: Family issues in the pathogenesis of anorexia nervosa. *Psychosom Med* 1982;**44**:43–59.
11. Rabkin JG, Struening EL: Life events, stress and illness. *Science* 1976;**194**:1013–1020.
12. Holmes TH, Rahe RH: The social readjustment scale. *J Psychosom Res* 1967;**39**:413–431.
13. Cohen F: Stress and bodily illness. *Psychiat Clin North Amer* 1981;**4**:269–285.
14. Meyer RJ, Haggerty RJ: Steptococcal infections in families: Factors altering individual susceptibility. *Pediatrics* 1962;**29**:539–549.
15. Boyce WT, Jensen EW, Cassel JC, et al.: Influence of life events and family routines on childhood respiratory illness. *Pediatrics* 1977;**60**:609–615.
16. Beautrais AL, Fergusson DM, Shannon FT: Life events and childhood morbidity: A prospective study. *Pediatrics* 1982;**70**:935–940.
17. Jacobs S, Ostfeld A: An epidemiological review of the mortality of bereavement. *Psychosom Med* 1977;**39**:344–357.
18. Osterweis M, Solomon F, Green M, (eds.): *Bereavement: Reactions, Consequences, and Care*. Washington, DC: National Academy Press, 1984.
19. Kraus AS, Lillenfeld AM: Some epidemiological aspects of the high mortality rate in the young widowed group. *J Chron Dis* 1959;**10**:207–217.
20. Parkes CM, Benjamin B, Fitzgerald RG: Broken heart: A statistical study of increased mortality among widowers. *Br Med J* 1969;**1**:740–743.
21. Helsing KJ, Szklo M: Mortality after bereavement. *Am J Epidemiol* 1981;**114**:41–52.
22. Kaprio J, Koskenvou M, Rita H: Mortality after bereavement: A prospective study of 95,647 widowed persons. *Am J Pub Health* 1987;**77**:283–287.
23. Lynch J: *The Broken Heart: The Medical Consequences of Loneliness*. New York: Basic Books, 1977.
24. Verbrugge LM: Marital status and health. *J Marr Fam* 1977;**7**:267–285.
25. Carter H, Glick PC: *Marriage and Divorce: A Social and Economic Study*. Cambridge, MA: Harvard University Press, 1970.
26. Bruhn JG: Effects of chronic illness on the family. *J Fam Pract* 1977;**4**:1057–1060.
27. Klein R, Dean A, Bogdanoff M: The impact of illness of the spouse. *J Chron Dis* 1968;**20**:241–252.
28. Ader R (ed.): *Psychoneuroimmunlogy*. New York, Academic Press, 1981.
29. Calabrese JR, Kling MA, Gold PW: Alterations in immunocompetence during stress, bereavement and depression: Focus on neuroendocrine regulation. *Am J Psychiatry* 1987;**144**(9):1123–1134.
30. Bartrop RW, Luckhurst E, Lazarus L, Kiloh LG, Penny R: Depressed lymphocyte function after bereavement. *Lancet* 1977;**1**:834–836.
31. Schleifer SJ, Keller SE, Camerino M, Thornton JC, Stein M: Suppression of lymphocyte stimulation following bereavement. *JAMA* 1983;**250**:374–377.

32. Linn MW, Linn BS, Jensen J: Stressful events, dysphoric mood, and immune responsiveness. *Psychol Rep* 1984;**54**:219–222.

33. Kiecolt-Glaser JK, Fisher LD, Ogrockl P, Stout JC, Spelcher CE, Glaser R: Marital quality, marital disruption, and immune function. *Psychosom Med* 1987;**49**(1):13–32.

34. Berkman LF: Assessing the physical health effects of social network and social support. *Ann Rev Pub Health* 1984;**5**:413–432.

35. Broadhead WE, Kaplan BH, James SA, et al.: The epidemiologic evidence for a relationship between social support and health. *Am J Epidemiol* 1983;**117**:521–537.

36. Cohen S, Syme SL (eds.): *Social Support and Health*. Orlando, FL: Academic Press, 1985.

37. Berkman LF, Syme SL: Social networks, host resistance and mortality: A nine year follow-up study of Alameda County residents. *Am J Epidemiol* 1979;**109**:186–204.

38. House JS, Robbins C, Metzner HL: The association of social relationships and activities with mortality: Prospective evidence from the Tecumseh Community Health Study. *Am J Epidemiol* 1982;**116**:123–140.

39. Ortho-Gomer K, Johnson JV: Social network interaction and mortality: A six year follow-up study of a random sample of the Swedish population. *J Chron Dis* 1987;**40**:949–957.

40. Blazer DG: Social support and mortality in an elderly community population. *Am J Epidemiol* 1982;**115**:684–694.

41. Zuckerman DM, Kasl SV, Osterfeld AM: Psychosocial predictors of mortality among the elderly poor: The role of religion, well-being, and social contact. *Am J Epidemiol* 1984;**119**:410–423.

42. Nuckolls KB, Cassel J, Kaplan BH: Psychosocial assets, life crisis and the prognosis of pregnancy. *Am J Epidemiol* 1972;**95**:431–441.

43. Norbeck JS, Tolden VP: Life stress, social supports, and emotional disequilibrium in complications of pregnancy: A prospective, multivariate study. *J Health Soc Behav* 1983;**24**:30–46.

44. Ramsey CN, Abell TD, Baker LC: The relationship between family functioning, life events, family structure and the outcome of pregnancy. *J Fam Pract* 1986;**22**:521–527.

45. Healthy People: The Surgeon General's report on health promotion and disease prevention. DHEW (PHS) Pub No. 79-55071. Public Health Service Washington, DC: Government Printing Office, 1979.

46. Baranowski T, Nader PR, Dunn K, Vanderpool NA: Family self-help: Promoting changes in health behavior. *Journal of Communication* 1982; Summer:161–172.

47. Sackett DL, Anderson GD, Milner R, Feinleib M, Kannel WB: Concordance for coronary risk factors among spouses. *Circulation* 1975;**52**:589–595.

48. Bewley BR, Bland JM: Academic performance and social factors relating to cigarette smoking by school children. *Br J Prev Soc Med* 1977;**31**:8–24.

49. Stunkard AJ, Sorensen TIA, Hanis C, et al.: An adoption study of human obesity. *N Engl J Med* 1986;**314**:193–201.

50. Garn SM, Cole PE, Bailey SM: Effect of parental fatness levels on fatness of biological and adoptive children. *Ecology of Food and Nutrition* 1976; **6**:1–3.

51. Hartz A, Giefer E, Rimm AA: Relative importance of the effect of family

environment and heredity on obesity. *Ann Human Genet* 1977;**41**:185–193.

52. Feinleib M, Garrison RJ, Fabsitz R, et al.: The NHLBI twin study of cardiovascular disease risk factors: Methodology and summary of results. *Am J Epidemiol* 1977;**106**:284–295.

53. Sutton G: Assortive marriages for smoking habits. *Ann Human Biol* 1980;**7**:449–456.

54. Venters MH, Jacobs DR, Luepker RV, Maiman LA, Gillum RF: Spouse concordance of smoking patterns: The Minnesota heart survey. *Am J Epidemiol* 1984;**120**:608–616.

55. Graham S, Gibson RW: Cessation of patterned behavior: Withdrawal from smoking. *Soc Sci Med* 1971;**5**:319–337.

55a. Price RA, Chen KH, Cavallii SL, et al.: Models of spouse influence and their applications to smoking behavior. *Soc Biology* 1981;**28**:14–29.

56. Ockene JK, Nuttall RL, Benfari RS, et al.: A psychosocial model of smoking cessation and maintenance of cessation. *Preventive Medicine* 1981;**10**:623–638.

57. Mermelstein R, Lichtenstein E, McIntyre K: Partner support and relapse in smoking cessation programs. *J Consult Clin Psychol* 1983;**51**:465–466.

58. Heinzelman F, Bagley RW: Response to physical activity programs and their effects on health behavior. *Pub Health Rep* 1970;**85**:905–911.

59. Doherty WJ, Schrott HG, Metcalf L, Iassiello-Vailas L: Effect of spouse support and health beliefs on medication adherence. *J Fam Pract* 1983;**17**:837–841.

60. Barbarin OA, Tirado M: Family involvement and successful treatment of obesity: A review. *Fam Sys Med* 1984;**2**:37–45.

61. Bryan MS, Lowenberg ME: The father's influence on young children's food preferences. *J Am Diet Assoc* 1958;**34**:30–35.

62. Stuart RB, Davis B: *Slim Chance in a Fat World: Behavioral Control Obesity.* Champaign IL: Research Press, 1972.

63. Brownell KD, Heckerman CL, Westlake RJ, Hayes SC, Monti PM: The effects of couple's training and partner co-operativeness in the behavioral treatment of obesity. *Behav Res Ther* 1978;**16**:323–333.

64. Pearce JW, LeBow MD, Orchard J: Role of spouse involvement in the behavioral treatment of overweight women. *J Consult Clin Psychol* 1981;**49**:236–244.

65. Saccone AJ, Israel AC: Effects of experimental versus significant other-controlled reinforcement and choice of target behavior on weight loss. *Behav Ther* 1978;**9**:271–278.

66. McKenney JM, Slining JM, Henderson HR, Devine D, Barr M: The effect of clinical pharmacy services on patients with essential hypertension. *Circulation* 1973;**48**:1104–1111.

67. Morisky DE, Levine DM, Green LW, Shaprio S, Russell RP, Smith CR: Five year blood pressure control and mortality following health education for hypertensive patients. *Am J Pub Health* 1983;**73**:153–162.

68. Levine DM, Green LW, Deeds SG, Chwalow J, Russel RP, Finlay J: Health education for hypertensive patients. *JAMA* 1979;**241**:1700–1703.

69. Haynes RB, Mattson ME, Chobanian AV, Dunbar JM, Engerbretson TO, et al.: Management of patient compliance in the treatment of hypertension: Report of the NHLBI working group. *Hypertension* 1982;**4**:415–423.

70. Lask B, Matthew D: Childhood asthma: A controlled trial of family psychotherapy. *Arch Dis Child* 1979;**54**:116–119.

71. Liebman R, Minuchin S, Baker L: The use of structural family therapy in the treatment of intractable asthma. *Am J Psychiatry* 1974;**131**:535–540.

72. Reiss D, Gonzalez S, Kramer N: Family process, chronic illness, and death. *Arch Gen Psychiatry* 1986;**43**:795–804.

73. Steidl JH, Finkelstein FO, Wexler JP, Feigenbaum H, Kitsen J, AS, Quinlan DM: Medical condition, adherence to treatment regime and family functioning: Their interaction in patients receiving long-term dialysis treatment. *Arch Gen Psychiatry* 1980;**37**:1025–1027.

74. Ruberman W, Weinblatt E, Goldberg JD, Chaudhary BS: Psychosocial influences on mortality after myocardial infarction. *N Engl J Med* 1984; **311**:522–557.

75. Koskevuo M, Kaprio J, Kesaniemi A, Sarna S: Differences in mortality from ischemic heart disease by marital status and social class. *J Chron Dis* 1980;**33**:95–106.

76. Horne RL, Picard RS: Psychosocial risk factors for lung cancers. *Psychosom Med* 1979;**41**:503–514.

77. Thomas CB, Duszynski BA, Shaffer JW: Family attitudes reported in youth as potential predictors of cancer. *Psychosom Med* 1979;**41**:287–302.

78. Anderson BJ, Auslander WF: Research on diabetes management and the family: A critique. *Diabetes Care* 1980;**3**:696–702.

79. Johnson SB: Psychosocial factors in juvenile diabetes: A review. *Journal of Behavioral Medicine* 1980;**3**:95–116.

80. Klus J, Habbick BF, Abernathy TJ: Diabetes in children: Family responses and control. *Psychosom* 1983;**24**:367–372.

81. Grey MJ, Genel M, Tamborlane WV: Psychosocial adjustment of latency-age diabetics: Determinants and relationship to control. *Pediatrics* 1980; **65**:69–73.

82. Koski ML, Kumento A: The interrelationship between diabetic control and family life. *Pediat Adol Endocrin* 1977;**3**:41–45.

83. Orr DP, Golden MP, Myers G, Marrerro DG: Characteristics of adolescents with poorly controlled diabetes referred to a tertiary care center. *Diabetes Care* 1983;**6**:170–175.

84. White K, Kolman ML, Wexler P, Polin G, Winter RJ: Unstable diabetes and unstable families: A psychosocial evaluation of diabetic children with recurrent ketoacidosis. *Pediatrics* 1984;**73**:749–755.

85. Shouval R, Ber R, Galatzer A: Family social climate and the health status and social adaptation of diabetic youth. *Pedia Adol Endocrin* 1982;**10**:89–93.

86. Fischer AE, Dolger H: Behavior and psychosocial problems of young diabetic patients. *Arch Intern Med* 1946;**78**:711–732.

87. Anderson BJ, Miller JP, Auslander WF, Santiago JV: Family characteristics of diabetic adolescents: Relationship to metabolic control. Diabetes Care 1981;**4**:586–594.

88. Khurana R, White P: Attitudes of the diabetic child and his parents towards his illness. *Postgrad Med* 1970;**48**:72–76.

89. Minuchin S, Baker L, Rosman BL, Liebman R, Milman L, Todd TC: A conceptual model of psychosomatic illness in children: Family organization and family therapy. *Arch Gen Psychiatry* 1975;**32**:1031–1038.

90. Minuchin S, Rosman BL, Baker L: *Psychosomatic Families.* Cambridge, MA: Harvard University Press, 1978.
91. Baker L, Minuchin S, Milman L, Liebman R, Todd T: Psychosomatic aspects of juvenile diabetes mellitus: A progress report. *Mod Prob In Paediatr* 1975;**12**:332–343.
92. Cederblad M, Helgesson M, Larsson Y, Ludvigsson J: Family structure and diabetes in children. *Pediat Adol Endocrin* 1982;**10**:94–98.
93. Clark NM, Feldman CH, Evans D, Millman EJ, Wailewski Y, Valle I: The effectiveness of education for family management of asthma in children: A preliminary report. *Health Educa Quart* 1981;**8**:166–174.
94. Gustafsson PA, Kjellman NI, Cederblad M: Family therapy in the treatment of severe childhood asthama. *J Psychosom Res* 1986;**30**:369–374.
95. Baranowski T, Nader PR, Dunn K, Vanderpool NA: Family self-help: Promoting changes in health behavior. *Journal of Communications* 1982;Summer:161–172.
96. Earp JL, Ory MG, Strogatz DS: The effects of family involvement and practitioner home visits on the control of hypertention. *Am J Pub Health* 1982;**72**:1146–1153.
97. Brownell KD, Heckerman CL, Westlake RJ, Hayes SC, Monti PM: The effects of couples training and partner co-operativeness in the behavioral treatment of obesity. *Behav Res Ther* 1978;**16**:323–333.
98. Saccone AJ, Israel AC: Effects of experimental versus significant other-controlled reinforcement and choice of target behavior on weight loss. *Behav Ther* 1978;**9**:271–278.
99. Wilson GT, Brownell K: Behavior therapy for obesity: Including family members in the treatment process. *Behav Ther* 1976;**9**:943–945.
100. Pearce JW, BeLow MD, Orchard J: Role of spouse involvement in the behavioral treatment of overweight women. *J Consult Clin Psychol* 1981;**49**:236–244.
101. Brownell KD, Kelman JH, Stunkard AJ: Treatment of obese children with and without their mothers: Changes in weight and blood pressure. *Pediatrics* 1983;**71**:515–523.

PROTOCOL
Implications of Research on Families and Health for Physicians

Assessment

1. Assess **stress** within the family by obtaining a genogram. Include:
   a. deaths of significant family members
   b. illness in the family
   c. recent divorce or separation
   d. chronic marital or sexual difficulties
2. Assess **coping** including:
   a. how well the individual patient and the family have dealt with stress in the past (obtained from the genogram)
   b. how they are coping with current stressors
3. Assess **resources**, including:
   a. sources of family and social support
      • informational support
      • emotional support
      • financial support
   b. availability and utilization of supports
   c. how helpful the patient and family perceive the supports to be
4. Assess **role of the health behavior** in the family:
   • What function or role does a particular health related behavior, such as smoking or diet, play within the family.
   • What will happen if the behavior or risk factor is changed? Ask "What would it be like for you and your family if you no longer . . . smoked? . . . were overweight?"

Intervention

1. Screening: When an unhealthy behavior or risk factor is detected, screen the entire family for the same risk factor, even when it is not genetically determined, including:
   a. smoking
   b. excess alcohol consumption
   c. elevated cholesterol
   d. obesity
   e. failure to use seatbelts
   f. drinking while driving
   g. hypertension
2. Educate the family as well as the patient about the risk factor or illness.

3. Intervene at the family level, when possible:
    a. Encourage both members of a couple to quit smoking, or all members of the family to reduce the cholesterol in their diets.
    b. Work to get the patient's spouse to support lifestyle changes or compliance with medication. Block tendencies for spouses to "police" or "nag" the patient.
    c. Encourage family involvement in the management of the illness, while supporting the patient's autonomy and ultimate responsibility for care.
    d. Refer severely dysfunctional families with chronic illnesses to a family therapist. Keep the focus of the referral on the diabetes, not on the family problems. Refer for "difficulty controlling diabetes" not "family dysfunction." (See Chapter 15 for more on families and chronic illness.)

CHAPTER 3

Family Systems Concepts
Tools for Assessing the Family in Primary Care

To provide family-oriented medical care it is important for a physician to be able to assess how a family's functioning plays a part in both the illness and the health of its members. Just as a physician must organize and evaluate the signs of physical illness in order to make an appropriate diagnosis, the same is true when considering the emotional, interactional, and historical processes that take place in a patient and his or her family. To do so without benefit of a conceptual framework for understanding the family can be overwhelming.

Doherty and Baird first conceptualized and labeled primary care family assessment and counseling in their landmark volume, *Family Therapy and Family Medicine*, in 1983 (1). Others in family medicine have developed screening instruments and assessment methods that can be useful in primary care such as the Family APGAR (2), the family circle (3), and PRACTICE (4). The family genogram (5,6) borrowed from the family therapy field is an essential tool for the assessment of families. (7).

Family assessment begins at the initial contact with any patient during a routine encounter and involves taking relational factors into account when considering medical problems. This minimal assessment may or may not lead to a family meeting to assess a situation in greater depth. Thus when a physician identifies marital problems, or hypothesizes a link between symptoms of different family members, he or she has made an assessment that may lead to a family meeting to further evaluate the situation (1,4). (See Chapter 5 for a discussion of how to convene the family.) Family-oriented primary care involves a continuum of family assessment from minimal (e.g., routine visits with individual patients) to maximal (e.g., calling a family conference), depending on the patient's needs.

Family Systems Concepts

In this chapter we will present family systems concepts and case illustrations that will help the physician: organize his or her thinking about families, identify how families are structured, recognize family interactional patterns and processes, and be aware of family development across time.

The Family

1. The Family as a System. Through the application of systems theory, we see the family as more than the sum of its parts. The family is organized by interpersonal structures and processes that enable it to be both stable and adaptable over time.
- Who are the members of the patient's family?
- When it comes to daily support, who does the patient consider as family?

2. Family Stability. Family stability is the interpersonal process by which the family strives to maintain emotional balance in the system (e.g., a mother who despite significant disability continues to care for her children).
- What does the family do to maintain balance and security for its members?
- If change occurs too quickly, what will happen to the family's stability?

3. Family Change. Family change is the interpersonal process by which the family adapts, alters, or becomes different.
- What does the family do to facilitate needed change?
- If change does not occur quickly enough, what will happen to the family?

4. The Relational Context of the Symptom. The presenting symptom is part of a large family and psychosocial context that can influence and be influenced by that symptom. For some acute, self-limited illnesses, a primarily biomedical intervention may be enough for any symptom. But for many medical problems the relational context is important to treatment.
- How do the patient's symptoms influence the family?
- How does the family influence the patient's symptom?

> Mr. Payne, a 42-year-old factory worker, came to see Dr. M because he had been experiencing more frequent chest pains over the prior two months. Mr. Payne had a history of chronic stable angina that had previously been well controlled with medication. Dr. M's medical evaluation revealed that his blood pressure, physical exam, and electrocardiogram had not changed. Dr.

M increased Mr. Payne's medication, ordered an exercise stress test, and scheduled him to return in one week.

At the follow-up visit, Mr. Payne reported that his chest pains were less frequent but still troublesome. Dr. M explained that the stress test was mildly abnormal but unchanged from his previous test, and recommended that he start taking a new medication. Mr. Payne was agreeable to Dr. M's plan but still appeared distressed. Dr. M began to explore what else was occurring in Mr. Payne's life. He learned that Mr. Payne's wife had started cleaning houses in the last six months to earn some extra income. Mr. Payne's son, Bob, 17, a high-school senior worked with his mother after school. Mr. Payne seemed irritated by how busy his wife was and how little time he had with his son. Mr. Payne felt his main support was his 21-year-old daughter, Mary, who lived and worked in a nearby town. Mary came home to visit on weekends. Three months ago Mary announced she was engaged. Although Mr. Payne liked Mary's fiance, he felt she was making a decision to marry prematurely. He worried about her future.

Dr. M said he was impressed with how family members cared for and helped each other. He suggested that the family come to an appointment together because they might be a resource to Mr. Payne and Dr. M.

Dr. M's discussion of Mr. Payne's family helped place the **symptom in a larger relational context.** The family's emotional balance **(family stability)** had been disrupted by numerous changes and anticipated changes: Mrs. Payne's new job, Bob's eventual graduation, and Mary's engagement. Mr. Payne was experiencing the stress of all these transitions and his symptoms may have been a signal that the family was also having difficulty navigating the changes **(family change).** Dr. M invited the family in to explore how the family's functioning as a whole might play a part in Mr. Payne's symptoms and their alleviation **(family as a system).**

Family Structure

5. Hierarchy. Hierarchy has to do with how power or authority is distributed within the family (8). Typically, parents have greater authority than children and thus are above them in the family hierarchy.
- Who is in charge in the family system?
- Is the family's hierarchy clear and appropriate (e.g., parents in charge of their children) or reversed (e.g., parents controlled by children)?

6. Boundaries. Boundaries define different functional subgroups in the family, such as the marital subgroup, the sibling subgroup, the grandparents, etc.
- What are the subgroups in the family?
- Are the boundaries between subgroups (e.g., parents and children) clear and appropriate or confused and problematic?
- How does the family deal with emotional closeness and distance?

7. Family Role Selection. Family role selection is the unconscious assignment of complementary roles to members of a family. The roles then function to maintain the stability of the family system (e.g., mother is in charge of discipline; father is the nurturer).

- What roles do family members play, and how do these roles relate to each other?
- Who is the family's expert on illness and health?
- Who is most often the "sick" member of the family?

8. Scapegoat or Noble Symptom Bearer. The scapegoat or noble symptom bearer is identified by the family as the source of its problems, accepts the family's blame, and through his or her symptoms also reflects the dysfunction of the family as a whole.

- Does the family have a scapegoat or noble symptom bearer?
- How do his or her symptoms reflect problems for the family as a whole?

9. Parentified Child. The parentified child is a child in the family, often the oldest, who performs the parental functions when one or both parents have abdicated the role (e.g., an oldest daughter does the cooking and child care because of the mother's chronic disabilities).

- Does a child in the family function as a parent?
- Have one or both parents abdicated their role?

10. Alliance. An alliance is a positive relationship between any two members of a system (e.g., a mother and father cooperating together).

- What are the important alliances in the family?
- How are alliances between family members viewed by other family members?

11. Coalition. A coalition is a relationship between at least three people in which two collude against a third (e.g., a parent and a child siding against another parent).

- What coalitions exist in the family?
- Who is siding against whom?

> Mr. and Mrs. Payne, Mary, 21, and Bob, 17, came to the family meeting called by Dr. M. After Dr. M shared his findings, Mary was the first family member to speak as she expressed her concern about her father's "longstanding" health problems. She blamed her mother for not taking better care of him. Bob quickly defended his mother, saying she had been working very hard and had a lot on her mind. Bob became upset with Mary for attacking their mother. Mrs. Payne told Dr. M that her husband had had health complaints for as long as she had known him. Mr. Payne then said that his chest pains were worse since the last doctor's appointment.

Dr. M could see that the **hierarchy** within the Payne family was reversed. Mary took charge of the family interaction (**parentified child**). She acted in a **coalition** with her father against her mother, much as Bob was in a **coalition** with Mrs. Payne against Mary during the meeting. A good working relationship **(alliance)** did not exist between Mr. and Mrs. Payne regarding Mr. Payne's health. This was due in part to the confused generational **boundaries** in the family which contributed to the distance between Mr. and Mrs. Payne. Instead of strong marital and sibling subsystems, both children functioned as protectors of their parents. Mr. Payne was the family's "sick" member; Mary acted as the expert on his health; Mrs. Payne was cast as the uncaring spouse; and Bob was her defender **(family role selection)**. Mr. Payne drew attention away from the family's conflicts by focusing on his chest pains **(noble symptom bearer)**.

Family Process

12. Enmeshment. Enmeshment characterizes a system in which members have few interpersonal boundaries, limited individual autonomy, and a high degree of emotional reactivity (e.g., mother insists on remaining with her adolescent son during his physical and answers questions for him).
  • Are family members overinvolved with each other?
  • Do family members "feel each others feelings"?
  • Do family members seldom act independently?

13. Disengagement. Disengagement characterizes a family system in which members are emotionally distant and unresponsive to each other (e.g., a husband does not tell his wife or children about any of his health problems).
  • Do family members have little emotional response to each other?
  • Are family members distant or isolated from each other?

14. Triangulation. Triangulation occurs when a third person is drawn into a two-person system in order to diffuse anxiety or conflict over issues of intimacy in the two-person system (e.g., rather than arguing with each other about personal issues, a mother and father express their marital discontent by arguing over parenting their son).
  • Do family members talk directly to each other about personal matters?
  • Or when emotional issues arise between two members, do they focus on a third family member?

15. Family Patterns. Family patterns are the ordered sequences of interaction that typify how a family functions (e.g., when one spouse pursues, the other spouse withdraws; when a father gets depressed, the family tries to cheer him up, but he gets more depressed, and they become frustrated).
  • What sequence of behaviors are being used to solve the family's dilemma?
  • Does this pattern make the situation better or worse?

• If worse, what other behaviors might interrupt the sequence or pattern?

> After commenting on his health problems, Mr. Payne told his wife how upset he was that she had shown so little interest in their daughter's marriage. Mr. Payne told Dr. M he discussed his wife's apparent disinterest frequently with his daughter who he described as "hurt."

Mr. Payne had developed a very close relationship with his daughter (**enmeshment**) which at times substituted for the emotional support he felt was missing from his wife. And rather than discussing his own feelings of neglect, Mr. Payne became angry at Mrs. Payne about her "lack of interest" in their daughter's plans to marry (**triangulation**). Dr. M recognized that whenever family members became upset with each other the focus of attention shifted to health issues or a third family member (**family pattern**).

The Family Across Time

16. The Family Life Cycle. The family life cycle is the normal process of family development beginning with marriage, pregnancy, launching of children, retirement and ending with death in which specific developmental tasks must be accomplished. (See Appendix 3.1)
   • In what developmental stage is the family?
   • What are the important tasks that need to be accomplished in this stage?

17. Family Projection Process. Family projection process involves the transmission of unresolved conflicts, issues, roles, and tasks from one generation to another (e.g., the men in each generation never go to physicians for health problems).
   • What unresolved issues from past generations may be affecting the family in the present?

18. Intergenerational Coalition. A coalition of two members from different generations against a third member of the family is an intergenerational coalition (e.g., a grandmother and granddaughter against a mother).
   • Is there evidence of family members from two different generations colluding against a third member?

> Dr. M commented on the many important changes that the family was facing—their son graduating, mother starting to work, and daughter planning to marry. Mr. and Mrs. Payne both agreed that these changes were affecting them. They were hopeful about their children's future but anxious, as well, about their leaving. Following this discussion Mr. Payne talked at length about his mother's death five years ago. Mrs. Payne said her husband had never gotten over the loss although he never discussed it with her. Mrs. Payne had never been close to her mother-in-law.

The Payne family was facing the "leaving home" stage in their development **(family life cycle).** Both children were leaving either for college or to get married within the next several months. This placed increasing pressure on the marital relationship as they faced an "empty nest." The anticipation of these changes or losses also reawakened Mr. Payne's unresolved grief over his mother's death **(family projection process).** Mrs. Payne's comments about her husband's grief and her own lack of attachment to her mother-in-law led Dr. M to hypothesize that perhaps Mr. Payne and his mother had been in close relationship that excluded Mrs. Payne **(intergenerational coalition).**

The case of Mr. Payne illustrates how family systems concepts can be used to better understand the interplay between a patient's symptoms and his or her family. Without such conceptual tools a family's interactions can seem confusing at best and frustrating at worst. And while not all the concepts apply to every family, family systems theory does provide a way for a physician to organize his or her thinking about any family. The information gathered by assessing a family as a system, its structure, process, and development across time, can be used to arrive at an effective treatment plan in collaboration with the patient and family.

References

1. Doherty W, Baird M: *Family Therapy and Family Medicine.* New York: Guilford Press, 1983.
2. Smilkstein G: The Family APGAR: A proposal for a family function test and its use by physicians. *J Fam Pract* 1978;**6**:1234.
3. Thrower SM, Bruce WE, Welton RF: The family circle method for integrating family systems concepts in family medicine. *J Fam Pract* 1982;**15**:451.
4. Christie-Sealy J (ed.): *Working With the Family in Primary Care: A Systems Approach to Health and Illness.* New York: Praeger, 1984.
5. Bowen M: *Family Therapy in Clinical Practice.* New York: Jason Aronson, 1978.
6. McGoldrick M, Gerson R: *Genograms in Family Assessment.* New York: W.W. Norton, 1985.
7. Jolly W, Froom J, Rosen M: The genogram. *J Fam Pract* 1980;**2**:251–255.
8. Simon F, Stierlin H, Wynne L: *The Language of Family Therapy: A Systemic Vocabulary and Sourcebook.* New York: Family Process Press, 1985.

Appendix 3.1
The Family Life Cycle

Family Life Cycle Stages	Developmental Tasks
Leaving Home	*Differentiate self in relation to family *Develop intimate peer relationships *Establish oneself in work
Couples and Pairing	*Form a committed relationship *Realign relationships with extended family to include partner
Pregnancy and Childbirth	*Make room for children in the family *Become parents while remaining spouses
Family with Young Children	*Form a parent team *Negotiate relationships with extended family to include parenting and grandparenting roles
Family with Adolescents	*Shift parent–child relationship to permit adolescent to move in and out of system
Adulthood and Middle Years	*Refocus on marital and career issues *Deal with disabilities and death in grandparents *Deal with own aging and mortality
Graying of the Family	*Maintain functioning in face of physiologic decline
Death and Grieving	*Deal with loss of spouse, siblings, and peers *Preparation of own death

*Adapted from Carter CA, McGoldrick M (eds.): *The Family Life Cycle: A Framework for Family Therapy*, New York: Gardner Press, 1980.

PROTOCOL
Family Systems Concepts

The Family

1. Family as a System
   - Who are the members of your patient's family?
   - When it comes to daily support, who does your patient consider as family?
2. Family Stability (Homeostasis/Morphostasis)
   - What does the family do to maintain balance and security for its members?
   - If change occurs too quickly, what will happen to the family's stability?
3. Family Change (Morphogenesis)
   - What does the family do to facilitate needed change?
   - If change does not occur quickly enough, what will happen to the family?
4. Relational Context of the System
   - How do the patient's symptoms influence the family?
   - How does the family influence the patient's symptoms?

Family Structure

5. Hierarchy
   - Who is in charge in the family system?
   - Is the family's hierarchy clear and appropriate (e.g., parents in charge of their children) or reversed (e.g., children in charge of their parents)?
6. Boundaries
   - What are the subgroups in the family?
   - Are the boundaries between subgroups (e.g., parents and children) clear and appropriate or confused and problematic?
   - How does the family deal with emotional closeness and distance?
7. Family Role Selection
   - What roles do family members play, and how do these roles relate to each other?
   - Who is the family's expert on health and illness?
   - Who is most often the "sick" member of the family?
8. Noble Symptom Bearer/Scapegoat
   - Does the family have a scapegoat or noble symptom bearer?
   - How do his or her symptoms reflect problems for the family as a whole?

9. Parentified Child
   • Does a child in the family function as a parent?
   • Have one or both parents abdicated their role?
10. Alliance
   • What are the important alliances in the family?
   • How are alliances between family members viewed by other family members?
11. Coalition
   • What coalitions exist in the family?
   • Who are the coalition members siding together against?

Family Process

12. Enmeshment
   • Are family members overinvolved with each other?
   • Do family members "feel each other's feelings"?
   • Do family members seldom act independently?
13. Disengagement
   • Do family members have little emotional response to each other?
   • Are family members distant or isolated from each other?
14. Triangulation
   • Do family members talk directly to each other about personal matters?
   • Or when emotional issues arise between two members, do they focus on a third family member?
15. Family Patterns
   • What sequences of behavior are being used to solve the family's dilemma?
   • Does this pattern make the situation worse? If so, what different behaviors might interrupt the sequence or pattern?

The Family Across Time

16. The Family Life Cycle
   • In what developmental stage is the family?
   • What are the important tasks that need to be accomplished in this stage?
17. Family Projection Process
   • What unresolved issues from past generations may be affecting the family in the present?
18. Intergenerational Coalition
   • Is there evidence of family members from two different generations colluding against a third member?

CHAPTER 4

Greasing the Wheels

Promoting a Working Alliance with Patients and Families

The relationship between families and their physician is the most powerful vehicle for influencing patients about issues regarding health and illness. Physicians influence their patients and patients influence their physicians. The doctor–patient relationship is an essential subsystem of the biopsychosocial approach to treatment. As such, it deserves special thought and consideration, and careful assessment when this alliance is problematic. The way the physician handles his or her part in the doctor–patient relationship can affect a patient's sense of well-being and the likelihood that a patient and family will cooperate with any given treatment plan, not to mention the physician's own sense of job satisfaction. For these important reasons, we will now turn to some pragmatic suggestions for promoting a constructive working alliance with patients and family members. We will focus on the physician's side of this equation because that is what we can alter. Three fundamental interviewing skills enhance the potential for an effective partnership to develop between physician and family: building rapport, structuring the interview, and converting resistance into cooperation.

Building Rapport

Early in an interview both physician and patient test each other. Physicians look for whether a patient will be a clear and reliable source of information about the presenting problem. Physicians also look for some sense of cooperation from the patient: Will the physician and patient easily understand each other and work together, or will this alliance require more attention to succeed? While physicians scrutinize their patients, the patients, of course, are checking out their physicians. First and foremost, patients generally assess the physician: Does the physician seem to ask the right questions, order the right tests, prescribe the right medicine, provide some information about the presenting complaint? Does the physician listen attentively and empathize with patient concerns? In this way the patient decides if the physician is competent and understanding.

During this phase of the interview, it is important to focus, almost exclusively, on building rapport. The term used by family therapists to characterize this early phase of rapport-building is **joining** (1). Joining with each individual patient and family member is like oiling an important piece of machinery. If it is well-oiled, the machine is likely to run smoothly and effectively when it is needed. If not, the machine will grind, make a lot of noise, and run inefficiently or sometimes not run at all. Joining, like oiling, is a maintenance task that in and of itself will not produce the desired outcome, but the absence of which threatens the outcome of the interaction.

Joining occurs most consciously in the socializing phase of an interview or conference. It begins with greeting, making contact, and establishing rapport with each person. From an individual perspective, this process involves searching for a common wavelength or language with which to communicate. Searching for commonality may involve commenting on the weather, on a common heritage, or inquiring about the patient's employment. It is finding a respectful way to make a connection, person to person, before beginning the central business of the interview. For example:

- Hello, Mrs. Jones, I'm Dr. Brown. How did you manage to get here today through all that snow?
- Hello, my name is Dr. Brown. Mr. Mancini? That's Italian isn't it? My wife's family came over from Italy.
- I'm glad to meet you, Mr. Hammer. I see from your chart that you are a carpenter. I did some construction work while I was in college. That's tough work.

It is in these beginning interactions that a physician may consciously or unconsciously use different parts of his or her own history or behavior to connect with a given patient. This may be done at the level of content, as in the above introductions, or it may be done at a process or nonverbal level. For example, with a depressed woman, the physician may speak in a low, soothing voice. With a loud, anxious man who just had a myocardial infarction, the physician may speak with strong conviction. With a particularly difficult patient, part of establishing rapport may involve matching behavior, such as sitting in the same position, using similar speech cadence, or mirroring some of the patient's gestures until the patient has relaxed enough to have productive exchange.

Once a connection has been formed, joining involves listening for the patient's health belief system, their cultural explanations for illness, and, especially, their personal diagnosis of the problem. Understanding the patient's position provides a starting point for negotiating a diagnosis (if you do not agree with their's) and collaborating on an effective treatment plan.

> PATIENT: I think I feel some lumps in my neck, Doctor. I want you to check them for me.
> DR: So you've noticed some unusual lumps in your neck. Is there anything particular you are concerned about?
> PATIENT: Well, sort of. My brother died of Hodgkin's disease several years ago, and I am afraid I may have the same thing.

This is a straightforward example of connecting with a patient's agenda and understanding her own diagnosis so that an acceptable treatment plan can follow.

When interacting with more than one person at a time, as in a family conference, joining also involves being wary of emotional triangles and family coalitions. (See Chapter 3 for an explanation of these concepts.) To be effective, it is important for the physician **to develop positive working alliances with both the patient and other family members**, rather than being drawn into coalitions with the patient against family members or vice versa.

> DR: Thank you, Mr. Howell, for coming in to help me understand your wife's recent problems sleeping.
> MR. HOWELL: I don't see how I can contribute. I'm sure my wife has already told you I snore, and she probably told you that's why she can't sleep. But, I doubt it. I've been snoring for years. Maybe if you just gave her sleeping pills, we could all get some rest.
> DR: Your viewpoint is certainly important to me. Perhaps we can all work together to solve this problem. I would like to hear both of your perspectives on this sleep disturbance.

Here, Mr. Howell assumed the doctor had already taken sides with his wife. This assumption is frequently made when a patient has a long-standing relationship with a physician that has not included other family members. For this reason alone, it is useful to **routinely meet family members early on when seeing a new patient.** Not only can you put faces to names when a patient discusses their family, but connections have already been made for future interactions. It can be awkward during an emergency, or in the midst of a serious problem, to have to join with unknown family members. In the above example, the physician focused on Mr. Howell early in the interaction and solicited his view of the problem. He let him know his views would be heard, that he would not be blamed, and that he might contribute to alleviating rather than worsening the problem. The physician then turned to give Mrs. Howell the same opportunity to be heard without blame or sidetaking.

In the next example, again the physician maintains a flexible position, a position from which he can empathize and support each person in turn.

> DR: Mr. and Mrs. Sweet, I appreciate you both taking the time to come in and discuss your son's recent difficulty keeping his sugars under control. As I've told Ralph, diabetes can be difficult to manage, and we need all the help we can get.
>
> MR. SWEET: Well, I think if my wife would feed the kid the right foods, we probably wouldn't have a problem. I tell her this, but she won't listen to me.
>
> MRS. SWEET: Why should I listen to you? You're never home to even know what he eats.
>
> DR: It's clear you both have a perspective that will be important to hear. You both are obviously concerned about your son or you wouldn't be here today. Let's begin with Ralph and hear what problems he feels he's having sticking to his diet.

The physician maintaining an alliance with each member of this family might result in a productive conversation in which the parents pull together to help their son stick to his diet. But, if Mrs. Sweet and Ralph consistently berate Mr. Sweet, this mother–son coalition might signal to the physician a need to either collaborate or refer to a family therapist. When triangles or coalitions persistently interfere with treatment, a new approach is necessary. Being able to negotiate difficult triangles or coalitions and develop constructive working alliances are important to building both patient's and family member's confidence in the competence of the physician. Not doing so can result in problematic interactions for the physician.

> Dr. C had enjoyed working with Mr. Bell over the years. In the last year Mr. Bell's daughter moved to town, in part to be closer to her aging father. Mr. Bell was mildly obese with moderate hypertension. His daughter began bringing him to his doctor appointments and soon was demanding that Dr. C monitor his medication more closely and give her father a "complete physical." While she was quite demanding and difficult to deal with, Mr. Bell remained content with his medical care, did not see additional tests as being important, and defended his doctor to his daughter. Framing Mr. Bell as "the patient" in his mind, Dr. C continued treatment as before and tried very hard to minimize or ignore the daughter's demands and protests.
>
> Unfortunately several months later Mr. Bell had a severe stroke, leaving him comatose until he eventually died. Mr. Bell's daughter had experienced Dr. C as cooperating with what she saw as her father minimizing his health

problems, and so she was furious and blamed Dr. C after the stroke occurred. This difficult relationship between the physician and his patient's family made decisions regarding care both complex and unpleasant, and made grieving after the patient's death complicated for both the daughter and the physician.

After this experience, Dr. C vowed to spend more time and energy forming an alliance with the patient's family members with the recognition that discounting them often backfires in the long run.

Establishing Leadership in the Interview

Providing leadership by orchestrating a well-organized interview also builds patient confidence in the physician's competence. A well-organized interview means more than just asking open-ended questions so a patient can express his or her feelings. It also means having goals for the interview, a structure and tasks to accomplish these goals, and a clear sense of the responsibilities inherent in both the doctor's and the patient's roles. With regard to these roles, Whitaker, a family therapist, conceptualizes the early stages of a psychotherapeutic relationship as involving struggles around structuring the interview and the initiative for change (2). His view is that the therapist must take responsibility for structuring the interview, recognizing that of necessity the patient is in control of the initiative for change. Whitaker believes that many major therapeutic impasses are the result of confusion over who is in charge of treatment and who is in charge of change. Adapting these concepts to the primary care context, we like to think of the physician as being in charge of the interview and the treatment plan, while recognizing that the family members are of necessity in charge of their own health and recovery. The way a physician chooses to structure an interview is central to the physician role and part of his or her contribution to the success of the treatment.

Ground rules for structuring an interview or conference can help the physician maintain control over the interview, prevent a family member from dominating the discussion, and make the most effective use of time. We think of the physician as needing to **direct traffic** in a group interview, requiring skills significantly different than what is needed in an individual interview. The following are general rules that help the physician conduct an effective interview:

1. Allow only one person to speak at one time. The physician needs to establish leadership during the interview or conference so he or she can protect each person's right to be heard.
2. Have each person use "I" statements. Insisting each person in the group speak only for him- or herself prevents any discussion from degenerating into blame and accusation.

> PATIENT TO HUSBAND: You're always on my back about my weight. No one
>   could lose weight living with your nagging.
> DR: Can you stick to the rule of only using "I" statements while we discuss
>   these difficult problems?
> PATIENT: Well, I'm having a hard time sticking to the diet we previously agreed
>   to.
> DR TO HUSBAND: Dieting is often a challenge for the strongest of us. When do
>   you see your wife doing well with her diet?

In this example the patient quickly moved to blame her husband for
her difficulties. By invoking the rule about "I" statements, the physician
was able to move the interview back to a nonblaming and more constructive path.

3. Emphasize strengths. Even in the most difficult interactions or
with the sickest of patients, some resource or strength can be noted and
utilized in treatment. This approach boosts people's self-esteem, recognizes positive gains, minimizes conflict, and encourages the family to
take as much responsibility as possible for the health of their loved ones.

> PATIENT: Well, I'm having a hard time sticking to the diet we previously agreed
>   to.
> DR TO HUSBAND: Dieting is often a challenge for the strongest of us. When do
>   you see your wife doing well with her diet?
> HUSBAND: Well, I do notice she seems to do quite well when I'm away on a
>   business trip.
> WIFE: I didn't realize you noticed. It's easier to eat well when you aren't here.
> DR: I'm very impressed, first, that you, Mr. Jones, were so observant. And then
>   it is clear, Mrs. Jones, that you are able to make some progress eating well
>   when you are on your own. Perhaps you'd like to talk together now about
>   how you could each use these good qualities to your advantage when you
>   are both at home, as is usually the case.

4. Model this behavior yourself. The physician, as leader of the interview or conference, sets the tone for the discussion in the way he or she
speaks. Using "I" statements, speaking respectfully to each person, and
maintaining a belief in the patient and family's ability to mobilize
resources to bring to bear on the illness or problem—all these behaviors
can be contagious.

Converting Resistance into Cooperation

Cooperation and resistance are interpersonal phenomena. Both are two-
way streets. It is difficult to cooperate with someone who is uninterested
or belligerent. It is also difficult to resist someone who refuses to fight.

In a primary care context, this means that both cooperation and resistance are some measure of the goodness of fit between the physician and the patient or family. We prefer the term "cooperation" over the term "compliance," because cooperation implies the collaborative, interpersonal nature of this exchange. Compliance, on the other hand, implies that the physician gives orders that the patient should obey. This authoritarian mind-set can lead to situations in which patients either lie or omit information to protect themselves, maintain the appearance of compliance, and protect their relationship with a valued physician. Cooperation implies an effort on both the doctor's and the patient's parts to express their own and understand the other's point of view.

Cooperation results from many factors, most especially, an established connection between the physician and the patient and family, and an agreed-upon and well-understood treatment plan.

> PATIENT: I understand I am to reduce my meal portions and avoid all sweet desserts to bring my diabetes under control.
> HUSBAND: Do you recommend the whole family change our diets?
> DR: How do you feel about that?
> HUSBAND: I feel I should to support my wife, but I'm also afraid I will end up resenting giving up foods I really like.
> PATIENT: I don't expect you to do that.
> DR: Many aspects of your wife's diet are part of good nutrition, so you may want to use this as an opportunity to change some of your family's eating habits. But, it is very important that family members not sacrifice too much or resentments will build. You and your wife can be creative and find alternative foods for her to eat when the rest of the family wants dessert.
> HUSBAND: I understand. We will work on this together. Her well-being is important to all of us.

Resistance occurs when the physician and the patient or family become involved in a struggle over treatment. This struggle may be obvious; it may be clear why the patient is not improving. Or, the struggle may be covert; the patient may not be improving and the physician may not realize the patient or family disagrees with the treatment plan and so is not implementing it fully. In the following example, there are hints from the husband that he is not fully supportive of the treatment plan and will leave its implementation solely to his wife.

> PATIENT: I understand I am to reduce my meal portions and avoid all sweet desserts to bring my diabetes under control.
> DR TO HUSBAND: How do you feel about that?
> HUSBAND: I don't like it, but I guess she has to do what "the doctor" says.
> DR: It is very important to get your wife's diabetes under better control. Losing weight is the most important thing she can do for her health.
> HUSBAND: This is up to her.

When working with resistant patients, there is a strong tendency to believe that lack of cooperation is a result of lack of information or misunderstanding. When a patient does not do as we ask, we may talk louder and longer, going over the same information about the same treatment plan over and over again.

> PATIENT: Well, Doc, I've been trying to watch my sweets, but my sugar just keeps going up and up.
> DR: Perhaps you should meet with the dietician again to review your diet.
> PATIENT: I've already seen her three times. I'm not sure it's helping.

When the patient education has been clearly transmitted once, or even twice, it is useful to hypothesize that "more of the same" is unlikely to be helpful and that the patient or family may be showing a lack of agreement or willingness to participate in the treatment plan as it is currently constructed (3).

> PATIENT: Well, Doc, I've been trying to watch my sweets, but my sugar just keeps going up and up.
> DR: You say you've been trying to watch your sweets. Has that been difficult?
> PATIENT: Well, to tell you the truth, Doc, my mother had diabetes. She had an occasional dessert on the side and she lived to a ripe old age. I'm her daughter, so I assume I can get away with it too. I just can't give up everything I enjoy, Doc.
> DR: I certainly wouldn't want that, either. Let's study your diabetes to see how much it is like your mother's. It may be, it may not be. Because your sugars are up, we have to be concerned that you can't get away with this as easily as your mother did, unfortunately. I'd like you to keep a diary for the next two weeks. Record what you eat every day, including the occasional sweets, and record your sugars. That way we can tell just how much you can treat your diabetes as your mother did. If there is a problem, then we'll need to talk about how to help to enjoy yourself, and give yourself special treats that aren't sweet. Maybe we could have your family come in and help us on that one.
> PATIENT: I hope it doesn't come to that, Doc, but I guess I have to face the music.

One common scenario that results in mysterious patient resistance occurs when the "customer," the person motivated and most interested in treatment, is not the patient (3). For example, the customer in a well-child check is most commonly the parent(s), but may be a grandparent who does not think the parent is handling a problem properly. The customer when a middle-aged man comes in for a complete physical may be the man, but it is often his wife who may be concerned that he is "working too hard." An adolescent with vague complaints may only be in the office because of parental pressure. In general, cooperation is greatest when the "customer" is involved in treatment. Resistance may occur when the patient and the customer are not the same person and the physician does not know that.

DR: How may I be of use to you today?
PATIENT: I've come in for a physical.
DR: Has something particular prompted you to get a physical at this time?
PATIENT: Oh, my wife's father died of a heart attack when he was about my age. My wife wants me to get my "ticker" checked out.
DR: What do you think about this?
PATIENT: I think my wife's a worry-wart. My heart's just fine. I run a mile every day.
DR: Why don't we go ahead and check you out, and maybe your wife could join us for the discussion of the results.
PATIENT: That's a good idea, Doc. She won't necessarily believe what I say.

Finally, the physician may experience resistance to treatment when he or she does not fully understand the meaning of the symptom to the patient or the family. As discussed in Chapter 1, some symptoms or illnesses in addition to causing pain or hardship may also serve some adaptive function for the patient. In these cases, the patient may fear at some level that giving up the symptom may be more painful than having the illness. This is a frequent problem with patients on disability or children who are school phobic. Is the gain from the illness greater than the fear of what the treatment might bring? Similarly, a woman whose workaholic husband only pays attention to her when she is ill may be quite ambivalent, consciously or unconsciously, about carefully following medical recommendations for treatment. These cases are certainly not routine. However, when a patient's or family's resistance to treatment persists, it is useful to explore the risks of a cure for this patient: "How would your life change if suddenly, overnight, you were cured of this problem?" "How would your significant relationships change?" In this situation it can be helpful to aid the patient or family in examining whether the cure is worse than the illness. In this way treatment can either proceed or change without peoples' ambivalences about change being expressed indirectly through resistance to treatment.

DR: Jane, I just don't understand why your sugars are so high. I am well aware that you understand the regimen you are supposed to be following. And I know you are a bright girl for being fifteen. Perhaps there is something we don't understand about your situation.
JANE: I don't know, Doc. It's a mystery to me.
DR: I wonder what would happen if suddenly, overnight, you were cured and no longer had to deal with this diabetes.
JANE: It would be heaven, Doc. All my problems would be solved.
DR: I wonder, how would it change your relationship with your parents.
JANE: Well, I guess they would have to interfere in some other part of my life.
DR: So, treating your diabetes is one area right now that you and your parents struggle over. They try to tell you what to do, and you are determined to do it your way.
JANE: That's right. It's my body.

DR: You do it your way, even if it's occasionally bad for you?

JANE: Well, maybe.

DR: How about if I invite your parents in to discuss your diabetes? Perhaps we could find a way for you to be in charge while still reassuring them you are going to be okay.

In this example treatment for diabetes in this teenage girl has become intertwined in her struggle for independence from her parents. When they advise or chide her about taking care of herself, she feels intruded upon and rebels. Trying to manage the treatment without understanding what function it has come to serve in this family is likely to fail.

Clear recognition of what one does and does not have control over as a physician is fundamental to establishing a collaborative, cooperative relationship with patients. While we can offer advice, prescribe medications, recommend treatment, and be persuasive with our patients, in the end we can only directly change ourselves. How our patients will choose to participate in what is recommended is their right and responsibility. In the process of treatment then, we must focus on our own behavior: on structuring the interview in the most useful way, on having the strongest treatment plan possible, on using the patient's and family's strengths and resources to help the patient heal, and on enjoying our work.

Physicians' Personal Issues as Contributions to Resistance

Physicians' personal experiences can be humanizing and result in increased empathy for patients and a wider range of strategies for patient care (4). (See Chapter 23 for a more in-depth discussion of these issues.) However, unresolved personal issues can negatively affect our ability to see patients clearly and to function optimally. This interference in physician functioning is the physician's contribution to resistance and can come from many sources. Cases may resemble our own current family situation in ways that cloud our judgment. A physician whose father just died of a sudden myocardial infarction may begin sending many more patients for catherization and argue strongly with patients who object. Patient situations may recapitulate our own unresolved family of origin issues (5,6). A physician whose mother was alcoholic may become unusually angry when dealing with alcoholic patients. And less exotic problems such as fatigue, illness, and general energy level can affect our ability to think clearly when a patient appears resistant to what we feel is clearly the correct medical course. Interactions with patients seen early in a given afternoon may influence us in ways that affect our treatment of patients seen later that afternoon (7).

Sometimes a patient's or family member's behavior so offends a physician's sense of values that the physician has difficulty forming or maintaining an alliance or developing any understanding of that person's offensive behavior. Cases of physical or sexual abuse or other criminal activity are common examples of situations many physicians find challenging in forming good working alliances with the patients involved. Even a mild suspicion of such problems, or some other breach of the physician's own code of ethics, can contribute to difficulty building therapeutic relationships between the doctor and the patient and family.

> Dr. R was a woman active in the feminist movement who enjoyed her obstetrical practice. She was very supportive and capable guiding women through the physical and emotional challenges of pregnancy, labor, and delivery.
>
> Mrs. Hernandez came to see Dr. R at 18 weeks of pregnancy. She spoke broken English, having just moved to this country after meeting her husband, becoming pregnant by him, and marrying him on a trip here to visit her relatives. The pregnancy went along smoothly, though Mrs. Hernandez was clearly stressed by all the changes she had encountered in such a short period of time. Dr. R saw her frequently and was as supportive as she could be.
>
> At 36 weeks, Mrs. Hernandez came in complaining that she was having some light intermittent bleeding that seemed to occur after her husband would insist they have intercourse. Upon questioning, Mrs. Hernandez acknowledged to Dr. R that she did not want to have sex at this point with her husband but that he disregarded her feelings. Dr. R had met Mr. Hernandez only briefly, but felt his behavior was reprehensible and unacceptable. She took out a prescription pad and wrote out a prescription stating Mrs. Hernandez was to engage in no sexual intercourse until after delivery for medical reasons.
>
> Mr. Hernandez had been vocal about his reluctance to attend his child's birth but he was in the room when Dr. R walked in to do the delivery. She felt herself bristle as she thought of how Mrs. Hernandez described his earlier behavior. Mr. Hernandez did not change Dr. R's impression as he spent the next few hours laughing inappropriately and making wisecracks while his wife endured her labor pains. He made it especially clear that this baby was to be a boy named after him. No girls' names were even considered. Dr. R was very cool and did not speak to him at all, continuing her supportive relationship with Mrs. Hernandez.
>
> Mr. Hernandez left the room during the last hour of labor. He reentered just as the baby was delivered: a girl. Dr. R continued to address only Mrs. Hernandez and the baby, telling the child "You have such a nice Mommy. She's going to take very good care of you." The next morning on rounds, Dr. R found Mrs. Hernandez somewhat depressed saying her husband had not yet visited, and she knew he wouldn't have left the hospital if the baby had been a boy.
>
> Sometime afterward, Dr. R discussed this experience with a colleague. She wondered how joining could ever occur with someone so obnoxious. The colleague raised several questions that helped her reconsider the situation: What motivated Mr. Hernandez' obnoxious behavior? What role did anxiety,

insecurity, and cultural values play in the scenario? In the end, would some alliance between the physician and the father have been helpful to the patient? Dr. R struggled with her own sense of values and her commitment and responsibility to help her patients.

Finally, interactions with colleagues can play a part in how we treat certain patients. Some cases brew controversy. If consultants are drawn into a struggle and become divided over the case, physician difficulty as well as patient resistance can intensify rather than decrease. For example, an oncologist may wish to give a 5-year-old with a malignant brain tumor every possible treatment available even when the side effects of the treatment are severe and the prognosis is not affected. The child's primary care physician in this situation may wish to consider stopping invasive treatments when the child appears certain to die. Because of his longstanding relationship with the family, they look to him for advice about treatment. In intensely emotional situations such as this, struggles between consultants and a primary care physician are common and can mimic the ambivalence the family has over whether to continue treatment.

Family systems consultations and Balint groups offer some of the best solutions to "physician resistance." Family systems consultations can occur when a physician has a systems-oriented colleague who is willing to trade consultations with difficult families. It is rare that another provider does not see a patient or family differently, enabling some new approach to treatment (8). Balint groups are also important vehicles for physicians to examine their own reactions to patients among trusted colleagues (9,10). Every primary care provider needs to have a system for dealing with the inevitable personal issues stimulated by our work. This process allows for the most creative and useful treatment to occur. It also allows challenging patients to facilitate our own growth, personally and professionally.

To conclude this chapter, we present 10 questions to help assess the physician–family alliance. This instrument assesses the likelihood that problems will emerge in the doctor–patient relationship that could impair or negatively influence treatment. Problems in the physician–patient or physician–family alliances can be a function of the patient, the presenting problem, and the approach of the physician. These questions primarily focus on the physician's contribution to building the alliance, clearly only half of the equation, but that half over which one has some control. This instrument will be useful in deciding which families require special attention in developing a therapeutic alliance.

References

1. Minuchin S, Fishman C: *Family Therapy Techniques.* Cambridge, MA: Harvard University Press, 1981.

2. Neill J, Kniskern D (eds.): *From Psyche to System: The Evolving Therapy of Carl Whitaker.* New York: Guilford Press, 1982.
3. Watzlawick P, Weakland J, Fisch R: *Change.* New York: W.W. Norton & Co., 1974.
4. Candib L, Steinberg G, Bedinghaus J, Martin M, Wheeler R, Pugnaire M, Wertheimer R: Doctors having families: The effect of pregnancy and childbearing on relationships with patients. *Fam Med* 1987;**19**:114–119.
5. Crouch M: Working with one's own family: Another path for professional development. *Fam Med* 1986;**18**:93–98.
6. Mengel M: Physician ineffectiveness due to family-of-origin issues. *Fam Syst Med* 1987;**5**(2):176–190
7. Seaburn D, Harp J: Sequencing: The patient caseload as an interactive system. *Fam Sys Med* 1988;**6**:107–111.
8. McDaniel S, Campbell T, Wynne L, Weber T: Family systems consultation: Opportunities for teaching in Family Medicine. *Fam Syst Med* 1988;**6**:391–403.
9. Balint M: *The Doctor, his Patient, and the Illness.* New York: International Universities Press, 1957.
10. McDaniel S, Bank J, Campbell T, Mancini J, Shore B: Using a group as a consultant, in Wynne L, McDaniel S, Weber T (eds.): *Systems Consultation: A New Perspective for Family Therapy.* New York: Guilford Press, 1986.

PROTOCOL
Assessing the Physician–Family Interaction

1. How do you assess this patient's level of cooperation, given his or her presenting problem(s)?
   (4) [ ] a cooperative patient with acute self-limited problems
   (3) [ ] a cooperative patient with stable, long-term problems
   (2) [ ] a cooperative patient with unstable, long-term problems in need of careful monitoring
   (1) [ ] an uncooperative patient with unstable, long-term problems in need of careful monitoring
   (0) [ ] a help-rejecting patient with numerous complaints

2. What is your involvement with the "customer" for treatment?
   (4) [ ] the customer, either patient or family member, participates actively in treatment
   (3) [ ] the customer is a family member with whom I've had some minimal contact
   (2) [ ] the customer appears to be a family member, but I have not had contact with that person
   (1) [ ] the customer may be the patient, but I am not sure
   (0) [ ] I do not know who the customer is

3. With which members of the family have you established rapport?
   (4) [ ] with everyone who is relevant
   (3) [ ] with the patient and some family members
   (2) [ ] with the patient only
   (1) [ ] with some family members, but not the patient
   (0) [ ] with no one

4. What does the patient and family want from you?
   (4) [ ] a collaborative relationship
   (3) [ ] information and support
   (2) [ ] advice
   (1) [ ] a quick cure
   (0) [ ] nothing

5. What do you expect from the patient and family?
   (4) [ ] active participation in treatment
   (3) [ ] to be receptive and cooperate
   (2) [ ] to do what I say and get better
   (1) [ ] to not take too much of my time
   (0) [ ] to go away

6. How is the family participating as part of the treatment team?
   (4) [ ] family is an active part of the treatment team
   (3) [ ] some important family participation
   (2) [ ] solicited some family participation, but not connected with most important family members

(1) [ ] I don't know the family, but feel they might be willing to par-
    ticipate

(0) [ ] I don't know the family, and doubt they'd be willing to partici-
    pate

7. How have you clarified responsibilities and established leadership
   as head of the family–physician treatment team?

   (4) [ ] I am in charge of treatment, the patient and family are in
       charge of their health and healing

   (3) [ ] the responsibilities are clear, but not always adhered to

   (2) [ ] the responsibilities are unclear or fuzzy

   (1) [ ] I have a vague sense of overresponsibility or irritation

   (0) [ ] the patient is in charge of treatment, somehow I feel in charge
       of the patient

8. Comparing this patient and family to your own current family:

   (4) [ ] my own experience helps me to be more effective with this
       family

   (3) [ ] this family does not resemble my own family, and I enjoy work-
       ing with them

   (2) [ ] this family does not resemble my own family, and I do not espe-
       cially enjoy working with them

   (1) [ ] I have some of the same illnesses or issues in my current fam-
       ily, and it is confusing and difficult to work with this patient
       and family

   (0) [ ] there seems to be some similarities, but I can't get a handle
       on it

9. Comparing this patient and family to your own family of origin:

   (4) [ ] my own experience helps me to be more effective with this
       family

   (3) [ ] this family does not resemble my family or origin, and I enjoy
       working with them

   (2) [ ] this family does not resemble my family of origin, and I do not
       especially enjoy working with them

   (1) [ ] I have some of the same illnesses or issues in my family of
       origin, and it is confusing and difficult to work with this
       patient and family

   (0) [ ] there seems to be some similarities, but I can't get a handle on
       it

10. With regard to this patient and family, the members of the medical
    treatment team are:

    (4) [ ] cooperating and coordinating treatment

    (3) [ ] cooperating about some aspects of treatment

    (2) [ ] communicating minimally

    (1) [ ] divided over treatment

    (0) [ ] in open warfare over this case

Physician–Family Alliance Score

0–10 Tidal wave predicted.

A family consultation is important and necessary.

If consultation fails, consider referral to a trusted colleague.

11–20 Rough waters ahead.

Family likely to be obstructive.

Consider requesting a consultation with a family-oriented colleague.

21–30 Light chop.

Physician–family alliance basically sound.

Family likely to cooperate and participate in treatment.

Proceed, but continue to try and improve the doctor–family relationship.

31–40 Smooth sailing.

Physician–family alliance strong.

Family participation dependable and constructive.

CHAPTER 5

Convening the Family

How, When, and to What End?

Bringing the family of a patient together for a family meeting or conference is a basic skill that is essential for family-oriented medical care. Why convene the family? Although one can obtain a considerable amount of information about the family from an individual patient, we believe that it is often essential to assemble the family to assess adequately the patient and family system. The extra time and effort involved in arranging family conferences is usually minimal and repays itself many times over. The health care provider can obtain a more thorough assessment of a specific problem, determine the impact on the family, negotiate a comprehensive treatment plan, and obtain the family's assistance in carrying out that plan.

Meeting with a patient and family encourages the physician to adopt a larger biopsychosocial perspective and to evaluate the family system. By asking other family members to come in, the physician implicitly recognizes that the problem affects more than just the patient. For some family members, this may be the first time anyone has acknowledged that they are suffering as well as the identified patient. During a family meeting, the patient has the opportunity to receive support and validation from other family members.

Families can be important allies to the physician in the evaluation and treatment process. The physician usually sees the patient for less than an hour every few weeks or months, while the family lives with the patient. **Family members can provide valuable information about the problem** and often have their own diagnoses and treatment plans.

Generally See Patient Alone		Family Conferences Desirable		Family Conferences Essential
Minor acute problems (e.g., common cold, contact dermatitis)	Routine self-limiting problems (e.g., influenza)	Treatment failure of regular recurrence of symptoms	Routine prevention/educational care (e.g., prenatal visits, routine child visits)	Chronic illness (e.g., hypertension) Serious acute illness (e.g., myocardial infarction) Psychosocial problems Life style problems (e.g., obesity) Death

FIGURE 5.1.   When to convene the family. From: Doherty W.A., Baird M. (2), reprinted by permission.

Hopkins medical clinics, 70 percent of the patients with hypertension wanted members of their families to learn more about hypertension. An intervention consisting of family education and support was designed and resulted in a significant reduction in blood pressure and mortality. Because of this success, the family intervention has been incorporated into the routine care of hypertensive patients at John Hopkins (7).

Incorporating new techniques and procedures, such as family conferences, into clinical practice requires a change in routine and the development of new skills. For physicians in training or those in practice who are developing a family approach to care, it is useful to establish certain circumstances for which the family is routinely convened. When this is done, a family conference becomes the rule at certain times, rather than the exception or something special. Similar to other practice routines (e.g., measuring blood pressures, Pap smears during pelvic exams), the family conference comes to be expected by patients, staff, and other health care providers. We suggest that the following situations require a routine family conference.

1. Hospitalization. This is often a time of crisis for a family. Admission to the hospital may have resulted from an acute and unexpected problem (e.g., myocardial infarction), an exacerbation of a chronic illness (e.g., asthma), or the downward course of a terminal illness (e.g., cancer). In any case, families are usually anxious, stressed, and wanting information and support. We recommend that the physician meet with the family as soon as possible after hospitalization to explain what has happened, the proposed treatment plan, and the patient's prognosis, and to answer questions.

For most medical problems, treatment continues after discharge from the hospital. A second meeting with the family and the inpatient treatment team toward the end of the hospitalization is useful to discuss discharge planning. Such a meeting would include the discussion of medication, physical and sexual activity, home services and treatments, and follow-up care. (See Chapter 21.) It is relatively easy to organize a family conference during a hospitalization because family members typically come to the hospital to visit the patient anyway.

2. Routine Pregnancy and Well-Child Care. Our practice is to encourage fathers and other significant support persons to come to all prenatal and well-child care. We insist that the father attend one prenatal visit during the first half of the pregnancy to discuss the pregnancy, one visit toward the end of the pregnancy to discuss labor, delivery, and their newborn, and one well-child visit during the first six months to discuss their baby and how the family is adjusting to this transition. When the father is absent, bringing other significant family members (especially the mother's mother) and friends is particularly important. This participation is considered an essential part of the medical care and is recorded in the chart. In addition, a home visit is routinely made two weeks postpartum to assess the family. (See Chapter 8 for a discussion of family-oriented pregnancy care and Chapter 9 for family-oriented well-child care.)

3. Death and Dying. At the time that the diagnosis of a terminal illness is made and then when a patient dies, it is essential to meet with the family. They are usually in a state of shock and grief and need information and support. Because of the strong emotions surrounding death in the family, there is often a high degree of denial, which can interfere with effective communication and the sharing of feelings. Death is often viewed as failure by the physician and may be accompanied by guilt. This may result in the physician avoiding the family at a time when it is most important to have contact. (See Chapter 14 for further discussion of working with grieving families.)

4. Diagnosis of a Serious Chronic Illness. Similar to hospitalization for an acute medical problem, the diagnosis of a serious chronic illness, such as diabetes, ischemic heart disease, or cancer, is often a time of crisis for families. Families must gradually accept the new diagnosis and learn to cope with it. This may lead to healthy adaptation (e.g., improved communication, commitment, and intimacy) or family dysfunction (e.g., over- or underinvolvement with the ill family member, overprotectiveness). A family assessment will help the physician determine how best to use the family as a resource in helping the patient cope with his or her illness as well as assist the family's adaptation. (See Chapter 15 on a family-oriented approach to chronic illness.)

After the physician has incorporated family conferences in the routine management of the situations listed above, he or she will find it useful to convene the family in numerous other situations, including poor compliance or control of a chronic illness, high utilization of medical services, somatization, and psychosocial problems, such as anxiety, depression, alcoholism, parent–child problems, marital difficulties, and sexual dysfunction. In addition, it can be very helpful and efficient to invite the family in for a meeting when they first register as patients. Such a meeting lets the family know that the physician is family-oriented and values the family's involvement in the health care of each member. Time can be saved by obtaining a genogram and family history from the entire family, rather than from each individual family member.

How to Convene the Family

Family members are usually eager and willing to attend family conferences with health care providers. This is particularly true when the family wants to receive information or share feelings about a family member's health problem. The following guidelines will help to ensure that all the appropriate family members attend. It may not be necessary to use all these approaches each time the family is convened. These are guidelines that can be adapted as necessary to particular circumstances during a clinical encounter. They are derived from our clinical experience working with families and the writings of others in family medicine (1,2) and family therapy (8–11).

1. Involve the family early. Start involving family members as early as possible in the management of a serious health problem, preferably during the first visit. Family members are often sitting in the waiting room and interested in participating. Routinely ask if any family members came with the patient, and if so consider inviting them in. At a minimum, take a minute to greet the family member at the end of the interview.

Avoid listening extensively to a patient's complaint about other family members before you have convened the family. Listen empathetically, but say something such as, "I am interested in helping you with this problem. In order to get a proper start, we need your family here to accomplish this." If the patient wishes to continue, gently suggest, "These issues may be better discussed at a later time."

2. Be positive and direct about your need to see the family: Expect the family to come in. "I need to meet with the father of your baby. Can he come in for your next prenatal visit?" A family meeting is like any other diagnostic test or therapeutic procedure. If the patient and the family are not convinced that the physician thinks it is important, they are unlikely to follow through. Explain that this is a routine procedure for this type of problem. "This is the way I like to work" or "I often find it useful to meet with other family members for at least a one evaluation session."

Avoid being ambivalent or giving mixed messages about the importance of a family conference. "Do you think it would be possible (or worthwhile) for your family to come in? I understand if they can't all make it." Patients pick up your confidence, or lack thereof, in any procedure you recommend.

3. Emphasize the importance of the family in caring for the patient. Tell the family that you need their help or opinion regarding the problem. "When one member of the family is having a problem, I find it helps to get the perspectives of other family members. People who know and care about each other often have a lot to contribute." Or "As a normal part of my work with patients, I like to involve family members as a resource." As a physician you can only observe the patient at a few points in time while family members see the patient every day.

If the problem is described only in individual terms ("I have chronic low-back pain"), ask how others in the family have responded to the problem ("What does your wife do when your back pain is severe?"). This inquiry enlarges the context of the problem and puts it in interactional terms. Other family members are often involved in some fashion, either influencing or influenced by the symptom. They may be in pain because of the problem or may be trying in an unproductive way to help the patient.

Avoid accepting the patient's word that another family member is unwilling to come in. First insist that the patient extend the invitation. Give the patient support and role-play with the patient asking the family to come in. If that fails, or appears it will fail, call the family member yourself.

4. Stress the benefits of a family meeting to the patient and the family. Acknowledge that the problem affects other family members and that the family can serve as a resource. "When one member is in pain, I often find that other family members are in pain as well. Bringing everyone in can result in more people receiving benefit from treatment."

Avoid blaming the family in any way. Don't imply there is a "family problem" or that the family is in need of therapy, even if you think there is a family problem and they do need therapy. The family may or may not be at a point where they agree with you. Recommending therapy or counseling can emerge in the family meeting or meetings when it is clear the family is ready and willing to negotiate about referral. (See Chapter 22 on making referrals.) These labels should not be used prematurely or in any way to be construed as blaming. Many families equate "therapy" with being "crazy" and will not want to participate with that implication.

5. Call the session a family meeting or conference, not family assessment, counseling, or therapy. Focus the purpose of the meeting on what the family identifies as the problem, not on your assessment of the problem. "I'd like the whole family to come in to discuss how best to manage Billy's bedwetting," not "I'd like to assess how family stresses (or problems) might be affecting Billy."

6. Give specific instructions for convening the family. Discuss exactly what the patient will say to the other family members and when necessary, role-play the invitation. Otherwise the patient may return home and announce to his or her spouse, "The doctor wants you to come in for my next visit because he thinks you are making me depressed." Instead, instruct the patient to say, "The doctor would like to hear your thoughts and ideas about my depression."

Offer to call other family members yourself, if needed. This may be necessary if the patient insists that family members will not come in, regardless of what he or she says to them. It is best to call the family members while the patient is in the office and knows what will be said.

Acknowledge the sacrifice that other family members will have to make to come in, and that you wouldn't ask them to do this unless you thought it was important. Specify exactly who you want to come and when you want them to come. Send a postcard to **remind the family of the meeting** or have your secretary call the day before the meeting.

Circumstances that Promote Reluctance and Resistance to Attending a Family Conference

Occasionally, a family resists coming to a family conference. The resistance may be overt: family members refuse to attend; or covert: they agree to come but do not show. Resistance can usually be predicted prior to the meeting and is diagnostic of dynamic difficulties in the family or between the family and the treatment system. (See Chapter 4 on promoting a working alliance.) This resistance most commonly occurs when there is a serious psychosocial problem (such as alcoholism, drug abuse, child or sexual abuse, sexual dysfunction). One of a number of dynamics may help to explain their resistance:

1. Significant marital or family conflict is present, and the presenting problem is part of the conflict. For example, the wife may be angry at her husband, believe that he drinks too much, and want their family physician to get him to stop.

2. Blame has been felt by family members for the problem in the past, and they are worried that they will be blamed again. For example, the father of a child with behavior problems may have been told previously that he has been too strict in his discipline of the child. If the physician fails to get the permission or collaboration of the patient for a conference, or implies any blame for the problem, other family members may be very resistant to coming in.

3. An exclusive relationship has been established by one member of the family with the physician, and other family members may feel excluded. For example, Mr. J. had been followed by his physician for his diabetes for years. At the time he developed impotence, his physician asked his wife to come in for the first time. She refused because she blamed herself for her husband's problem and was afraid his physician would also blame her.

In each of these situations, family members assume that the physician has heard the patient's version of the problem and has accepted it as the Truth.

Dealing with Resistance

When resistance to a family conference is apparent the following approaches can be helpful:

1. Don't accept the patient's initial response that his or her family refuses to come in. The patient may be nervous and want to protect and exclude other family members, but with support be willing to do what is needed. (This circumstance is much like the cancer patient who initially refuses chemotherapy out of both fear and denial but slowly accepts the illness and requests treatment.) Inquire how the patient made the request. After getting the patient's permission, call the other family members directly.

2. Sometimes the patient fears how other family members will respond to the request to discuss a problem. **Listen carefully** to the realistic difficulties of taking this step.

> PATIENT: This problem doesn't involve my husband. He would never come in. He doesn't believe in counseling.
> PHYSICIAN: Your husband can help me to better understand your problem. I suspect that he cares for you enough to be willing to come in to help you.
> PATIENT: My parents would be mortified if they knew about all of this. I don't want them to know.
> PHYSICIAN: Most parents appreciate the opportunity to help one of their children. They may be quite worried about you and benefit by discussing their concerns.
> PATIENT: My children are too young to understand any of this. It would only frighten them.
> PHYSICIAN: It can be frightening to discuss these problems openly with your children. However, I am certain that your children are aware that something is wrong. It is more frightening for them when they are left in the dark and are allowed to imagine the worst.

3. State that you are "stuck" and cannot help the patient without seeing the rest of the family (2). Firmly request that they come in. "There is simply no way I can help your daughter unless I have your husband's help. He needs to come in for the next appointment."

4. Don't argue when trying to persuade a resisting family member to come in. Agree with him or her as much as possible and try to use the explanations for refusal to come as reasons to come.

a. If the family member is in conflict with the patient, stress how important it is for you to hear the other side of the story.

> HUSBAND: Listen Doc! My wife doesn't listen to anything I have to say, and I certainly don't want to come in and hear her blame me again for all of her problems.
>
> PHYSICIAN: I don't want you to listen to her blame you either, but I do want to hear your side of the story. I have discussed some of this problem with your wife, but I am certain that the situation is more complicated than she sees it. Your perspective of her problems would be very helpful to my efforts to try to help her.

b. If family members claim that they are not involved in the problem or that it is none of their business, explain how important it is to have a neutral family member to help you out with the problem.

> MOTHER: My daughter is an adult now, and I try to stay out of her affairs. This is her problem, and it doesn't involve me.
>
> PHYSICIAN: I can see that you have helped your daughter to be independent and allowed her to deal with these problems on her own. To help your daughter cope with her difficulties, I need the help of someone who knows and cares about her, but has not gotten overinvolved in her problems. Do you think you could help me with this?

c. If the family member says that the problem is with the patient and not with the family, explain that meeting with the family will help you to assist the patient.

> SISTER: This is not a family problem. My brother has been drinking for years, and we did everything we could to help him. He has to stop blaming others for his problems and face up to them himself.
>
> PHYSICIAN: I agree that your brother needs to confront his alcoholism and get treatment for it. I would like to help him get treatment, but I need you and the rest of the family to help me. At least you can fill me in on what tricks he uses to deny and hide his drinking, and what hasn't worked in the past, so I don't waste my time trying them again.

5. Make a home visit. This is a very powerful and effective move to get reluctant family members in. It demonstrates a genuine and serious concern for the family and willingness to meet them on their own turf. After such a visit and appropriate joining, the family will rarely refuse to reciprocate by coming in for a family conference. In addition, a home visit allows the physician to evaluate the home situation and observe the family in their own environment. (See Chapter 20 for further discussion of home visits.) This can provide a more comprehensive and valid overall assessment of the family.

When the Family Doesn't Come In

1. Meet with the family members who have come for the family session. Thank them for their time and interest, but express the importance of consulting with the missing family members before proceeding.

Assess why all the invited family members did not come in for the family session. Be wary of excuses such as "My husband couldn't get time off from work today," or "Jimmy can't miss any more school than he has already." These explanations may be quite legitimate, but if the family really believes that meeting is important, they usually can get time off or be excused from work or school to attend.

Find out specifically which family members the patient invited, how they were asked, and what their responses were. Ask those who have come why the missing family members did not want to attend, and what it would take to get them to come.

2. Plan with the family how to proceed. This will depend upon the nature and urgency of the problem, which and how many of the important family members have come for the family conference. Options include:

    a. **Reschedule the family meeting.** If key members of the family are not present for the family conference (such as the father in a parent–child problem), or the problem is thought to result in part from dysfunctional family dynamics (substance abuse or psychosomatic illness), it usually is preferable to reschedule the session than meet without these family members. For example, if the physician meets only with the mother and child with a behavior problem, the message to the father is not only that he does not need to take part, but that his involvement is unimportant. If the father is distancing from the family and there is marital discord, as there can be in parent–child problems, meeting with the mother without the father will only make matters worse.

When crucial family members do not come to the session, meet briefly with those present to obtain their advice in getting the other members of the family in. **Call** missing family members directly by phone during the session to assess why they did not come in and to help get their cooperation for a meeting.

    b. **Meet with the family that has come.** In some circumstances, such as at the time of hospitalization, or immediately after a death, the physician must meet with whichever family members are present. It is important to determine which family members did not come, so they can be contacted if necessary at a later time. Again it may be useful to directly call some missing family members during the session.

An essential component of family-oriented health care is meeting with entire families or subgroups of families when indicated. These meetings may be for routine care, discussing a new diagnosis, discharge from the hospital, treatment planning, dealing with noncompliance or assisting with psychosocial problems. Despite the emphasis on the importance of the family in family medicine, many physicians lack the conviction or the skill to convene families effectively. This difficulty can be addressed by routinely meeting with families in the above circumstances. Following a protocol will improve success in convening families so that the physician becomes more comfortable with family meetings and uses them more frequently.

References

1. Christie-Seely J: *Working With the Family in Primary Care.* New York: Praeger, 1984.
2. Doherty W, Baird MA: *Family Therapy and Family Medicine.* New York: Guilford Press, 1983.
3. Schmidt DD: When is it helpful to convene the family? *J Fam Pract* 1983;**16**:967–973.
4. Kushner K, Meyer D, Hansen M, Bobula J, Hansen J, Pridham K: The family conference: What do patients want? *J Fam Pract* 1986;**23**:463–467.
5. Kushner K, Meyer D, Hansen JP: Patients' attitudes toward physician involvement in family conference. *J Fam Pract* 1989;**28**:73–78.
6. Kushner K, Meyer D: Family physicians' perceptions of the family conference. *J Fam Pract* 1989;**28**:65–68.
7. Morisky DE, Levine DM, Green LW, Shapiro S, Russel RP, Smith CR: Five year blood pressure control and mortality following health education for hypertensive patients. *Am J Public Health* 1983;**73**:153–162.
8. Bauman MH: Involving resistant family members in therapy. In Gurman AS (ed.): *Questions and Answers in the Practice of Family Therapy.* New York: Brunner/Mazel, 1981.
9. Garfield R: Convening the family: Guidelines for the initial contact with a family member. In Gurman AS (ed.): *Questions and Answers in the Practice of Family Therapy.* New York: Brunner/Mazel, 1981.
10. Starr S: Dealing with common resistance to attending the first family therapy session. In Gurman AS (ed.): *Questions and Answers in the Practice of Family Therapy.* New York: Brunner/Mazel, 1981.
11. Stanton MD, Todd TC: Engaging "resistant" families in treatment: Principles and techniques in recruitment. *Fam Proc* 1981;**20**:261–293.

PROTOCOL
Convening the Family

When to Convene the Family

1. Routinely convene the family in the following circumstances:
   a. During hospitalization (on admission and at time of discharge)
   b. Routine obstetrical and well-child care
   c. Terminal illness and death
   d. Diagnosis of a serious chronic illness
2. Consider convening the family in other circumstances, including:
   a. diagnosis of a serious illness
   b. compliance problems
   c. poor control of a chronic illness
   d. high utilization of medical services by an individual or family
   e. somatization
   f. anxiety or depression
   g. substance abuse
   h. parent–child problems
   i. marital or sexual difficulties

How to Convene the Family

1. Involve the family in the patient's medical care as early as possible. Routinely ask patients if any family members came with them and invite those family members in for part of the visit.
2. Be positive and direct about your need to see the family: Expect them to come in for the family conference. Explain that it is a routine procedure.
3. Emphasize the importance of the family as a resource in caring for the patient. Tell the family that you need their help or opinion.
4. Stress the benefits of a family meeting to the patient and family. Acknowledge that the problem affects all members of the family.
5. Give specific instructions to the patient on who to invite, and how to invite them.

Avoid

1. Being ambivalent or uncertain about the importance of a family conference.
2. Accepting the patient's word that family members are unwilling or unable to come in.

3. Blaming the family in any way.
4. Suggesting that there is a family problem or that the family needs help in the form of therapy.

Dealing with Resistance to a Family Conference

1. Don't accept the patient's initial response that his or her family refuses to come in. Inquire how the patient made the request.
2. Elicit the patient's fears concerning how family members will respond to the request to discuss the problem.
3. State that you are "stuck" and cannot help the patient without seeing the rest of the family.
4. Don't argue. Try to use the patient's explanations for the family refusing to come as reasons for the importance of the meeting.
5. Make a home visit.

When the Family Doesn't Come In

1. Meet the family members who have come and assess why all those invited did not come in.
2. Plan with the family how to proceed, and whether to:
   a. reschedule the family meeting, if crucial family members are missing or
   b. have the conference with the family members who are present.
3. Call the missing family members directly.

CHAPTER 6

Conducting a Family Conference
A Cornerstone for Family-Oriented Care

Much has been recommended and written about seeing the family together in the medical setting (1–3). However, the specifics of conducting a family conference have yet to be spelled out. That is the purpose of this chapter. We will offer a concrete, step-by-step guide to conducting a family conference in a medical setting. It is not the only way to conduct a family conference, but is one effective way to conduct a family conference.

This guide to conducting a family conference is an integration of procedures from a variety of approaches. We draw from the family therapy literature (4,5) and the family medicine literature (6,7) to produce a format that addresses the issues involved in interviewing a family in a primary care medical setting. The conference is not family therapy, or even necessarily family counseling. The interview format is generic. It can be used for the diversity of reasons a family conference is called, such as facilitating lifestyle changes, grief work, improvement with compliance, referral, or as a precursor to primary care counseling. It is a blueprint for helping family members communicate about issues of concern to them and to you, their physician. It draws on the family's resources to establish a collaborative plan between them and the medical system.

General **goals for leading a family conference** generally include the following:

1. Socialize and **join** with the family. Get to know each member. Accommodate to the style of family members. Create an environment in which each family member feels safe and supported.

2. Organize the group so that communication is clear; **establish goals** for the conference that are clear, mutual, and attainable.
3. Gather information and **facilitate discussion** from each person present about the issue of concern; **transmit information** about the medical issues involved, as is appropriate.
4. **Identify resources** and supports that are available to the family.
5. **Establish a plan** that allows the family to collaborate with you in addressing the issues of concern.

Our guide for a family conference is a compendium of specific tasks designed to accomplish these five goals. It is oriented toward a family interview or a network session of family, friends, and involved professionals, although it can easily be adapted for a couple or a family-oriented individual session. (See Chapter 5 for issues around convening the family, i.e., who to ask and how.)

We begin with a section on preconference preparation and end with postconference tasks. A successful session depends on attention to information already known about the patient and family that can lead to the development of appropriate goals and strategies for the conference. Likewise, after the conference, it is essential to evaluate whether the goals of the conference were met, review the information gathered, and record this information and the treatment plan efficiently in the chart so that treatment can proceed most effectively.

Preconference tasks
    A. Set the stage
    B. Review the genogram
    C. Develop hypotheses
Conference tasks
    Phase 1. Socialize
    Phase 2. Develop goals
    Phase 3. Discuss the problem or issue(s)
    Phase 4. Identify resources
    Phase 5. Establish a plan
Post-conference tasks
    X. Revise the genogram
    Y. Revise hypotheses
    Z. Write up the conference report

Although these phases are clearly demarcated, and assigned approximate time frames for clarity and pacing, the actual process of conducting a family conference demands a good measure of sensitivity to the natural flow from one phase to another. Phases can overlap or take place concurrently in an actual session.

Steps for Conducting a Family Conference

Preconference tasks

A. Set the Stage

The goal of this first phase of preconference preparation is to make contact with the patient and family and to plan for the family conference. This planning may occur as the result of a concern expressed during a regular patient visit or it may be initiated during a phone conversation.

1. Choose your contact person. It is important to choose the appropriate contact person as this person will set up the conference successfully, or unsuccessfully. Typically, the contact person should be the patient if he or she is a capable adult. If not, the contact person may be a patient's son or daughter—if the patient is elderly and mentally incompetent, or some other responsible party.

2. Establish a rationale. The conference can be for the purpose of discussing the prognosis for an illness, gathering information, providing support to a family coping with a difficult illness, answering questions, or any reason why a physician might want to communicate with a family or a family with a physician. The stated rationale should be clear, purposeful, and be nonthreatening to the contact person and the family. For example, "I'd like to meet with the rest of the family, the people most important to you, to discuss the dietary changes necessary with your type of diabetes."

3. Establish who in the patient's network will attend. Review family, friends, and other involved professionals to decide with the patient who is relevant to the issue of concern, and who to invite.

4. Set the appointment. Mail a reminder or call the relevant parties to confirm the appointment.

B. Review the Genogram

The goal of this second phase of preconference preparation is to review what is currently known about the patient and their family with regard to the issue of concern for the family conference.

1. Prepare or revise the genogram, based on information in the chart and your contact with the patient. The genogram should represent the most up-to-date picture of the patient and the family. Information depicted should include names, ages, marital status, children, households, significant illnesses, dates of traumatic events such as deaths, and occupations. It can include emotional closeness, distance, or conflict between members, significant relationships with other professionals, and any other information important to the case. Putting together a genogram may reveal repeating dysfunctional emotional patterns, common medical problems, and other important considerations in the process of evaluation and treatment planning. (See Appendix 1 at the end of this chapter for a summary of standard genogram symbols.) McGoldrick and Gerson (8) give a complete review of standard symbols, as well as helpful hints in creating and revising genograms.

   2. Note the patient and family's life cycle stage. The family life cycle stages give a framework for predicting individual and family developmental issues that may be influence the symptom or issue of concern. See Appendix 1, Chapter 3, for a description of the family life cycle stages. Identify at least three generations and note their developmental issues. For example, the family of a man recovering from a myocardial infarction may be facing the following life cycle issues:

patient – contemplating retirement
wife – going through menopause
teenage son – leaving home for college
couple – "empty nest" syndrome
patient's mother – failing health, nursing home placement being considered

C. Develop Hypotheses
The goal of this third phase of preconference preparation is to develop initial hypotheses about the issue of concern and how the family is functioning to deal with the concerns. These hypotheses will help guide the exploration of issues in the family conference.

   1. Set your own goals for the interview. For example, in a family conference held just after the death of a family patriarch, goals might be to answer remaining medical questions, to facilitate the grieving process for the survivors, and to support the new leaders in the family. In a family conference held to assess the treatment of a noncompliant juvenile diabetic, goals might be to assess the functioning of the parents with regard to the medical regime, assess the relative independence of the adolescent from his parents, review other stressors in the household, and complete any necessary patient or family education about diabetes.

   2. Develop tentative hypotheses to test in the meeting. These hypotheses will be expanded and revised as new information is gathered throughout treatment. Begin with the life cycle stage of the family, relevant and current medical problems, and the issue of concern. Build hypotheses using other data, such as the emotional tone conveyed by the contact person (e.g., flat affect after a death), or how a family has dealt with similar issues in the past (e.g., excellent coping early in a crisis followed by a deterioration in functioning). An example might be hypothesizing an acute grief reaction in a middle-aged man with chest pain and no biomedical findings when the symptoms occurred soon after the funeral of his best friend. Typically, hypotheses are generated after setting the appointment with the contact person. With a particularly difficult patient or family, you may wish to sit down, review the chart, and develop hypotheses before inviting the family in.

3. Develop a strategy for conducting the conference. Include specific questions, observations, or tasks that will facilitate data-gathering and help test the hypotheses. The strategy will help prevent muddled thinking and drifting about in the session. Having developed initial hypotheses and a working strategy, be careful to remain open to information that supports alternative hypotheses and to the unique needs of this particular family.

The Five Phases of a Family Conference

Phase 1. Socialize (approximately 5 minutes)
The goal of this first phase of the family conference itself is to welcome the family, to get to know them better, and to help them become more comfortable in the setting of the conference.

1. Greet the family. Introduce yourself to the contact person and to the other adults in the household. Shake hands and greet each member of the family. Use formal names for adults, at least initially; be sure to greet and make contact with all children attending, regardless of age. Invite the family members to sit where they wish. This information may be used to hypothesize about who is close to whom, etc.

2. Orient the family to the room. Inform them of any colleagues behind observation mirrors or students sitting in on the conference. Show children where toys or blackboards are located. If you are audio- or videotaping, show the equipment to the family and obtain oral permission from adult members. Signatures on the consent form can be gathered at the end of the conference.

3. Talk with each family member. Begin by briefly introducing the agenda for the meeting. This is a restatement of the rationale used in convening the family–e.g., "We are here today to discuss your father's death." Follow this with the comment: "It would help me if I first got some more information about each of you." It is very important *not* to delve into problem identification, problem-solving, or expression of important feelings prior to the completion of this phase.

Request demographic information from each of them such as their age, work/school activity, education, length of marriage, etc. Try to find something in each person that is interesting. Attend to and reflect individual and family strengths. Take the opportunity to be human and generally less intimidating to the family.

While talking to the family, remember to give special attention and respect to the adult leader/spokesperson of the family. Make special efforts to engage those in the family who are distant or uncomfortable. Note each family member's language and nonverbal behavior. Attempt to generally match this style and language in as natural a way as possible to facilitate communication.

For some families who are especially large or especially uncomfortable, this phase may need to be expanded to 10 minutes, perhaps spending less time on the problems or the plan. Examples might be when you have not met a family before, when you suspect family members may worry you will side with the patient against them, or when someone feels blamed.

Phase 2. Set the Goals (approximately 5 minutes)
The purpose of this second phase of the family conference is to establish the group's goals for the session.

1. **Ask the group, "What would you like to make sure we accomplish today?"** Solicit ideas from each person who wishes to speak.
2. **Translate each goal so it is clear, concise, and realistic.** For example, "Today we'll focus on Donna's recent depression and how we can all help her," or "Today we've agreed to focus on your upcoming move and how to handle your son's diabetes, given the new situation."
3. **Sometimes it is useful to write the goals up on an easel or blackboard** so everyone can see and participate.
4. **Propose any goals you feel are important** that the family has not mentioned. Be careful not to propose goals the family is not yet ready to deal with. Take your cue from the family's reaction to your suggestions.
5. **Set priorities among the goals.** If there are more than two or three, suggest the other goals be addressed at a later time.

Phase 3. Discuss the Problem or Issue(s) (approximately 15 minutes)
The goal of this third phase of the conference is to exchange information with the family.

   1. Solicit each participant's view of the issue or the problem.
Allow the family to discuss with each other their shared concerns or differences. "Often family members have different views about what the problem is. Today I would like to hear from each of you about how you see the problem." Address each member of the family, usually beginning with the adult who appears most distant to the issue at hand. For example, with a child behavior problem, you might address the father first because you have not had contact with him to date about this and because the mother has complained he is uninvolved with the child. Help family members to be more concrete and specific by asking. "How is this a problem for you?" "When did this first become an issue?," etc. Explore the involvement of others in this issue: "Have you been given advice from other people about this problem?" "What do you think of

their advice?" Include questions about previous treatments and other professionals involved.

Ask about other recent changes in the family that could impact on the issue of concern, such as moves, illness, death, occupational shifts, marriages, divorces, or births. While keeping focused on the issue at hand, be aware of changes in the family system that influence and are influenced by the presenting concern.

Observe repetitive family interactional patterns. Final treatment plans should not go against these patterns, unless specifically planned for and negotiated. Some process reminders are:

- Encourage family members to be specific; ask for examples.
- Help family members to clarify their thoughts.
- Maintain an empathic and noncritical stance with each person.
- Affirm the importance of each person's contribution.
- At this point, do not offer advice or interpretations even if asked.
- Block interruptions from others if persistent.
- Note, but do not emphasize, disagreements among family members.

2. Encourage the family and the patient to ask any questions they might have of you. Use this time to share any other information the family needs to have.

3. Ask how the family dealt with similar problems or issues in the past.

Phase 4. Identify Resources (approximately 10 minutes)
The goal of this fourth phase of the conference is to recognize the available resources to bring to bear on the issue(s) of concern.

1. Identify family resources and strengths. List family members that are available to the patient. Ask participants to volunteer strengths they perceive in the patient and the family. "It is clear to me you all have a lot going for you even though you are stressed at the current time. What do you feel this family (and/or this patient) does really well?" Record the strengths on an easel or a blackboard. The family often resists this exercise out of embarrassment, but it is powerful both because it is supportive and because it can diminish unnecessary or less effective services outside the family.

2. Identify medical resources. Identify specialists, nursing services, mental health services, and other allied health professionals that might be helpful to the patients or family. Help the family members to specify clearly their expectations of physicians, medical staff, and other help care providers. Answer any questions and clarify any misconceptions about what can and cannot be provided.

3. Identify community resources. Include nutritional services, homemaker services, community support groups, etc.

Phase 5. Establish a Plan (approximately 10 minutes)
The purpose of this last phase of the conference is to clarify each person's role in carrying out a mutually agreed upon treatment plan.

1. At the end of the conference, ask the family about their involvement in the next step. "What is your plan for proceeding?"

2. Negotiate a formal or an informal contract with the family regarding their concerns, and have each person repeat back what they will contribute.

   a. Establish what each family member will do.
   b. Clarify what you will do.
   c. Discuss primary care counseling or referral at this point, if relevant.
   d. Make an appointment for follow-up, if appropriate.

For example, "Today we agreed that Mrs. W. will monitor her own diet with regard to her hypertension. Mr. W. will ask her once a week how she is doing and take her out to a special dinner if she feels she has had a good week on the diet. Joe and Johnny agreed to leave these issues in their parents' hands."

3. Ask if family members have any questions.

4. Have family members sign video release and release to obtain records, if needed.

5. Thank everyone for coming and conclude the conference.

Postconference tasks

X. Revise the Genogram.
This task involves recording on the genogram any new information or previous misconceptions that emerged in the family conference.

Y. Revise Hypotheses.
Use the information gathered in the family conference to revise and refine the preconference hypotheses and plan for future treatment.

Z. Write Up the Conference Report.
Several family assessment formats suggested for use in primary care can be adapted as outlines for conference write-ups, such as the **PRACTICE** form (9) or the Resident Consultation Evaluation Form (7).

Whatever the format, a conference report should include:

1. **Attendance**
   a. Who attended the session
   b. Who was important but did not attend, and why

2. Problem list
   a. Issues of concern to the family
   b. Other issues of concern to you
3. Global assessment of family functioning, including
   a. Family structure
   b. Family process (see Chapter 3 for an in-depth discussion of concepts involved in assessing family structure and family process)
   c. The family life cycle stage and the relevant developmental challenges of that stage
4. Family strengths and resources
5. Treatment plan
   a. Medical regimen
   b. The roles to be played by the patient and the family members.

Family conferences offer an opportunity for the family-oriented physician to gather a wealth of information about the patient, and for the family to pose their questions and concerns to the medical care team. The preceding format makes the family conference a manageable and efficient component of family-oriented primary care.

References

1. Doherty W, Baird M: *Family Therapy and Family Medicine.* New York: Guilford Press, 1983.
2. Christie-Seely J (ed.): *Working with the Family in Primary Care.* New York: Praeger, 1984.
3. Crouch M, Roberts L (eds.): *The Family in Medical Practice.* New York: Springer Verlag, 1987.
4. Haley J: Conducting the first interview, *Problem-Solving Therapy.* San Francisco: Jossey-Bass, 1987.
5. Weber T, McKeever J, McDaniel S: A beginner's guide to the problem-oriented first family interview. *Fam Proc* 1985;24:357–364.
6. Talbot Y: Families–the "How." *The Family in Family Medicine: Graduate Curriculum and Teaching Strategies.* Kansas City, MO: Society of Teachers of Family Medicine, 1981.
7. McDaniel S, Campbell T, Wynne L, Weber T: Family systems consultation in family medicine. *Fam Syst Med* 1988;6:391–403.
8. McGoldrick M, Gerson R: *Genograms in Family Assessment.* New York: W.W. Norton and Co., 1985.
9. Christie-Seely J: PRACTICE–A family assessment tool for family medicine, in Christie-Seely J (ed.): *Working with the Family in Primary Care.* New York: Praeger, 1984.

Appendix 6.1
Genogram Format

A. Symbols to describe basic family membership and structure (include on genogram significant others who lived with or cared for family members – place them on the right side of the genogram with a notation about who they are.)

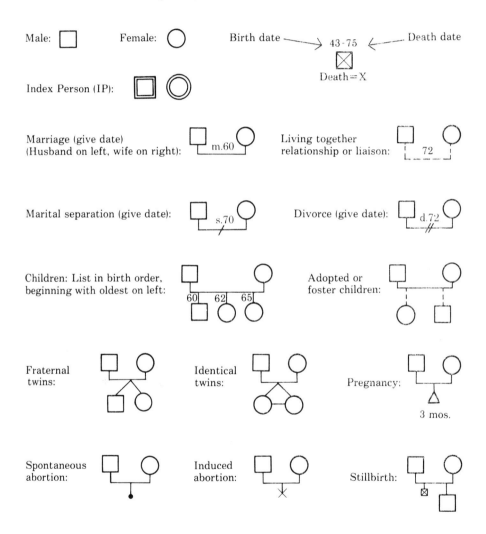

Members of current IP household (circle them):

Where changes in custody have occurred, please note:

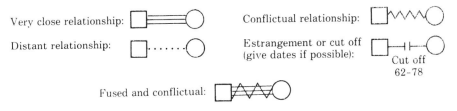

B. Family interaction patterns. The following symbols are optional. The clinician may prefer to note them on a separate sheet. They are among the least precise information on the genogram, but may be key indicators of relationship patterns the clinician wants to remember:

Very close relationship:

Distant relationship:

Conflictual relationship:

Estrangement or cut off (give dates if possible):
Cut off
62–78

Fused and conflictual:

C. Medical history. Since the genogram is meant to be an orienting map of the family, there is room to indicate only the most important factors. Thus, list only major or chronic illnesses and problems. Include dates in parentheses where feasible or applicable. Use DSM-III categories or recognized abbreviations where available (e.g., cancer: CA; stroke: CVA).

D. Other family information of special importance may also be noted on the genogram:

    1) Ethnic background and migration date
    2) Religion or religious change
    3) Education
    4) Occupation or unemployment
    5) Military service
    6) Retirement
    7) Trouble with law
    8) Physical abuse or incest
    9) Obesity
   10) Smoking
   11) Dates when family members left home: LH '74.
   12) Current location of family members

It is useful to have a space at the bottom of the genogram for notes on *other key information*: This would include critical events, changes in the family structure since the genogram was made, hypotheses and other notations of major family issues or changes. These notations should always be dated, and should be kept to a minimum, since every extra piece of information on a genogram complicates it and therefore diminishes its readability.

PROTOCOL
Conducting a Family Conference

Preconference Tasks

A. Set the stage
   1. Choose your contact person.
   2. Establish a rationale.
   3. Establish who will attend.
   4. Set the appointment.
B. Review the genogram.
   1. Prepare the genogram
   2. Note the family's life cycle stage.
C. Develop hypotheses
   1. Set your own goals for the interview.
   2. Develop tentative hypotheses about the family and their concerns.
   3. Develop a strategy for conducting the interview.

Phases of a Family Conference

Phase 1. Socialize (approximately 5 minutes)
   1. Greet the family.
   2. Orient the family to the room.
   3. Join with each family member.
Phase 2. Set the goals (approximately 5 minutes)
   1. Solicit goals for the session from each person who wishes to speak.
   2. Make each goal clear, concise, and realistic.
   3. Add any goals you feel are necessary.
   4. Prioritize the goals.
Phase 3. Discuss the problem or issue(s) (approximately 15minutes)
   1. Solicit each person's point of view.
   2. Encourage the family to ask questions of you.
   3. Ask how the family dealt with similar past problems.
Phase 4. Identify resources (approximately 10 minutes)
   1. Identify family strengths.
   2. Identify medical resources.
   3. Identify community resources.
Phase 5. Establish a plan (approximately 10 minutes)
   1. Solicit the family's plan.
   2. Contract with the family regarding their concerns, including referral or reappointment if necessary.

3. Ask for any remaining questions about the plan.
4. Conclude the family conference.

Postconference Tasks

X. Revise the genogram.
Y. Revise the preconference hypotheses.
Z. Write up the conference report, including
    1. Attendance
    2. Problem list
    3. Assessment of family functioning
    4. Family strengths and resources
    5. Treatment plan

Health Care of the Family in Transition

CHAPTER 7

Working with Couples in Primary Care

The Backbone of the Family Treatment System

Couples, whether traditional or nontraditional, are the backbone of family life. They are the unit that produces, nurtures, and raises the next generation. They are connected both to the past through their parents and to the future through their children. They are sometimes the patients and often the customers for the health care of their families. While physicians occasionally see couples for primary care, marital, or relationship counseling, issues having to do with couples more generally permeate the delivery of primary care.

To open the section on "Health Care of the Family in Transition," we begin this chapter with a family life cycle perspective on couples. Suggestions presented here on implementing a developmental perspective can then be applied to the other points of transition discussed in subsequent chapters of this section. Following the life cycle perspective, we discuss contacts with the physician made by newly committed couples. Then we turn to more general issues of working with couples in primary care, specifically the relevance of the couple to the provision of health care, common relational patterns between couples around health and illness, and issues around divorce and health care. We conclude this chapter with guidelines for working with couples in primary care.

A Family Life Cycle Perspective for Couples

The developmental milestones involved with pairing, from dating to marriage, parenting, retirement, and finally death, each have health considerations. Contraception, pregnancy, and the diseases of later life typically bring a couple, individually or together, into the health care system. Any presenting complaint needs to be considered in light of relevant developmental challenges for a couple in order to assess the relationship that might exist between the symptom and current family life cycle issues. For example, a young woman, Mrs. Jones, presented with low back pain. Mrs. Jones' work was mothering both an infant and a toddler. It was important for comprehensive, effective treatment of this patient to have a session in which both Mr. and Mrs. Jones discussed ways to increase the support and decrease the physical and emotional stresses and strains common to the family life cycle stages of early parenthood.

One way to implement a developmental family life cycle perspective in primary care is to ask oneself the following questions when seeing any patient:

* **Where in the life cycle are the three generations of this family:**
  What is happening with the parents?
  What is happening with the grandparents?
  What is happening with the children?

* **Are the life cycle stages in phase or out of phase?**
  For example, a couple who marries in order to become independent of their parents is marrying before resolving identity or "leaving home" issues and so is out of phase. Similarly out of phase is the couple who becomes pregnant before marrying. This couple typically has not resolved commitment issues prior to becoming parents. Out-of-phase families are at higher risk for physical and emotional symptoms because of the many simultaneous developmental challenges they must face.

* **What developmental challenges predominate for the family?**
  For example, approaching retirement Mr. and Mrs. Short had little time for planning their new life together because they were spending so much time and energy trying to manage and care for Mrs. Short's elderly mother with Alzheimer's. Only after working with their physician to place their deteriorating parent in a nursing home were they able to make constructive plans about how they might spend their retirement time.

* **How are the relevant developmental challenges related to the presenting complaint?**

> Soon after her mother was placed in a nursing home, Mrs. Short presented in the office with "chest pains." After diagnosing anxiety-based symptoms, Dr. P explored Mrs. Short's concerns about placing her mother and then invited Mr. Short to come to a subsequent session. At the conjoint session, Mr. Short was able to be supportive and help his wife accept that she could no longer take care of her mother. The couple was then able to discuss plans for how they

might spend their retirement time while still staying in the area so Mrs. Short could visit her mother. At two-month follow-up, Mrs. Short's symptoms had not recurred.

(See Chapter 3, Appendix 1, for a listing of the family life cycle stages and the issues relevant to those stages.)

New Couple Visits

The early developmental challenges of a newly committed relationship, whether it is a marriage or some other live-in commitment, involve the couple's bonding with each other, creating a new family that takes first priority in their lives, and renegotiating relationships with their families of origin. (All in-law jokes turn on the difficulties inherent in this challenge.) Traditionally, physicians have participated in the coupling ritual through the premarital visit that included blood tests required to obtain a marriage license. Today, states vary with regard to whether they require blood tests for venereal disease (or AIDS), so all couples are not required to see a physician before they marry. However, for those that are required, or those that wish to verify they are committing to a "healthy" person, visits early in a couple's relationship (and later visits such as annual physicals or regular GYN checks) offer an opportunity to promote communication and consideration of the developmental issues ahead of the couple.

Rarely at this stage do couples wish to discuss or be counseled about the wisdom of their choice of mates (1). (Such counseling is like trying to stop a speeding locomotive with your hand.) These discussions are probably unwise, and may alienate the couple unless one member has explicitly requested to talk about it. Instead, the physician can explain, "As your family physician, I find it very useful to find out a bit about both of your backgrounds, including your family histories, pertinent medical problems and your plans for the future. This will assist me in caring for both of you."

This family-of-origin approach to a 20–30 minute visit allows the physician to join with the couple and facilitate discussion of important developmental issues in a way that the couple may find useful. It involves constructing a genogram with the couple that symbolically joins the two individuals' families, as will occur if they marry. In drawing the genogram it is easy to generate discussion about significant emotional issues, such as whether the couple has received parental "permission" to commit or marry. Lack of parental support may predict future marital problems (2,3). Other issues about how the family handles marriages may be significant or interesting to the couple, such as whether their parents had the blessing of their own parents, how siblings' marriages have fared, and any history of divorce or other relationship dysfunction in the extended family. Information about the history of disease in the two families should be included on the joint genogram. The physician may ask about current use of contraception and expectations about having children. The same family-of-origin format can be used productively with couples in nontraditional relationships, such as gay couples. With these patients, it is important to explore the additional issue of how their families and other supports view their sexual orientation as well as their choice of a partner. Visits with new couples can be concluded with suggestions regarding the frequency and format for future health care.

Joan and Jim came in to see Joan's physician, Dr. M, to get their blood work done prior to applying for a marriage license. After a nurse drew their blood, Dr. M sat down and drew their genograms together on a large sheet of paper. This discussion revealed that Jim had been married before and had one son, Jimmy, age 10. This was the first marriage for Joan. Dr. M asked Jim what he felt was successful in his first marriage that he would like to bring into this new marriage, and what he intended to make different. Joan then discussed her concerns about becoming a stepmother and part-time parent, and what she had done to solidify her relationship with Jimmy prior to the marriage. Dr. M asked about "permission" to marry and found that Jim's parents had supported the union all along, while Joan's parents had initially resisted lending their support because of Jim's first marital failure. However, Joan reported that as her parents spent more time with Jim their affection for him grew, as did their confidence that the two of them could have a successful relationship. The interview concluded with a discussion of Joan's desire to have a baby soon after the marriage. Dr. M promised to discuss the implications of this for the couple and for their relationship with Jimmy at a prepregnancy visit after the wedding.

A family life cycle approach to this or any other couple would include a consideration of the effect of this developmental milestone on other members of the family.

Dr. M was aware of Joan's parents' early disapproval of their relationship because Joan's mother, Mrs. Webb, had come in 3 months previously, complaining of tension headaches. After Dr. M reassured her she had no obvious neurologic problems, Mrs. Webb began discussing her worries about her youngest daughter marrying a divorced man. No one in her family had ever been divorced, and Mrs. Webb worried this relationship was a set-up for unhappiness and failure. Mrs. Webb also acknowledged that she was going to miss her daughter when she moved out and wondered who would fill the gap. Dr. M suggested Mrs. Webb go home and discuss her concern with Mr. Webb, perhaps while on a dinner date, and that the two of them spend more time with Jim and Joan to observe this relationship and discover whether her worries were well-founded. A follow-up visit revealed fewer headaches.

The Relevance of Couples to the Provision of Health Care

Once a couple is married (or committed to a long-term relationship), their relationship is impacted by the health care system when one of them seeks care. The question is: when is it relevant for the health care provider to be concerned about the couple rather than just the individual patient? Traditional medicine routinely deals with couples only at such times as when one person has a sexually transmitted disease and the "contact" needs to be treated. However, many more opportunities occur to use the marital or relationship system to assess and treat illness, improve health, and perhaps even save the physician some time. The following are roles that are common for spouses or partners to play in coping with illness:

* **The partner as caregiver.** Frequently if an adult is sick, that person's partner or spouse is the primary informal caregiver. For a man recovering from an MI after hospitalization, his wife is typically his "nurse." For a woman with Alzheimer's disease, her husband is typically the person to help orient her, assist her memory, and guide her through the day. He may also be the person to give out her medications. Both because of proximity and because of the strong relationship between couples, it is useful for the physician to network with the information caregiver to monitor treatment, assess the patient's progress, and support the family in managing any illness or trauma.

* **The partner as customer.** When a patient in the office is vague or seems to be unconcerned about this visit to the doctor, it is often because someone else sent him or her. With couples that someone is most often the patient's partner. Middle-aged men who request a "complete check-up" are commonly sent by their wives who feel they are overworking or not paying attention to their health. The customer for treatment, the person who wants the patient assessed or treated, is sometimes crucial to understanding the presenting complaint.

> For example, Mrs. White, a patient with early and undiagnosed Alzheimer's disease, came in for a physical. When Dr. D, her physician, asked why she decided to have a check-up, she said, "I don't know. My husband seems to think something is wrong with me." Mrs. White was unclear about why she was seeing her doctor. The customer for treatment was clearly her husband.

* **The partner as informant.** At times a patient is unable to provide reliable information, or any information at all. For those times, a connection with the patient's partner is essential for the decision-making that is central to medical care.

> After talking to Mrs. White, Dr. D realized he needed to confer with her husband. At Dr. D's invitation, Mr. White joined them from the waiting room. He told Dr. D that his wife had become more and more forgetful in the last several months. Mr. White said he decided to schedule his wife for a physical when she left the stove on after cooking one night several weeks ago.

* The partner as consultant. The patient's partner is often useful in the assessment of an illness or problem. A partner may be willing to provide information that the patient has avoided mentioning or has not noticed. A partner may give another perspective, a second opinion to that of the patient, when the diagnosis is unclear or mysterious.

> In the case of Mrs. White, the patient had denied any significant problems so Mr. White's consultation was essential to the assessment process. Mr. White also offered that his wife's mother had had Alzheimer's Disease and wondered if this could be the same thing.

* The partner as participant in treatment. Some medical issues impact directly on a relationship and so, in some sense, require the partner to participate in treatment. Any major lifestyle change, such as stopping smoking, drinking, or changing diets, affects the larger family, and research has demonstrated that the family influences these lifestyle changes. (See Chapter 2.) Contraception is another clear issue that affects both members of a couple. In these cases, it is most efficient to involve the partner in the treatment process as early as possible.

> For Mrs. White, involvement of her husband in the treatment plan was essential. For example, Dr. D was able to manage the problem of Mrs. White waking up in the middle of the night and wandering by getting Mr. White to sleep on the outside of their bed. That way, if Mrs. White awoke and tried to get out of bed, her husband woke up and was able to take care of her.

* The partner as part of the problem. Blatant relationship or marital problems clearly fall in this category. There are also occasions when a couple's relationship may interfere with medical treatment in more subtle ways, for example, when a wife does not change her cooking habits after her husband has been diagnosed with coronary artery disease. Or, with drinking problems, when a husband excuses his drunk wife's behavior long past when he should. At these times, involvement of the spouse is especially important to the long-term success of any treatment. (See Chapter 12 on working with couples with relationship problems.)

> With Mr. and Mrs. White, these problems emerged after Mr. White complained that his wife had left the stove on. Mrs. White became very angry and said, "Ever since that day, my husband won't let me do a thing. He treats me

like a child that has to be watched every minute. I can't even make my own bed." Mr. White acknowledged his fear and concern had led him to take on all household chores. "It's just easier for me to do everything," he said. Clearly some tasks were important for Mr. White to manage; however, he felt perhaps he had to do virtually everything at this point to be safe. Dr. D was able to alleviate some of the strain for the couple by helping to negotiate what was safe for Mrs. White to do and what was not.

* Illness as a burden for the partner. Serious acute or chronic illness or severe trauma are very stressful for a patient's partner, and can lead to significant physical and mental health problems for that person.

> Dr. D noticed in speaking to Mr. White that he looked quite fatigued and somewhat sad. In response to the question "How are you doing?," Mr. White explained that he felt overwhelmed by the physical demands of caring for his wife and the emotional stress of seeing her deteriorate. After encouraging him to share these feelings, Dr. D asked Mr. White to schedule a check-up for himself and referred him to an Alzheimer's family support group and to a social worker to obtain home services.

Providing a spouse like Mr. White with information and support can be an important part of preventive medicine in terms of the marriage, the spouse's own health, and the spouse's role as caregiver and informant for the patient. When a patient is terminal or dies, the partner is clearly affected and may require attention him- or herself.

Common Relational Patterns Between Couples Around Illness

Families all have health belief systems that determine their behavior at times of illness. Couples often pattern themselves around what they saw their parents do, or what they wish their parents had done, when they have to cope with illness. Healthy couples are flexible and able to take many different roles with each other. Either member of the couple is able to be in the sick role or in the role of caretaker during an illness. Rigid roles can lead to marital strain or dysfunction and affect the sick person's ability to become healthy again. The following are common relationship patterns that occur for couples having difficulty dealing with having an ill member.

* Sick–healthy pair. This adaptation, with one sick member and one healthy member, can be one of the most functional if both members of a couple are allowed to play each role as necessary. If the roles are rigid, the couple will have difficulty when the "healthy" member of the pair becomes ill.

In one couple, for example, the husband was seen as sickly because he had many childhood illnesses and that was his role in his family of origin. The wife, on the other hand, was seen as strong because she took care of her younger siblings during her childhood. When the wife was diagnosed with breast cancer, both members of this couple had difficulty doing what was necessary. The wife denied to herself that the lump in her breast could be anything significant. After her surgery, the husband came down with a cold and felt unable to visit his wife or do the necessary household chores.

* **Sick–caregiving pair.** This adaptation can also be healthy if it is flexible and not driven by either partner's need to be special (through being sick or through being a caretaker). If the pattern is rigid, the caregiving spouse may encourage the sick spouse to be more dependent than need be so that each partner derives secondary gains from the illness.

For example, one wife babied her husband during the six months after his MI. She suggested he retire immediately, stop smoking, and generally take it easy. She was so concerned that he not strain himself that she answered all his phone calls, and friends (or his physician) had to relay their messages to him through her. Her overinvolvement resulted in serious marital strain.

* **Sick–distant pair.** In this pattern one partner copes with the stress of the spouse's illness by pulling away and turning to work or other people during the time of the illness. The healthy version of this adaptation occurs when the distancing spouse distracts himself with other people or activities but remains connected to the patient in important ways. When this pattern is dysfunctional, the distancing spouse may deny the partner's illness altogether or refuse to spend time with the partner until he or she recovers.

For example, after one woman was diagnosed with epilepsy, her longtime boyfriend began stopping off after work at a local bar. He spent more and more time drinking with his friends at the bar, leaving his girlfriend to call on her mother when she did not feel well.

* **Competing spouses.** These couples have symmetrical rather than complementary relationships that are based on similarity rather than difference. While healthy, each member may push the other in a positive way to be all he or she can be. Some of these couples adapt to illness through competitive or dueling symptoms. They can play an ever-ending game of "If you think you feel bad, you should know how I feel . . . ." This is an unfortunate adaptation, even if the symptoms are relatively benign, because both members experience themselves as needy and neither member feels able to nurture the other.

* **Shared illness.** Some couples are extremely dependent on each other. Prior to illness, this pattern may function fine. If an illness

threatens their interdependence, a dysfunctional adaptation may occur. Somatic fixation is a problem shared by many couples. Some even focus on the same organ functions in a kind of folie aux deux.

> For example, a man became convinced he had contracted chlamydia after having an affair, though tests were unrevealing. Soon his wife developed exactly the same symptoms as her husband, believing he had passed on his "infection" to her. The illness was a common focus that in fact functioned to bring the couple closer after the distance that resulted in the affair.

* **Coalitions around illness.** Sometimes illness intensifies already existing relationship patterns in a family (4,5). Prior to illness, families may function without normal limits. The presence of illness can exert pressure on relationships, making family dysfunction more likely.

> For example, in one family the couple agreed that the woman would be in charge of raising the children while the father worked to support the family financially. When one of the children became sick with severe asthma, the mother became quite concerned and worried over the child night and day. She stayed in the hospital with the child, then doted on him when he returned home for recuperation. This pattern persisted long after the child returned to health. The mother remained overinvolved in his life and the father grew more and more distant from both his child and his wife. If any arguments occurred, the mother always took the side of the child against her spouse. Eventually the family had to be referred for family therapy.

Divorce and Health Care

Approximately two out of five couples who are married today will end their marriage in divorce (6). Divorce is a stressful experience, repercussions of which may be felt in the primary care physician's office. Either or both members of the pair may look to the physician for support or guidance during periods of severe marital stress. For those with a high degree of conflict, a marital separation may provide some relief. However, the dissolution especially of a long-term relationship requires a realignment of relationships in the nuclear family, the extended family, and the wider support system. During this time healthy people become situationally "crazy" and unhealthy people have that much harder time of it. People are likely to have an increase in psychological symptoms, somatic symptoms, and perhaps even disease. (See Chapter 2 for a review of the research in this area.) In addition to the biomedical treatment of illness, many divorcing people may benefit from supportive, pragmatic primary care counseling if they are not already involved in psychotherapy. (See Chapter 9 for a discussion of issues related to the primary health care of children from a divorced family, and Chapter 12 for a discussion of primary care marital counseling.)

Divorce presents special issues in working with individuals and couples around their health care. Divorce offers some individuals new opportunities for happiness, and may in the long run improve their health. However, it can also introduce complexity and stress, especially for a family with children, and these factors can affect health and illness.

Guidelines for Working with Couples in Primary Care

1. Most important, **treat as a "couple" any relationship the patient defines in that way**, whether it be a marriage, a live-in relationship, or a homosexual relationship. The definition of couple for the purposes of primary care should be functional rather than legal. The reality is that much diversity exists in the way people choose to live their lives. A physician may miss relevant health information (such as HIV status) if he or she does not remain open-minded to the possibilities. Sometimes the "couple" most relevant to health care is not a romantic couple. For example, in a teenage pregnancy the grandmother may be as or more important than the father of the baby. Other examples of this phenomena also exist.

> Mrs. Wisp was a 28-year-old divorced mother of two. She and her current boyfriend and her children live in a house with another family composed of a mother, father, and three children plus the father's father. Mrs. Wisp had little money and said she welcomed this family's generosity. Because of Mrs. Wisp's recent depression, her physician, Dr. B invited all the members of the household in for a conference. During this meeting it became clear that the executive pair for this household was Mrs. Wisp and her longtime friend, Mrs. Barrel. They were the most important people to each other, having supported each other while men came and went in their lives. It was this pair that made most of the families' decisions. It became obvious that Mrs. Barrel was a key person in Mrs. Wisp's general health care as well and was central to any attempts to alleviate her depression.

2. **Develop the art of maintaining simultaneous strong alliances with two related people.** Several basic principles can help to facilitate this process:

* **Do not talk at any length about a partner who is absent.** Instead, invite them in to participate in the conversation. (See Chapter 4 for recommendations on inviting partners to a session.) This prevents destructive triangling and other potential problems, such as the physician coming to be seen as a better spouse, or better listener, than the spouse him- or herself.

* **Build rapport with each person present.** Be sure to make contact with each member of the pair within the first several minutes of the

interview. This is especially important if you have a more in-depth relationship with one person than with the other.

* **Validate each person's point of view as real and meaningful to that person.** Couples, especially when under stress, often talk as if only one person's point of view can be valid. In fact, most often, each person's point of view makes good sense when viewing the world through their eyes. The doctor–patient and doctor–family alliance depends on empathizing and being able to understand each person's perspective. By staying connected with each person, regardless of conflict, the physician models these same skills for the family.

* **Do not collude or keep important secrets with one against the other.** Often statements such as "Do not ever tell my wife I told you this, but . . . " are warning signals for present or future dysfunction in a family. If a secret is revealed, it is important to consider whether the secret is contributing to dysfunction in the couple. It is also important to consider whether the patient revealing the secret was, in a sense, requesting help in revealing the secret to other significant people. Making statements such as "Please do not ask me to keep a secret that I may feel is negatively affecting your health" can be important in establishing your neutrality in interpersonal conflict and your commitment to both individual and family health. This issue can become quite sticky around such issues as affairs, HIV status, previous pregnancies or abortions, etc. Success working with couples in these situations means working with the patient around why it is a secret and providing the patient with the support and encouragement necessary to inform the partner if the secret is harmful in any way.

> MR. WOOD: Doc, I want you to know my father had Huntington's Chorea but I've never had the guts to tell my wife. I've kept it a secret because I don't want her to worry. I worry enough for the two of us.
> DR. O: I understand how hard that must be for you to wait and wonder if you will get the same disease as your father. I know you want to protect your wife from the concern she would feel if she knew of this problem. At the same time, I myself worry that because she doesn't know she is unable to support you about this. You are unable to be as close as you could be if you shared this problem together. I also worry that if the worst should happen and you should get the disease that Mrs. Wood will not have had the opportunity to prepare herself for it.
> MR. WOOD: Well, I hadn't really thought of it that way. My mother said I should tell her, but I didn't want to think of my wife having to go through what my mother did. But, even if it were a good idea, I couldn't bring myself to tell her.
> DR. O: Why don't you think it over? If you decide it is important to tell her, and I think it is, I would be happy to meet with both of you to answer her questions regarding the disease.
> MR. WOOD: Would you just tell her, Doc, if I asked her to come in and see you?

> DR. O: No, I won't tell her myself. That's for you to do. But I would be happy to be there and offer support and information.

3. When working conjointly, **use the interview to model and teach good communication skills**. The following four straightforward suggestions can make a session with a couple therapeutic, independent of what is discussed, because the couple will gain experience in respectful communication.

* **Model respectful listening.** Balancing questions to both members of a couple and patiently listening to each of them communicates respect for both parties. For couples who take each other for granted, have dysfunctional communication, or just never learned to listen, this can be very useful.

* **Allow only one person to speak at a time.** This simple principle creates an environment where people can listen to each other. It is amazing how often people routinely speak over each other. In their hurry to be understood they clearly communicate a lack of interest in what their partner has to say. Physicians, in a discipline that shoulders a lot of tasks that need to be done in a short period of time, run a high risk of contributing to this problem themselves.

* **Reflect back individual's statements** to communicate empathy, understanding, and allow for correction. Again, this simple technique ensures understanding between people. For the physician, it is crucial for ensuring accurate diagnosis and being sure the patient understands the treatment plan. For the couple, it is essential for clear communication and intimacy.

* **Balance the interview so each partner is able to present his or her point of view.** Do not allow one partner to dominate the conversation. It is important to create space for each person to speak. Most couples look to the physician to provide this structure in an office visit.

> DR. O: I am glad you were able to come in today. I understand, Mrs. Wood, that your husband told you of his father's disease. I would be happy to answer either of your questions today about Huntington's Chorea.
>
> MRS. WOOD: I am very worried, Doc. When do you think my hus- band will become sick?
>
> DR. O: We are unsure whether your husband has the disease, Mrs. Wood. He may never become sick. If he does, it is likely to happen in the next ten years.
>
> MRS. WOOD: Well, he told me that, but I guess I wanted to hear it from you. What is the disease like?
>
> DR. O: Mr. Wood, you haven't said anything yet today. It took a lot of courage and confidence in your wife to share this information with her. I'm impressed with how much you each care for each other. Rather than my answering your wife's question, why don't you tell her what you know, and then I'll add to that when you're done.

4. **Assess what role or roles the partner is playing with regard to the illness** and, when relevant, utilize the partner in that role to facilitate the treatment plan.

• **Support the caregiver.** Involve him or her in the treatment plan, but watch for and try to prevent overfunctioning or burnout in this person.

• **Invite the customer to at least part of all interviews.** The customer has the most investment in treatment, is usually a great ally, and often is instrumental in implementing a treatment plan.

• **Interview any important informant.** The spouse can offer a wealth of information about the patient's history, symptoms, and current functioning.

• **Utilize the partner as consultant.** Ask for suggestions, diagnoses, and reactions to treatment plans. The spouse is an expert on the patient and on what the couple can effectively manage.

• **When the spouse or partner plays any kind of major role with regard to the illness**, give him or her a role as a participant in the treatment plan.

• **When the partner is part of the problem**, develop a strategy to block the problematic behavior. If it persists, refer for family therapy.

• **Monitor the partner** for fatigue, symptoms, depression, and other signs that the patient's illness is becoming an intolerable burden for him or her.

5. **Assess the way the couple interacts around the illness.** Monitor relational patterns such as sick–healthy, sick–caregiving, sick–distant, competing, shared illness, and coalitions. Watch for rigidity to develop in the individual or the couple's behavior. Frequently, primary care counseling can provide the support needed to introduce more flexibility in the way the couple is handling an illness. If that is not successful, referral to a family therapist is necessary. (For other suggestions regarding establishing conditions for good communication, see Chapter 6 on conducting a family conference.) Couples provide a fundamental and practical working unit for treating many of the problems that bring patients into primary care. Couples are often caregivers for each other and so offer a natural team to link up with the medical provider. This teamwork becomes especially important in managing pregnancy and child health care, as the next chapters illustrate.

References

1. Friedman E: The family model in church and synagogue: A systems approach to pre-marital counseling; in Berger M and Jerkovic J (eds.): *Family Therapy in Context: Practicing Systems Therapy in Community Settings.* New York, Jossey-Bass, 1984.

2. Boszormenyi-Nagy I, Sparks G: *Invisible Loyalties.* New York, Harper and Row, 1973.
3. Stanton MD: Marital therapy from a structural-strategic viewpoint, in G. Sholevar (ed.): *Handbook of Marriage and Marital Therapy.* New York, Medical and Scientific Books, 1981.
4. Penn P: Coalitions and binding interactions in families with chronic illness. *Fam Syst Med* 1983;**1**:2:16–25.
5. Sheinberg M: The family and chronic illness: A treatment diary. *Fam Syst Med* 1983;**1**:2:26–36.
6. Glick PC, Norton AJ: Marrying, divorcing, and living together in the U.S. today. *Pop Bull* 1977:**32**:5.

PROTOCOL
Working with Couples in Primary Care

Family Life Cycle Approach

* Where in the life cycle are the three generations of this family?
* Are the life cycle stages in phase or out of phase?
* What developmental challenges predominate for the family?
* What do the relevant developmental changes have to do with the presenting complaint?

New Couple Visits

A. Use a family of origin approach in the interview with the couple.
  1. Do not overtly question their choice of mates.
  2. Construct a genogram with them that joins their two extended families.
  3. Explore parental support for the marriage or new commitment.
  4. Review the family history of success in committed relationships.
  5. Review the family history of disease and dysfunction.
B. Suggest a format for future health care.
C. Consider the effect of this relationship on any extended family members in your practice (especially if they are symptomatic).

Guidelines for Working with Couples in Primary Care

A. Treat as a "couple" any relationship the patient defines in that way.
B. Develop the art of maintaining simultaneous strong alliances with two related people.
  1. Do not talk at any length about a partner who is absent.
  2. Build rapport with each person present.
  3. Validate each person's point of view as real and meaningful to that person.
  4. Do not collude or keep important secrets with one against the other.
C. Use the interview to model and teach good communication skills.
  1. Model respectful listening.
  2. Allow only one person to speak at a time.
  3. Reflect back individual's statements to communicate empathy, understanding, and allow for correction.

    4. Balance the interview so each partner is able to present his or her point of view.

D. Assess what role or roles the spouse is playing with regard to the illness and, when relevant, utilize the spouse in that role to facilitate the treatment plant.

    1. Support the caregiver.

    2. Invite the customer to participate in treatment.

    3. Interview any important informant.

    4. Utilize the spouse or partner as a consultant.

    5. Give the partner a role as a participant in the treatment plan.

    6. If the partner is part of the problem, develop a plan to block the problematic behavior or refer for family therapy.

    7. Monitor the partner for signs that the burden of the illness is becoming problematic or intolerable.

E. Assess the way the couple interacts around the illness. Watch for rigidity in the couple's relational patterns around the illness, such as sick–healthy, sick–caregiving, sick–distant, competing, shared illness, and coalitions.

F. Consider primary care counseling or referral for family therapy if patterns become too entrenched and dysfunctional.

The Birth of a Family

A Family-Oriented Approach to Pregnancy Care

Participating in the care of a couple's pregnancy and the birth of a baby is one of the most rewarding experiences for family-oriented physicians. Physicians have an opportunity to have a major impact on patients and their families during this critical stage of family development. During pregnancy, the physician has extended contact with the family and usually becomes a trusted consultant (1). Families rely on their physician for most of their information about the pregnancy (2). Family-oriented pregnancy care builds upon traditional obstetrical care, providing an integrated approach that attends to the psychosocial needs of the woman and the family as well as the biomedical aspects of the pregnancy. In addition to the rewards of attending deliveries, the family-oriented physician who practices obstetrics can have a more varied and challenging practice and provides more pediatric, gynecological, and surgical care than those who do not practice obstetrics (3).

Research has shown that family stress, family supports, and aspects of family interaction can influence the course of pregnancy, including obstetrical and perinatal complications and birth weight. (See Chapter 2.) Unfortunately, traditional prenatal care is based upon a medical model that does not address the health of the family, but is primarily devoted to screening for problems and complications of pregnancy. Insufficient attention is paid to promoting health. The father is rarely invited to actively participate in the pregnancy that involves his developing child. Failure to include the father in the intimate experience of prenatal care runs the risk of establishing a very close "quasisexual" relationship between the mother and the often male physician, who may be pulled into the role of a substitute spouse (4). The exclusion of fathers supports traditional sex roles in which the mother is the producer and nurturer of children, and the father is the economic provider. Feeling excluded and isolated, the father may have difficulty bonding with the newborn and participating in the child's care, and the mother may feel overburdened. Traditional obstetrical care is fragmented and discontinuous, with obstetricians caring for mothers through the postpartum period, and pediatricians caring for babies from the time of birth. Family-oriented care spans this critical period of transition by providing care for the pregnancy and the expanded family.

> At the six-week well-child check, Mrs. Smitten was concerned about her infant's fussiness and poor weight gain. Because Dr. L. had cared for the family during their pregnancy, he was aware of the many stresses with which the family was coping: the father's recent layoff from work, the three-year-old daughter's regression back into diapers, and the failing health of the paternal grandfather who had moved into their home during the pregnancy. After observing breastfeeding, Dr. L. was reassured that the infant had a good suck, but was not getting much milk and so became quickly frustrated. Dr. L. asked Mrs. Smitten to return the following day with her husband to discuss how to break the vicious cycle which had developed: family stress was interfering with the normal milk let-down reflex which led to a hungry, cranky baby and an upset and disheartened mother which further inhibited her milk let-down.
>
> With Dr. L.'s assistance, the couple developed the following plan:
>
> 1. Mr. Smitten would look for temporary respite care for his father.
> 2. Mrs. Smitten would ask her mother to help with some of the chores around the house.
> 3. Mr. Smitten agreed to bottle feed the baby at night so his wife could have a full night's sleep.
> 4. During nursing, Mr. Smitten would take care of their three-year-old daughter, while Mrs. Smitten, after unplugging the telephone and putting on some soothing music, would breast feed the baby alone in the nursery. Dr. L. prescribed some nasal Oxytocin to use for a brief period to help stimulate the milk let-down response.

This case illustrates the basic goal of family-oriented pregnancy care which is not only to deliver the healthiest possible baby, but to help parents make the adjustments needed to provide the best possible care for their new child. In addition to monitoring the pregnancy for complications, the family-oriented physician strives to educate and support the family during this time of transition. He or she encourages the active participation of both mother and father in the pregnancy, labor, delivery, and child care, and assists the family in renegotiating roles and relationships within their family and with extended family members. This chapter will review the developmental issues that families face during this period of the family life cycle and offer specific suggestions for implementing a family-oriented approach throughout pregnancy, childbirth, and the newborn period.

Developmental Issues in Pregnancy and Childbirth: The Birth of a Triangle

The birth of the first child is a critical period of transition for all families. The couple must accommodate a new member to become a three-person family. For many couples, the birth of their first child is considered the beginning of the family. It is also a time in which the couple reassesses their commitment and responsibility not only to each other but to the new child. The couple must make room in their relationship for the new infant, while maintaining the intimacy and sexuality of their marriage. The dyad becomes a triad, and the triangle illustrates the complexities of these new relationships. In addition to new parent–child relationships, there are opportunities for alliances (e.g., parents working together to care for the child) and risks of coalitions (one parent and child against the other parent). With the addition of each new child, the family constellation is forever changed (5).

The birth of a first child affects the extended family as well. Everyone moves up a generation: parents of the couple become grandparents; sisters and brothers become aunts and uncles. Combrinck-Graham (6) calls this a centripetal phase in which the family comes closer together, and the connectedness or cohesion between family members strengthen, while interpersonal boundaries become diffuse. Becoming parents encourages couples to reflect on their relationships with their own parents, and offers opportunities for reworking these relationships. Subsequent pregnancies and the delivery of additional children have similar developmental challenges. Many parents report that while having two children is a joy that adds to the family, it is often experienced as more than twice the work of one, and puts additional stress on the family requiring further role negotiations.

While most families successfully negotiate the transition of a new child and continue healthy family functioning, problems can develop that lead to persistent dysfunctional patterns in the family. One common problem can occur when the mother establishes a close relationship with her infant that excludes the father. Feeling left out, the father becomes more involved outside the family, either in work or another relationship. The mother than feels abandoned by her husband and pulls closer to her infant away from her spouse, and a vicious cycle develops. Another dysfunctional pattern is the couple that abandons their husband and wife roles to be parents. These couples stop spending time alone together. All activities involve the child with a decrease in marital intimacy. Couples with shaky relationships to begin with, especially those who have not accomplished the developmental tasks of the previous stages of the family life cycle, are at the greatest risk for these dysfunctional patterns to develop. For example, the adolescent who becomes pregnant, leaves her parents' home and gets married, has neither separated emotionally from her parents nor established an intimate relationship with her husband. The girl's mother usually helps with the child-rearing, the husband is excluded from this sphere, and the long-term stability of the marriage is threatened.

A family-oriented approach to pregnancy and delivery can be beneficial regardless of whether a couple is married, or the family is nontraditional, such as gay couples. Even in pregnancies where the mother has no further contact or relationship with the biological father and plans to raise the baby alone, there are usually important family members or friends involved. In some of these cases, it may be this person, most commonly the mother's mother, who becomes primarily responsible for raising the infant. Thus, encouraging the active participation of these important people in the care of the pregnancy can have long term benefits.

Prepregnancy: Family Planning

As discussed in the previous chapter, it is ideal to meet with a couple during routine health care visits to help understand their relationship and their approach to health care issues. This is particularly important for matters pertaining to family planning and contraception, since these directly involve both members of the couple. Routine gynecological exams are an ideal opportunity to invite the woman's partner in to discuss birth control and plans for children. When a woman or a couple expresses the desire to become pregnant and start a family, one can offer an appointment for the couple to come in and discuss their plans.

At a routine gynecological visit or during a prepregnancy visit, several issues should be covered.

1. **Encourage the couple to discuss their ideas and plans regarding pregnancy and children.** Do they both want to start a family now? If there is a reluctance on the part of either partner, encourage them to discuss this together.

2. **Evaluate the extended family and their attitudes about pregnancy.** What are their own families' feelings about their plans? Have they put pressure on them to have children? Has the couple discussed it with them?

3. **Briefly assess where the couple is in the family life cycle and how they have negotiated the tasks of previous stages.** Have both members of the couple been able to develop a balance in which both are able to maintain connections with their families while also being able to commit to their partner? Is the pregnancy being used to leave home, to get married, or to improve a marriage? If this is the case, it can be helpful to get the couple to acknowledge this explicitly and discuss how successful this plan will be.

Jenny, a high school senior, came to see Dr. M for a pregnancy test. She had forgotten to take her birth control pills for several days during the previous month and was now several days late with her period. She was the youngest of five children and was the only one still living with her parents. Her 20-year-old boyfriend Jim brought her to the appointment, so Dr. M invited him into the exam room to discuss the situation. Jenny expressed the desire to keep the baby if she were pregnant and to move in with Jim. However, Jim doubted his ability to support a family and inquired about abortion.

The couple appeared relieved when the pregnancy test was negative. Together, they decided that it was not a good time to have a baby and agreed to continue using contraception at least until they got married or were living together. Jim offered to help Jenny to remember her birth control pills and to use a condom if she forgot.

4. **Review biological and psychological risk factors.** Is there anything in the woman's health history that might present a risk in pregnancy (e.g. medication, smoking, drug and alcohol use)? If so, counseling the woman to stop medication, drugs, or smoking prior to pregnancy is crucial. This is an excellent time to promote healthy behaviors in the family. Women who previously have been unable or unwilling to stop smoking or reduce their alcohol intake, may do so for the benefit of their planned child. Partners can either help or hinder these behavior changes. Risk factors, especially smoking, are often shared by couples (see Chapter 2), and it is more difficult for a woman to stop smoking if her partner smokes. Furthermore, the partner's support has been shown to have a very positive influence on smoking cessation. Thus it is crucial to elicit the partner's support for behavioral changes.

First Trimester: Initial Prenatal Visit

For the woman, the first trimester of a pregnancy is a time of introspection and adjustment to bodily changes, including unpleasant symptoms such as morning sickness (7). It is also a time of change in the couple's relationship. The couple must begin to deal with the increased commitment that a pregnancy represents. For most couples, there is some degree of ambivalence about the pregnancy. For some, there may be serious questions about continuing the pregnancy.

During the pregnancy, a comprehensive, biopsychosocial evaluation of the pregnancy, the woman, and the family should be performed. Some of this is accomplished during the first prenatal visit, but other information can be obtained throughout the pregnancy. If the issues presented in the last section have not been discussed previously with the couple, they should be covered during prenatal visits. In addition, the following areas should be discussed during the first prenatal visit.

1. **Explore whether the pregnancy was desired or planned, and whether there are any thoughts of terminating the pregnancy.** "What are your plans for this pregnancy?" Until you know this information, be careful not to congratulate the woman. If the woman is uncertain about continuing the pregnancy, discuss the options with her.

2. **Find out what social supports the mother has (e.g., father of child, parents, sibs, friends), and how these people feel about the pregnancy.** "What does your boyfriend think about your pregnancy?" "What has your mother's reaction been?" Tell the woman that you look forward to meeting these important people later in the pregnancy.

3. **Invite the father of the baby to all prenatal visits.** If the father is not at the initial visit, inquire whether he is in the waiting room, and ask him to join you. Insist on meeting with the father, or other support person if the father is not involved, at least twice during the pregnancy; early on to deal with pregnancy issues and toward the end to discuss labor, delivery, and the postpartum period.

> Jean came to her first prenatal visit with Dr. C when she was 16 weeks pregnant. The pregnancy had been planned by her (she had stopped using her diaphragm), but she had not yet told her husband Peter. She explained that Peter did not think they could afford a second child. When Dr. C asked Jean to invite her husband to her next appointment, she said she did not think that he could get the time off from work nor would he be interested in coming. "He wasn't involved with my first pregnancy," she explained, "and besides, I'm not sure I wanted him to come to my doctor's appointments."

Getting "Reluctant" Fathers In

Fathers are usually eager and willing to participate in prenatal care. However, a woman will occasionally say that her partner is "reluctant," unwilling, or unable to attend any prenatal sessions. Although rigid work schedules sometimes prevent fathers from coming in, it may signal lack of involvement in parenting or some type of marital distress. In these cases, it is particularly important to get the father in as early as possible, and to assess the marital relationship and its impact on the pregnancy.

1. **Involve the father early on in the pregnancy.** As the pregnancy proceeds, if a woman comes in alone she develops an exclusive relationship with the physician, making the father feel more excluded and less likely to come in. **Avoid** listening extensively to any complaints about partner before you have met him.

2. **Expect the father to come in** by being direct about your need for the father to participate in prenatal care. Expect him to come in. "I need to meet with the father of your baby. Can he come in for your next

prenatal visit?" Explain that this is a part of routine prenatal care. **Avoid** being ambivalent or giving mixed messages about the importance of the father coming in, such as "Do you think your partner would like (or be able) to come in?" Patients pick up your confidence, or lack thereof, in any procedure you recommend.

3. **Emphasize the important role of the father** in the care of the pregnancy. Tell the woman that you need her partner's help or opinion. **Avoid** accepting the patient's word that her partner is unwilling to come in. This can be a projection of her own reluctance or protectiveness. **Stress the benefits** of the partner's involvement to the patient and the pregnancy. **Avoid** blaming the mother or father in any way. Don't imply there are "marital problems" or that the couple is in need of therapy even if you think the marriage is in trouble. This can increase the couple's defensiveness or fear of coming in.

4. **Offer to call** the partner yourself if needed. This may be necessary if the patient insists that he will not come in, regardless of what she says to them or cannot come because of work. It is best to call the partner while the woman is in the office and can hear what is being said.

5. **Request that the father come in for one prenatal visit only**, just to listen, without asking him to participate. Within a few minutes of such a visit, reluctant fathers typically will want to participate.

> JEAN: And besides, I'm not sure I want him to come into my doctor's appointment.
> DR. C: I hear your concern. However as a family physician, I routinely meet with fathers during the pregnancy and would like to meet Peter as soon as possible. I think it is very important for a father to be involved in the care of his developing child.
> JEAN: Well, he never helps with the child he already has, so I don't know why he would consider getting involved before the next one's even born?
> DR. C: Would you like him to help out with your daughter more at home?
> JEAN: Why of course, what woman wouldn't? But he's too busy with his work.
> DR. C: In my experience, fathers who get involved during the pregnancy feel more committed to the family and help out more after the child is born. What if we invite him in for just one of your prenatal visits, and see how it goes?
> JEAN: Maybe for one visit, if you can find a time he can make it.

Meeting with the Couple

In prenatal care, the primary patient remains the pregnant woman, and family members are important sources of support for the woman. If the physician has an established relationship only with the woman, the father may feel like an outsider. When meeting with the couple during the pregnancy, time must be taken to establish a good relationship with the father, while still maintaining a positive relationship with the mother.

1. **Establish rapport with the father at the very beginning of the visit.** Thank him for coming in, acknowledge what an important role he has in the pregnancy, and how you will need his help. Find out about his work, and demonstrate interest in some aspect of his life.

2. **Acknowledge the father's importance throughout the pregnancy and after delivery.** Refer to THEIR pregnancy and THEIR child. Use him as consultant and ask him how he thinks the pregnancy is going. Encourage the couple to attend prenatal classes together.

3. **Encourage the father to attend prenatal visits whenever possible, and to listen to the fetal heart beat.** If one has a doptone stethoscope with two headsets or a speaker, couples enjoy listening to the fetal heart beat for a few minutes together. Both can be taught how to feel the uterus and where the baby is situated.

> DR. C: Hello, Peter, I am delighted that you could come in today. Did you have to take some time off from work to come in?
> PETER: Yeah, I had to leave my shift early today.
> DR. C: I see. What kind of work do you do?
> PETER: I'm the supervisor at one of the darkrooms at Kodak.
> DR. C: That must be challenging work. I appreciate the effort it took to get here. As I told your wife, I believe that the father plays a very important role in the care of his developing child, and I'd like to get your thoughts on how Jean's and your pregnancy is going.
> PETER: Well, I'm not really sure. She doesn't tell me much. I am concerned that she hasn't been eating very well recently.
> JEAN: I'm surprised you even noticed.
> DR. C: Well, let's talk about it. Jean, I think you should tell Peter how you have been feeling and how the pregnancy has been going in general. Then, if it is all right with Jean, the two of you can listen to the heartbeat together.

4. **Suggest that the father also have a physical check-up.** Fathers commonly have symptoms that mimic some of the symptoms of pregnancy, such as nausea, abdominal bloating, or increased urinations, called Couvade Syndrome (8). A physical examination not only gives the physician an opportunity to evaluate any physical and psychological symptoms and establish a relationship with the father, but also lets the father know that his physical health is also important. Young men tend to avoid physicians, so a check up during their spouse's pregnancy is a good time to do routine health screening (e.g., blood pressure, cholesterol) and review health risks (e.g., smoking, substance abuse). Becoming a parent may make some men more attentive to their own health.

5. **When there are signs of marital conflict, it is important to keep the initial and subsequent visits focused on prenatal care.** Avoid discussing marital problems or doing "marital counseling" as this

is likely to result in either the husband or the wife not returning for future appointments. By helping the couple work together to deliver a healthy baby, improvements in their relationship will occur that often generalize to other aspects of their marriage, without having to directly confront marital problems. Sometimes, such couples will acknowledge and request help for these problems, and a referral for marital therapy can be made. (See Chapter 12.)

Second Trimester: Subsequent Prenatal Care

The second trimester (13–27 weeks) is often a period of calm and increased closeness between the couple. Morning sickness usually has resolved and the woman feels physically and emotionally well. This is the time when the couple can enjoy pregnancy and feel that they really are going to have a child together.

1. **Elicit the couple's concerns and fears about the pregnancy**, especially regarding possible complications of labor or delivery, pain during labor, and birth defects. This is best done prior to 16 weeks when screening for neural tube defects (maternal serum alpha-fetoprotein) or Downs Syndrome (amniocentesis) is discussed. The couple may not have discussed these fears with each other, because of concerns about increasing their partner's anxiety or that their own fears won't be understood. Bringing these fears out in the open allows the partners to be supportive of each other. Acknowledge and normalize these fears and discuss any exaggerated or unwarranted fears. "All couples have fears about the baby's development and whether the baby will be normal, what concerns do both of you have?" One woman was concerned that her husband who worked as an X-ray technician was bringing home radiation that would harm her pregnancy, but was afraid to mention this to him because she thought he might have to quit his job.

2. **Have the couple go together for any necessary tests**, especially ultrasound. For many couples, a stronger bond develops with the baby when they can actually see it with ultrasound and receive a picture. Fathers can be trained how to do some of the routine prenatal care at home such as blood pressure checks, urinalyses done at home, and kick counts.

3. **Construct a genogram** with particular attention to pregnancy and childbirth experiences, as well as the presence of genetically transmitted diseases. Has anyone in previous generations died during childbirth? Assess how previous generations have dealt with pregnancy and childbirth, as these patterns often repeat themselves over several generations. For instance, are there any family themes regarding marriage (e.g., "men are not to be trusted"), pregnancy (e.g., children leave home by getting pregnant), or children (e.g., "they help keep marriages together")?

4. **Invite important family members and friends to prenatal visits.** Encourage the woman's mother to come for at least one visit. She is often the most important family health expert, especially regarding pregnancy and childbirth. In many families, beliefs about pregnancy and childbirth are passed on from mother to daughter for many generations, especially concerning nutrition and breastfeeding. Comments or advice from the extended family may conflict with medical recommendations (e.g., "no more than 20 pounds weight gain during pregnancy," "mother should stay in bed for two weeks after delivery") or lead to unnecessary anxiety (e.g., "women don't survive Caesarian births").

It is important to establish an alliance with this family expert and to work collaboratively, instead of competitively, with her as much as possible.

> Peter accompanied his wife to several additional prenatal visits and attended the refresher prenatal class with her. While obtaining a more detailed genogram of the family, Dr. C learned that the first few years of their marriage had been very difficult. Shortly after they were married, Peter started business school and Jean became pregnant. For several months after the birth, Jean's mother lived with them to help care for the baby. More recently, when Jean complained to her mother about how busy Peter was with his work, her mother suggested that she might be happier if she had another child to take care of.
>
> After learning this, Dr. C invited Jean's parents to join the couple for a prenatal visit. At the session, all four agreed that the arrangement after the first pregnancy had not been satisfactory. After the first couple of weeks, Jean had resented her mother's advice and help; Peter felt excluded from the family; Jean's mother thought she was being taken advantage of; and Jean's father felt abandoned by his wife. After discussing plans for the upcoming delivery, Peter decided to take two weeks off from work to be home after the delivery. Jean's parents agreed to help care for their three-year-old granddaughter and to assist with the new baby when their daughter asked for help.

5. **Discuss sexual issues of pregnancy** with the couple, including the safety of intercourse throughout pregnancy and the use of different positions. Normalize changes in libido that occur in both men and women during pregnancy. Toward the end of the pregnancy, discuss future birth control options with the couple.

6. **Begin discussing breastfeeding early on**, and provide information about its benefits to the baby and the family. Find out whether other members of the couple's extended families have nursed their children and what advice they have given.

7. **Encourage the couple to take a mini vacation** or "second honeymoon" alone together during the second trimester. Suggest that the father schedule a minimum of one or two weeks of paternity leave for the time of delivery. Have the couple discuss which family members or friends may be available to help during the first few months after birth.

8. **Find out what the couple has told or plans to tell the other child(ren) about the pregnancy.** By the time that the pregnancy is showing parents should tell other children. During the third trimester, invite the other children in to a prenatal visit to discuss the "new baby" and listen to the fetal heart beat.

9. **Discuss with the couple whether and how they want their children involved in the labor and delivery.** Generally children under five years old have difficulty understanding what is occurring and may become quite frightened. Older children need careful preparation, often provided by hospitals with family birthing centers, if they are going to be present at the delivery. Children at a delivery should always be accompanied by an adult family member or friend who can attend to their needs throughout the labor and delivery (9).

10. **Help parents anticipate sibling rivalry and regressions in development of siblings of the new baby** (e.g., bedwetting, thumb-sucking) and suggesting ways the parents can deal with these problems. These can include giving special attention and privileges to the older child, having the older child give a gift to the newborn, and finding special ways in which the older child can help with the baby's care, such as helping with diaper changes.

Third Trimester: Anticipating Labor and Delivery

The third trimester is usually a time of anticipation and anxiety concerning labor and delivery and the new baby. The ninth month never goes fast enough for the woman. Acknowledging and normalizing the impatience and anxiety during this period can be very helpful for couples. At this time one should review the typical events of labor and delivery and elicit the couple's desires regarding the use of a family birthing center (if available), episiotomy, pain medication, and different labor positions. Have the couple discuss what ways the father can be supportive to his partner during her labor. Options regarding breast feeding and circumcision should be discussed. While the health advantages of breast feeding, and the absence of medical indications for circumcision should be presented, the decisions of the couple should be respected and supported. These decisions are often based as much, or more, on cultural or religious tradition than on medical reasons. For example, the physician should not suggest bottle feeding is bad or that circumcision causes unnecessary pain, if those choices match the couple's well thought out preferences.

The primary goal during labor and delivery is to promote a normal childbirth with minimal interventions. Encourage families to use a family birth center, when available. Family birthing centers can offer many of the advantages of home birth with the technology and emergency care available if needed. The homelike atmosphere of these centers helps to demedicalize the birth process and to reduce the anxiety of both mother and father. A home visit during early labor can allow the woman to remain at home until she has entered the active phase of labor or prevent unnecessary trips to the hospital for false labor.

Labor and Delivery

1. **Avoid interventions** such as enemas, fetal monitoring, IVs, medication, and artificial rupture of membranes unless clearly indicated. Research has demonstrated that these interventions carry some risks (10). Encourage the father to take an active role in assisting during labor. It is often necessary to have the labor nurse and father negotiate what roles they will have—who will rub the woman's back, encourage her to push, etc.—or labor nurses may take over, leaving the father feeling helpless and neglected. Long labors can be extremely exhausting for both members of the couple, so having additional family members at the labor can provide more support for the mother and allow family members spell each other.

2. At the time of delivery, **the father's role should depend upon the needs and desires of the woman**. During difficult or long second stages of labor, he may need to support his partner at the head of the bed. If this is not needed, some fathers enjoy helping to deliver the baby's head or to cut the umbilical cord (11). Put the newborn directly on the mother's chest, skin to skin, shortly after birth if baby is stable, and encourage nursing as soon as desired. Early mother–infant contact has been shown to improve bonding (12), and early breastfeeding reduces the need for oxytoxics.

> Jean ruptured her membranes at home four days after her due date, and within several hours was in active labor. Shortly after settling into the birthing center, she delivered a 9 pound baby boy without an episiotomy or laceration. Peter cut the umbilical cord and helped the nurse with the baby's first bath. An hour later, Jean's parents brought their granddaughter into the birth center to see her parents and new baby brother.

3. **If complications arise during labor or delivery, it is important to explain clearly to the couple what is happening.** They usually will be very frightened and assume the worst (i.e., that the baby is dying) unless told otherwise. Choose consultants who have good communication skills and will work with the family. If a Caesarean section is required, many hospitals now allow the father to be present in the operating room. If the baby requires resuscitation, the father should be allowed to be present and observe (out of the way). Even when the outcome is bad, fathers are reassured by observing everything done for the infant.

4. At the time of birth, parents are usually anxious to be told that the baby is normal. This is best done by **examining the baby at the bedside and explaining the normal findings to both parents**. When birth anomalies are present, parents should be told immediately, but the overall health of the baby should be stressed. "Your baby appears to be very healthy. However he has a cleft lip that can be corrected surgically." Going into detail about the problem is not useful at the time of delivery, but is best left to later when the parents can attend to and remember what is said.

Fourth Trimester: Adjusting to a New Baby

First time mothers are usually anxious about their ability to breastfeed their infants and deserve lots of encouragement.

1. **Encourage feeding on demand and rooming-in, and avoid supplementing breastfeeding with formula or glucose water.** If the mother is having difficulty with breastfeeding, observe a feeding to see what the problems are. Find out whether her mother breastfed her, and, if possible, use her as a consultant. Unfortunately, a generation ago fewer women breastfed, so the grandmother may be just as anxious about it as the mother. A sister, sister-in-law, or close friend who has successfully nursed or even a group such as the La Leche League can provide advice and support.

2. **Encourage siblings to visit when the mother and infant are in the hospital.**

3. At the time of discharge from the hospital, be certain to meet with both the father and mother. **Conduct the newborn's discharge physical at the mother's bedside,** explaining normal findings again to the couple. Many first time parents are reluctant to handle the newborn for fear of injuring the infant. Having the couple participate in the examination, feeling the fontanels, and lifting the unswaddled child in their hands, can help them feel more comfortable with infant care.

Review postpartum and newborn instructions, and explore ways in which the father can participate in care of the child. For couples that breastfeed, the mother can pump her breasts for at least one bottle a day and the father can do one feeding at a convenient time. Keeping the baby adapted to a bottle allows the mother and couple greater independence. Birth control and the resumption of sexual activity should be discussed with the couple.

4. **At two weeks, a home visit is an excellent and enjoyable way to assess how the infant feeding is going and the new family is coping.** In addition, it avoids exposing the infant to patients at the physician's office with colds and other infections, and accommodates to the belief of

some cultures that the mother should not leave the house during the first several weeks after birth. At this time, there are usually very few biomedical issues to deal with and only a limited examination is needed. During the visit, check on how the siblings are doing.

During this period, the family-oriented physician should support the couple's own parenting skills and avoid giving too much advice. For example, mothers often ask how much formula the infant should be taking or whether he or she is getting enough breast milk. Rather than calculating how much formula based upon the infant's weight or age, encourage the couple to learn to assess whether the infant has had enough and is satisfied. This approach does not require a calculator, and it supports the parents' judgment and reduces their dependence upon health experts. With each success, their confidence will generalize to other areas of parenting. (Well-child care is discussed in Chapter 9.)

> Arriving at home for the two-week well-child check up, Dr. C. was met by the entire family, and a neighbor who "wanted to meet a doctor who really made home visits." After briefly examining the baby, Dr. C. joined the family for tea while they discussed how they were adapting to the new addition. Peter said he enjoyed staying home for the two weeks, but now he was eager to get back to work. Jean's parents liked getting to know their granddaughter better, and being consultants to the couple. Jean appreciated the help and support of her family and felt much more confident about her judgments and abilities as a mother.

One physician summed up the importance of pregnancy and delivery to the family when he said, "The family begins with the relationship between a man and a woman, but it is really not a family unit until a child is born. Therefore the events immediately preceding and surrounding the birth of a child have great social importance for family development" (13). A family-oriented approach that cares for the social, emotional, and biological needs of the entire family during pregnancy and birth provides a stage for promoting a healthy family throughout the life cycle.

References

1. Klein M: Contracting for trust in family practice obstetrics. *Can Fam Physician* 1983;**29**:2225–2227.
2. Prindham K, Schutz M: Preparation of parents for birthing and infant care. *J Fam Pract* 1981;**13**:181–188.
3. Mehle LE, Bruce C, Renner JH: Importance of obstetrics in a comprehensive family practice. *J Fam Pract* 1976;**3**:385–389.
4. McDaniel SH, Naumburg E: Gender issues: Family Medicine's family secret. *Fam Med* 1988;**20**:408–410.
5. Midmer D, Talbot Y: Assessing post-partum family functioning: The Family FIRO model. *Can Fam Physician* 1988;**34**:2041–2048.

6. Combrinck-Graham L: A developmental model for family systems. *Fam Proc* 1985;**24**:139–150.
7. Friederick MA: Psychological changes during pregnancy. *Contemporary OB/GYN* 1977;**9**:27–34.
8. Lamb GS, Lipkin M: Somatic symptoms of expectant fathers. *Am J Maternal Child Nursing* 1982;**7**:110–115.
9. Clark L: When children watch their mothers deliver. *Contemporary OB/GYN* Aug 1986:69–78.
10. Klein M, Lloyd I, Redman L, et al.: A comparison of low risk women booked for delivery in two different systems of care. Part 1: Obstetrical procedures, and neonatal outcomes. *Br J Obstet Gyneacol* 1983;**90**:118–122.
11. Block RA: We've let 1500 fathers deliver their own babies. *Medical Economics* Aug 9, 1982, p. 181.
12. Klaus MH, Kennel J: *Maternal-Infant Bonding*. St. Louis, CV Mosby Co., 1976.
12. Newton M: *Cybele Report* 1981;**2**:3.

PROTOCOL
Family-Oriented Pregnancy Care

Prepregnancy

1. Encourage the couple to discuss their ideas and plans regarding pregnancy and children.
2. Evaluate the extended family and their attitudes about pregnancy.
3. Briefly assess where the couple is in the family life cycle and how they have negotiated the tasks of previous stages.
4. Review biological and psychological risk factors.

First Trimester

1. Explore whether pregnancy was desired or planned, and whether there are any thoughts of terminating the pregnancy.
2. Find out what social supports the mother has (father of child, parents, sibs, friends), and how these people feel about the pregnancy.
3. Invite the father of the baby to all prenatal visits.
   a. Involve the father early on in the pregnancy.
   b. Be positive and direct about your need for the father to participate in prenatal care.
   c. Emphasize the importance of the father in the care of the pregnancy. Stress the benefits of the partner's involvement to the patient and the pregnancy.
   d. Offer to call the partner yourself if needed.
   e. Request that the father come in for **one prenatal visit only**, just to listen, without asking him to participate.
4. Meeting with the couple
   a. Establish rapport with the father at the very beginning of the visit.
   b. Acknowledge the father's importance throughout the pregnancy and after delivery. Use him as a consultant and ask him how he thinks the pregnancy is going.
   c. Encourage the father to attend prenatal visits whenever possible and to listen to the fetal heart beat.
   d. Suggest that the father have a physical check-up.
   e. When there are signs of marital conflict, keep all visits focused on prenatal care and avoid discussing marital problems or doing "marital counseling."

Second Trimester

1. Elicit the couple's concerns and fears about the pregnancy, especially regarding possible complications of labor or delivery, pain during labor, and birth defects.

2. Have the couple go together for any necessary tests, especially ultrasound.

3. Construct a genogram with particular attention to pregnancy and childbirth experiences, as well as the presence of genetically transmitted disease.

4. Invite important family members and friends to prenatal visits. Encourage the woman's mother to come for at least one visit.

5. Discuss sexual issues of pregnancy with the couple, including the safety of intercourse throughout the pregnancy and the use of different positions.

6. Begin the discussion of breastfeeding early on, and provide information about its benefits to the baby and the family.

7. Encourage the couple to take a minivacation or "second honeymoon" alone together during the second trimester. Suggest that the father schedule a minimum of one or two weeks of paternity leave for the time of delivery.

8. Find out what the couple has told or plans to tell the other child(ren) about the pregnancy.

9. Discuss with the couple how they want their children involved in the labor and delivery.

10. Help parents anticipate sibling rivalry and regressions in development of siblings of a new baby (e.g., bedwetting, thumbsucking) and offer some suggestions to the parents to deal with these problems.

Third Trimester

1. Anticipate and educate the couple about labor and delivery.

2. Discuss ways for the father to be supportive to the mother during labor and deliver.

3. Make preliminary decisions about:
   a. where to labor and deliver
   b. pain medication
   c. breast feeding
   d. circumcision

Labor and Delivery

1. Encourage families to use family birthing centers, when available.

2. Avoid interventions such as enemas, fetal monitoring, IVs, and medication unless clearly indicated. Encourage the father to take an active role in assisting during labor.

3. If the delivery is uncomplicated, encourage the father to assist as much as he likes, such as helping to deliver the baby's head or to cut the umbilical cord. Encourage nursing as soon as it is desired.

4. Explain clearly to the couple what is happening, especially if complications arise. Allow the father to be present for a Caesarean section if it is required.
5. Examine the baby at the bedside and explain the normal findings to both parents. When birth anomalies are present, inform parents immediately, but stress the overall health of the baby.

Postpartum

1. Encourage feeding on demand and rooming-in, and avoid supplementing breastfeeding. If the mother is having difficulty with breastfeeding, observe a feeding to see what the problems are.
2. Encourage siblings to visit when the mother and infant are in the hospital.
3. Conduct the newborn's discharge physical at the mother's bedside, and have the couple participate in the examination.
4. At two weeks, make a home visit to assess how the infant feeding is going and the new family is coping.

CHAPTER 9

Supporting Parents
Family-Oriented Child Health Care

Parents often view the physician as the person to whom they can turn not only for Johnny's runny nose but his developmental and behavior difficulties as well. In fact, a majority of pediatrician's time, estimated by some as high as 85%, is spent dealing with psychosocial and developmental issues that arise during well-child and acute care visits (1,2). Since most of these requests for assistance are not severe enough to warrant referral, primary care physicians need to develop an effective approach to working with parents regarding their concerns about their children. We advocate a family-oriented approach that expands the traditional biomedical, anticipatory guidance model to take into account the context of the child.

In the traditional anticipatory guidance model for physician involvement in child health care the physician uses his or her knowledge of child development and child developmental milestones to educate and guide parents in raising their child (1–4). The physician helps parents to deal with everyday health and behavior concerns and anticipate future changes or difficulties. The physician also uses his or her knowledge and skills to intervene when the child's health is at risk. In this model, the physician is available to parents as both a medical and child-rearing expert.

Our concern about the traditional model of anticipatory guidance is that its application is often a rather routine checklist approach to covering important developmental issues. This approach in and of itself does not place the child's development in context, in relation to his or her parents and siblings. It often does not take into account a particular family's strengths and weaknesses, strengths and weaknesses that should determine the level of intervention, if any, that is needed from the physician. We are also concerned that the traditional approach can place inappropriate expectations on the physician to be an expert parent, a better parent than any of his or her patients. It encourages the physician to assume the role of surrogate parent and give advice, whether needed or not, on everything from toilet training and proper selection of toys to child-proofing one's house. This approach by itself unduly medicalizes many aspects of childrearing and inadvertently encourages parents to believe they need expert medical advice to do their job.

In a family-oriented approach to child health care, the physician and parents, as well as other important child health care givers, such as grandparents, are partners in child health care. Both the family and the medical system have areas of expertise and need to collaborate to provide the best care for the child. **The physician's first job is to support the parents being in charge of their child's overall health care.** The physician is an expert on medical matters and, when needed, functions as an authoritative childrearing consultant. The physician uses his or her knowledge to educate, guide, and intervene, but utilizes parents' strengths and resources, guiding or intervening as much or as little as the parents need or request. In this way, the physician maintains an authoritative role in child health care and uses this role to support and foster a sense of confidence and competence in the parents.

In this chapter we will address how to implement a family-oriented approach to child health care by discussing dimensions of child health care, psychosocial assessment issues, and guidelines for family-oriented child health care.

Dimensions of Child Health Care

A physician's contacts with a family for child health care cannot always be neatly divided into well-child and acute care. It is not out of the ordinary for a "normal" well-child visit to be focused on a parent's unexpected concern ("Why isn't my baby gaining weight faster?") or an acute care visit to reveal only mild symptoms in the child but important concerns in the parent ("I'm feeling overwhelmed caring for my child"). One study has indicated that in one-third of acute child care cases the parent seeking care for his or her child was coming for reasons other than the primary complaint (5).

It is important in any child-health-care visit to understand not only the nature of the child's symptoms but what they mean to the parents and what the parents are requesting of the physician. For that reason we view these visits as having two dimensions, one pertaining to the child and the other pertaining to the parent. These dimensions interact to form four different configurations. (See Fig. 9.1.)

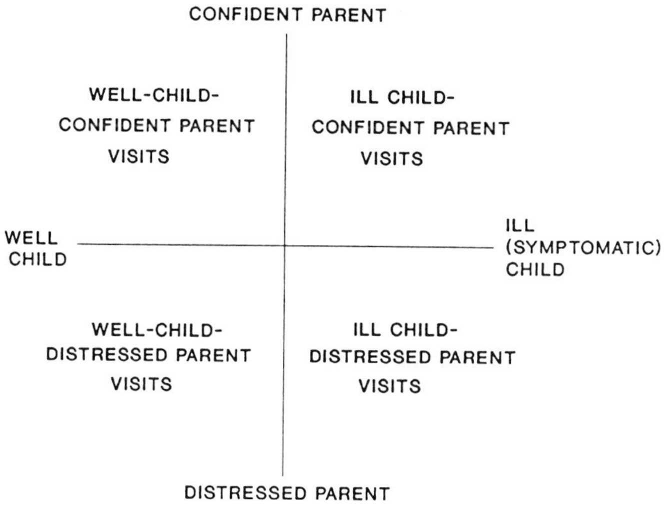

FIGURE 9.1   Dimensions of Child Health Care

1. **Well-Child–Confident-Parent Visits.** In these visits, the child is healthy and developing well, and parents are feeling confident in their parenting.

> Mrs. Gleason brought Joey, age 10 months, for a well-child visit. Mrs. Gleason reported that their daughter, age 4, was adjusting well to having a baby brother, and that Mr. and Mrs. Gleason were feeling good about how things were going. Dr. B examined Joey who was developing at a normal rate.

2. **Well-Child–Distressed-Parent Visits.** In these visits, the child is healthy and developing well but the parent has specific concerns, such as feeding, toilet training, or the use of pacifiers.

> Mr. and Mrs. Tanner brought Emily, age 2, for a routine well-child visit. Dr. N. examined Emily and found she was in good health. Dr. N. asked if Mr. and Mrs. Tanner had any concerns. Mrs. Tanner said they were having a lot of difficulty getting Emily to stop using a bottle and didn't know what to do.

3. **Ill-Child–Confident-Parent Visits.** In these visits, the child is sick and the parent feels confident to handle the illness, but needs reassurance that he or she is doing a good job as a parent.

> Mr. Conway brought Mike, age 4, to the doctor's office with a sore throat and swollen glands. Mr. Conway said his wife had stayed home from work with Mike the day before, but when Mike woke up with a temperature of 102 degrees today, they decided to make an appointment. Mr. Conway had arranged to be home with Mike for the day but wondered if an antibiotic was needed or if he and his wife should be doing something more.

4. **Ill-Child–Distressed-Parent Visits.** In these visits the child is ill and the parent is distressed not only about the child but about his or her own ability to manage the situation as a parent. These visits may also involve a child being brought to the doctor's with mild symptoms by a parent who has his or her own personal concern. ("Sometimes I don't know what to do next" or "I've been feeling very tired lately"). A more subtle variation of this category is the parent of a very symptomatic child who does not appear concerned but is actually denying his or her distress rather than truly feeling confident. These parents also need extra support from their physician.

> Mary brought Rachel, age 3, to see Dr. V because Rachel had symptoms of a cold. Mary, a single parent, reported that her daughter had started day care two months prior to the visit and seemed to be "sick all the time." Mary had started a new job and said she felt at her "wit's end" over Rachel's colds. Mary wondered if she was doing something wrong.

Understanding how the child and parent dimensions interact helps the physician clarify the multiple factors that may be involved in any visit. The physician is then better able to respond to the concerns related to both dimensions.

> Mrs. Jackson brought her son, 6, to the doctor's with a runny nose and a low grade fever. Dr. L determined that the boy had a cold and the parents had been treating him appropriately with liquids, Tylenol, and bed rest. Mrs. Jackson, though, was still distressed about her son's "congestion." Upon further questioning, Dr. L learned that the Jackson's oldest child had had serious pneumonia at the same age. When Dr. L said there was nothing to indicate pneumonia, Mrs. Jackson breathed a sigh of relief.

Having taken both the child and parent dimensions into account, Dr. L recognizes this to be an ill-child–distressed-parent visit and is better able to address the presenting complaint as well as the concern of the parent. The interplay of child and parent dimensions in an office visit illustrates the importance of considering psychosocial factors in child health care. In the next section on psychosocial assessment we will discuss child and family development as well as how child health concerns can be related to other family difficulties.

Psychosocial Assessment in Child Health Care

Gaining information on child, parent, and family functioning need not be a time-consuming task in the already overburdened schedules of primary care physicians. Much valuable information can be gained by exploring a few questions with the parent who has brought the child for a visit. In the long run it may actually be a time saver. Without a clear picture of the multiple factors that may contribute to a pediatric visit, the physician may not be able to respond adequately to the needs of both the parent and child. This may lead to numerous follow-up phone calls and well-child–distressed-parent visits until the whole agenda of the original visit has been addressed. By assessing psychosocial factors early the physician may be able to intervene in constructive ways that also save him or her time.

There are three valuable questions to explore in child health care psychosocial assessment:

1. **What are the developmental issues facing the child and his or her parents?** The physician's frame of reference for assessing child development and behavior is based on cumulative professional knowledge rather than anecdotal or personal experience alone. It is important for the physician to use such knowledge to both assess the child's growth and functioning and identify when parents have inappropriate expectations of their child. In the latter situation, gathering more information before intervening is usually the safest approach.

> MRS. RUSH: Doctor, Jennifer is 15 months old and she shows no interest in the potty at all. I've explained to her that big girls should not be using diapers but she doesn't understand. My husband thinks I'm on her too much about it.

In this well-child–distressed-parent visit, the physician realizes that a concern that may arise for some parents near their child's eighteenth month is toilet training (6). He sees that Jennifer has no physiological problem and appears to be a happy child. Mrs. Rush may be premature in her worry about Jennifer. Jennifer does not have the cognitive ability at 15 months to understand her mother's explanation of the importance of toilet training (7). She may not be physically prepared either as evidenced by her inability to take her pants off. Furthermore, she may not be ready emotionally for the responsibility and reward of using the "potty." The physician sees that there is an incongruity between Jennifer's level of development and Mrs. Rush's expectations. Rather than giving her advice prematurely, the physician explores the situation further.

2. **What life cycle tasks are facing the family at this time?** A child's development is part of the larger process of the family development. In the case of the Rush family, Mr. and Mrs. Rush and their new child are moving from one stage in the family life cycle, The Newly Married Couple to another, The Family with Young Children. (See Chapter 3, Appendix 3.1, for a description of all the family life cycle stages.) The Rushes are working to integrate a new member into what had previously been a dyadic relationship.

For families with young children the major tasks include: (a) adjusting the marital relationship to accommodate new family members; (b) taking on parenting roles; and (c) realigning the parent's relationship to their parents who now are grandparents. This is a time in the family life cycle when all three generations are drawn closer together while at the same time trying to redefine their relationships (8). In child health care assessment it is important to explore this larger developmental context.

> DR. S: This is a time of tremendous change for you and your husband. How has it affected the two of you?
>
> MRS. RUSH:P Most of the time I feel overwhelmed. I don't even know how my husband feels. We hardly ever see each other. By the time he's home from work, I'm ready to go to bed.
>
> DR. S: It sounds pretty strenuous for both of you. Are your parents or your husband's parents around?
>
> MRS. RUSH: His parents are out-of-state. Mine are nearby but sometimes they help too much. I mean, I feel like no matter what I do I should have done it differently.

Owing to the pressing demands of parenthood, the Rushes have not had time to renegotiate their relationship as husband and wife. Mrs. Rush's parents are naturally pulled closer to their daughter to help out, but their involvement often feels like criticism. Mrs. Rush feels overwhelmed, inadequate, and alone. Her concern about her daughter's toilet training may reflect the family's difficulty navigating normal changes in the family life cycle. Since it is not clear how Mr. Rush feels, Dr. S suggests that the Rushes hold off on potty training for now and invites Mrs. Rush to the next appointment. This will give Dr. S an opportunity to further assess as well as support them as a parenting team.

3. **Is the child's health or behavior difficulty related to other problems in the family?** Sometimes a child's illness is related to worry about a grandparent, school concerns, sibling rivalry, the stress of moving or loss. A child's difficulties may play a part in supporting the parents' marriage. For example, a child's health or behavior problems may give a couple with an unstable marriage a common focus of concern. With each new demand the couple may pull together for the sake of their child's health despite problems that may exist in the marriage. In that way the child and his or her difficulties may function as the glue which keeps the parents together. It has also been theorized that one of the ways couples can deal with marital discord is to "project" the conflict onto their children (9–12). The most typical pattern is for the mother to become overinvolved with a child while the father either encourages the overinvolvement by maintaining distance, or challenges it by battling with the mother over parenting questions. In either case the marital problems do not have to be addressed. Child-related difficulties may

receive exclusive attention and become the means by which marital dissatisfaction is also expressed. These patterns can represent quite serious dysfunction, or can be a mild concern, as in the example below.

> DR. S (TO MR. RUSH): What concerns do you have about Jennifer?
>
> MR. RUSH: None. I don't think there is a problem. No one in my family was toilet trained this young. She's just a baby. It's my mother-in-law who seems to be pushing this.
>
> DR. S (TO MRS. RRUSH): What do you think?
>
> MRS. RUSH: I'm not sure what to think. My mother is concerned.
>
> MR.RUSH: She always seems to be involved in our affairs.
>
> DR. S: How do the two of you feel the toilet training should be addressed?
>
> MR. RUSH: I don't think there's a big hurry, do you (to Mrs. Rush)?
>
> MRS. RUSH: No, I don't either. I guess I just needed to hear what you thought.
>
> DR. S: I think you're both correct. Different generations choose different times to toilet train. The important thing is that the two of you be together. It seems that when you have the chance to work together these decisions are easier to deal with.

Dr. S recognizes that marital stress over the involvement of Mrs. Rush's mother may predate the birth of Jennifer. He also hypothesizes that marital discord may be fueling Mrs. Rush's overconcern about Jennifer's toilet training. Interestingly, the focus on Jennifer has brought the couple together in order to make a decision. Dr. S supports the parents' capacity to work together and make good parenting decisions. Building an alliance with the couple around this issue will make it easier to address any future marital problems should the need arise.

In this case example we have illustrated not only the various aspects of assessment but also how the physician can use this assessment process to both involve other family members and support their competence to solve the presenting problem. The family-oriented physician functions less as the exclusive problem solver and more as a facilitator and consultant in the problem-solving process. In the next section we will discuss specific guidelines for implementing a family-oriented approach to child health care.

Guidelines for Family-Oriented Child Health Care

Child health care provides one of the best opportunities for a physician to implement a family-oriented approach to primary care. The physician has access to at least one parent on a regular basis for well-child and periodic acute care for many years. This gives the physician the chance to approach primary care in a way which supports parents and utilizes their strengths in the health care of their children. Following are some guidelines for implementing a family-oriented approach:

1. **Whenever possible invite both parents to child health care visits.** Although both parents don't always need to attend, the physician's invitation communicates respect for the importance of both parents' roles in their child's health care. In more serious or conflictual situations the physician may communicate the necessity of both parents being involved in order for an effective treatment plan to be developed. (See Chapter 10 for a discussion of working with parents on child behavior problems.) But even in routine visits it can be valuable to either have both parents come in periodically or have them alternate bringing their child for visits. This helps the physician develop a good working relationship with the mother and father so that, when and if other critical situations arise, the physician and parents have already established a foundation for collaboration.

If the mother has brought the child, then an invitation to the father can be extended through her:

> DOCTOR: Mrs. Bailey, your child is doing very well and it sounds like things are going well at home, too. One of the things I do as a normal part of my practice is to involve both parents whenever possible. Sometimes both parents come with their child; sometimes parents alternate accompanying their child. It's very valuable for me to get to know you both because you are the experts on your child. It also gives us a chance to work together for your child's ongoing health. So I'd like to invite your husband to come in whenever it can be arranged.

2. **Discuss the parents' view of how the child is developing.** This gives the physician a chance to learn the parents' view of how they feel their child is or should be developing. From a family viewpoint, it is also an opportunity to explore the impact of child-rearing on parents and significant others. Whether a physician is seeing one parent or both parents, valuable questions to pose include:

- How do you feel your child is doing?
- What is most rewarding in parenting your child (or children)?
- What is most challenging in parenting your child (or children)?
- What adjustments are you having to make in your marital relationship and daily routine due to the demands of parenting?
- How has the birth of this child had an impact on other family members, especially siblings and grandparents?

3. **Use your knowledge of parenting in a consultative rather than expert role.** Very often parenting and health concerns arise that call for the physician to offer suggestions based on his or her knowledge and training. As previously argued, we believe that the physician should be judicious in giving advice to parents, and when it's necessary to do so, take care not to undermine their authority. For that reason we feel the physician should think of his or her role at such points as consultative in nature (13). This allows him or her to play an important advisory

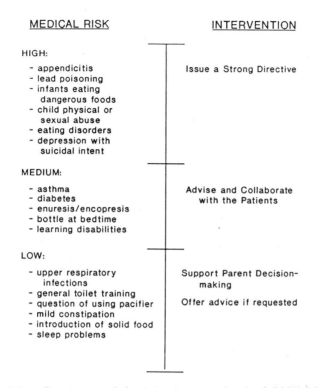

MEDICAL RISK   INTERVENTION

HIGH:

- appendicitis   Issue a Strong Directive
- lead poisoning
- infants eating
  dangerous foods
- child physical or
  sexual abuse
- eating disorders
- depression with
  suicidal intent

MEDIUM:

- asthma   Advise and Collaborate
- diabetes   with the Patients
- enuresis/encopresis
- bottle at bedtime
- learning disabilities

LOW:

- upper respiratory   Support Parent Decision-
  infections   making
- general toilet training
- question of using pacifier   Offer advice if requested
- mild constipation
- introduction of solid food
- sleep problems

FIGURE 9.2.   Continuum of physician intervention in child health care.

function in most situations without taking on a hierarchically superior position to the parents vis à vis their child.

The strength with which a physician should intervene will depend on the **health risk** involved. When a parent raises the issue of toilet training, the physician may see the health risks as **absent** or **mild**, and he or she may support the parents in making their own decisions. If the parents are discussing sending their child to bed with a bottle of milk, the physician may view the health risk as **moderate** and explain the danger to their child's teeth and gums while supporting the parents in developing a plan to help their child go to sleep without a bottle. If parents report feeding their infant child hot dogs or peanuts, the physician may perceive the health risk as potentially **severe** and make his or her recommendations actively and strongly. (See Fig. 9.2.)

Once the health risk has been assessed and the decision about how to intervene has been made, remember to use clear, concrete, understandable language in making any suggestions. Boyle and Hoekelman (14) report that interaction with a physician can be intimidating for parents and the use of technical language can be a contributing factor. By using layman's language a physician can help parents feel more comfortable.

4. **Support the parents in developing possible solutions.** Parents
have primary responsibility for carrying out medical treatment in most
child health care situations. For that reason it is important to encourage
parent involvement in treatment planning, and whenever possible support parents in developing their own solutions to child-health-care dilemmas. Even in severe risk situations (e.g., eating lead-based paint) which
call for strong physician interventions, it is important to discuss the parents' questions and concerns and, when appropriate, incorporate their
ideas into the plan. In many situations the physician's main intervention
may be to engage the parents in discussing and formulating their own
solutions. These discussions may range from helping parents decide
when to introduce solids into their child's diet to clarifying how their
child will receive medication when both parents are working all day.

Before the visit is concluded it is valuable to review the plan that the
parents have devised in consultation with the physician. This may involve
having parents restate the plan of action, clarify the areas of responsibility for the parents and the physician, and specify what follow-up will occur.

5. **When necessary, set up a separate appointment to further
address any remaining concerns.** Bass and Cohen (5) have shown
that in child health care visits there is often a difference between the
ostensible and actual reason for the appointment. A parent whose son
has cold symptoms may also be coming because he or she generally feels
overwhelmed with parenting responsibilities. Typically, no real
dichotomy exists between ostensible and actual reasons for a medical
visit; it is usually a matter of there being multiple reasons for most
visits. A parent may not only be concerned about his or her child's symptoms but about the anxiety a grandparent may have about the child or
the history of a similar illness in the family. It is important for the physician to explore the possibility of multiple factors in any visit.

If a child's illness provides an opportunity for the parent to ask for help
of a different kind, it is important to respond to the parent's concern
directly so the child will not have to be ill for the parent to get help in
the future. When an agreeable plan has been developed to address the
parents' presenting concern about their child, the physician can suggest
a separate appointment to further discuss any remaining concerns of
the parents. Offering such an appointment shows respect for the parents' concern and provides an opportunity to further assess and join
with the family.

In the following case Dr. M illustrates many of the guidelines for
family-oriented child health care.

> Mrs. Johnson brought eight-month-old Judy, the Johnson's first baby, for a
> well-child visit. During the course of the exam Dr. M asked how Mrs. Johnson
> felt Judy was doing and learned that Judy had been having some difficulty
> sleeping in the last month. She had been getting up three times a night and

Mrs. Johnson wondered if something was wrong. Dr. M asked if Mr. Johnson was concerned about Judy. She said her husband was losing sleep, as well, and didn't know what to think.

Dr. M completed his exam of Judy and reported to Mrs. Johnson that Judy was developing very well. Dr. M then asked Mrs. Johnson to further discuss the impact of Judy's sleep pattern on her and her husband. Mrs. Johnson said it had been "pretty awful." She and her husband often spent most of the night worrying and feeling they must be doing something wrong. Dr. M said he was sure there was no physiological problem. He then asked if there had been any other changes recently. Mrs. Johnson said Judy's birth had been the "one big change" in their lives and reported that everything else was going fairly well. Dr. M said that often a child's sleep, or lack thereof, created concerns for conscientious parents. Dr. M said he often met with parents who were dealing with these kinds of concerns and offered to meet with Mr. and Mrs. Johnson. Mrs. Johnson felt that would be helpful. They set up an appointment for the following week.

Dr. M asks about recent life changes in order to learn about losses, job stress, family illnesses, marital difficulties, or other issues that may play a part in the Johnsons' concerns. Dr. M realizes that there are several factors involved in this visit: Judy's overall health and development, her sleep pattern, the effect of Judy's sleep pattern on her parents, and the Johnson's concern about what to do. Dr. M's assessment is that this is a well-child–distressed-parent case. As the medical expert, Dr. M assures Mrs. Johnson that there is no physiological cause for Judy's sleep pattern. He then uses this as an opportunity to meet with both parents to support them as a coparenting team.

During the meeting with Mr. and Mrs. Johnson, Dr. M learned that both parents got up at night whenever Judy stirred or cried. They picked her up frequently to comfort her and worried that she might not feel well. The Johnsons said they had been trying to have a child for six years and just wanted to "do things right." Dr. M emphasized again that there was no physiological problem, but that infants often enjoyed the comfort their parents offered by picking them up when they cried. Dr. M said this did not create problems for the baby but could often be stressful or exhausting for the parents. When that was the case, Dr. M said he suggested letting the child cry longer so that the baby could get used to comforting him- or herself. Although this could make things worse for several nights, it was not dangerous for the child to cry and in a few days he or she tended to sleep better. Dr. M then asked the Johnsons what they felt they should do. The Johnsons discussed Dr. M's suggestion and decided it was worth a try. Mr. and Mrs. Johnson determined how long they were willing to let Judy cry and how they would alternate checking on her if the need arose. Dr. M supported their plan and suggested they call to let him know how it was going.

This chapter has focused on the physician's role of supporting parents being in charge of the broad range of child health care concerns that may be thought of as "normal." At times this means the physician uses his authoritative role as medical and child development expert to provide consultation and direction to distressed parents; at other times, the physician intervenes less and supports the parents establishing directions they deem appropriate. In either case the emphasis is on collaboration and empowering parents.

In the next chapter we will discuss child behavior problems that are more extreme in nature. These may involve both high health risk and high parental distress. Parents in these situations feel stuck; they have tried all the solutions they know to try and are unsure what to do or where to turn. While parent–physician collaboration is still the key, the physician will find it necessary to intervene more actively with these problems while still respecting the parents' authority regarding their child.

References

1. Christopherson ER: Anticipatory guidance on discipline. *Ped Clin North Am* 1986;**33**(4):789–798.
2. Brazelton TB: Anticipatory guidance. *Ped Clin North Am* 1975;**22**:533–544.
3. Solnit AJ: Psychotherapeutic role of the physician, in Green M, Haggerty R (eds.): *Ambulatory Pediatrics.* Philadelphia, W.B. Saunders Co., 1977, pp 197–207.
4. American Academy of Pediatrics: Guidance for health supervision. American Academy of Pediatrics, 1985.
5. Bass LW, Cohen RL: Ostensible versus actual reasons for seeking pediatric attention: Another look at the parental ticket of admission. *Pediatrics* 1982;**70**(6):870–874.
6. Talbot Y: Behavior problems in children, in Christie-Seely J (ed.): *Working With the Family in Primary Care: A Systems Approach to Health and Illness.* New York, Praeger, 1984.
7. Flavell JH: *The Developmental Psychology of Jean Piaget.* New York, D. Van Nostrand Co., 1963.
8. Combrink-Graham L: A developmental model for family systems. *Fam Proc* 1985;**24**(2):139–150.
9. Bowen M: Theory in the practice of psychotherapy, in Guerin PJ (ed.): Family Therapy. New York, Gardner Press, 1976, pp. 42–90.
10. Bowen M: *Family Therapy in Clinical Practice.* New York, Jason Aronson, 1978.
11. Kerr ME: Family systems therapy and therapy, in Gurman AS, Kniskern DP (eds.): *Handbook of Family Therapy.* New York, Brunner/Mazel, 1981, pp. 226–266.
12. Minuchin S: *Families and Family Therapy.* Cambridge, MA, Harvard University Press, 1974.
13. Wynne LC, McDaniel SH, Weber TT (eds.): *Systems Consultation: A New Perspective for Family Therapy.* New York, The Guilford Press, 1986.
14. Boyle WE, Hoekelman RH: The pediatric history. In, Hoekelman RH, Blatman S, Friedman S, Nelson N, Seidel H (eds.): *Primary Care Pediatrics.* St. Louis, MO, C.V. Mosby Co., 1987, pp. 52–62.

PROTOCOL
Supporting Parents in Child Health Care

Psychosocial Assessment in Child Health Care

1. What are the developmental issues facing the child and his or her parents?
2. What life cycle tasks are facing the family at this time?
3. Is the child's health or behavior difficulty related to other problems in the family?

Dimensions to Consider in Child Health Care

1. Well-child–confident-parent visits.
2. Well-child–distressed-parent visits.
3. Ill-child–confident-parent visits.
4. Ill-child–distressed-parent visits.

Guidelines for Family-Oriented Child Health Care

1. Whenever possible invite both parents in child health care visits.
2. Discuss the parents' view of how the child is developing.
   - How do you feel your child is doing?
   - What is most rewarding in parenting your child (or children)?
   - What is most challenging in parenting your child (or children)?
   - What adjustments are you having to make in your marital relationship and daily routine owing to the demands of parenting?
   - How has the birth of this child had an impact on other family members, especially siblings and grandparents?
3. Use your knowledge of parenting in a consultative rather than expert role.
4. Support the parents in developing possible solutions.
5. When necessary, set up a separate appointment to further assess any remaining concerns.

When Parents Get Stuck
Working with Parents on Child Behavior Problems

Parents often wrestle with the behavior problems of their children, with varying degrees of success and failure. Parents usually deal with such problems adequately, either by themselves or with the help of other family members or friends. But when they feel stuck in their attempts to resolve their child-related difficulties, parents often turn to a professional, primarily their physician, for help (1). Many times the primary care physician can provide the necessary help (2), but some parent concerns, as will be discussed later, require referral to a family therapist or other mental health professional.

Some of the most common child difficulties that parents discuss with their physician include problems of daily routine (refusing to eat, problems with bedtime, toilet training), aggressive or resistant behavior (fighting, tantrums), overdependent or withdrawing behavior (separation anxiety, fears), hyperactivity or restlessness, and children's habits that are undesirable to the parent (thumbsucking, playing with genitals too much) (3). By the time such child behavior problems are brought to the physician's attention the parents have usually tried numerous approaches and are feeling very frustrated. The parents may feel they have failed or that they are to blame for their child's problem. The physician may be tempted to accept the parents' doubts about their own competence and try to solve their dilemma for them. However, having taken such a position, the physician may feel as overwhelmed as the parents. On the other hand, if the physician succeeds, his or her success may only confirm the parents' feelings of inadequacy.

We believe that one of the physician's most important jobs is to **help parents identify their own strengths and utilize those strengths in addressing the problem they are having with their child**. It is valuable and necessary to discuss what the parents have done well and how it is reflected in their child. Even the act of requesting help, which is often experienced as an admission of failure by parents, can be framed as evidence of good parenting and a desire to do the very best for their child. By communicating this to the family the physician helps create confidence in the parents and also protects him- or herself from taking too much responsibility for solving the problem.

Working with families when parents feel stuck requires the physician to be planful, active, and ready to make suggestions that will help parents use their assets more effectively in addressing their child-related problem. Other authors have excellent suggestions for dealing with many specific child behavior problems. (See Ref. 2.) Our purpose in this chapter is to provide an overall framework for making those specific approaches work. Guidelines for accomplishing this task will be provided. We will conclude with suggestions for managing child behavior problems during office visits.

Working with Parents on Child Behavior Problems

Getting Started

MRS. MINNOCCI: Doctor, I've tried everything I know to get my 7-year-old, Mark, to stop having his little fits, but nothing I do makes any difference. He just ignores me; sometimes he even tries to hit me if he doesn't get his way. Half the time I end up in tears. My husband thinks I'm too easy on Mark and is about ready to give up on both of us.

1. **Meet with the parents, the child (or children) and other important child caretakers.** Typically the physician will meet with the mother and father, but in some cases a grandparent or even a close friend may care for the child and be a valuable asset in addressing the problem. Meeting with both parents gives the physician the opportunity to assess the family further, develop a working relationship with the parents, and mobilize parent resources to deal with the difficulty. By working exclusively with the parent who brings the child for the visit, the physician may be excluding the other parent from decisions that are best made by the parents together. In this way the physician may begin to function like a coparent rather than an authoritative child-rearing consultant.

Physicians working with families of separation and divorce should involve both parents in resolving their child's behavior problem whenever possible. There is growing evidence to indicate that the involvement of the noncustodial parent is a significant factor in the emotional adjustment of children after divorce (4–6). It may be difficult to have former spouses come into the office together, but it is not unreasonable to request that they do so for the sake of their child. At a minimum, the physician should meet both parents separately if a conjoint appointment cannot be made. By establishing contact with both parents the physician avoids any unhealthy coalitions with either parent and demonstrates respect for each of them and for their distinctive roles with their child.

In the Minnocci family the other significant child caretaker is the father:

> DR. O: It sounds like both you and your husband are working very hard to do the best for your son but what you are doing is not working and you are feeling very frustrated.
>
> MRS. MINNOCCI: That's right.
>
> DR. O: It seems to me this deserves more time than we have today. So I would like to suggest that you and your husband come back with Mark next week when we can meet for about 45 minutes. In the meantime, I would like both of you to observe Mark's behavior and begin to think about how you would like it to be different.

2. **Clarify what the parents would like to change.** It is valuable to begin by asking the parents what they would like to change. This approach addresses the problem in a way that focuses on constructive change rather than on a litany of failures.

> DR. O: What would you like to change with regard to your son?
>
> MRS. MINNOCCI: I want him to stop behaving like a baby.
>
> MR. MINNOCCI: He's got to stop these tantrums.
>
> DR. O: If he stopped the tantrums, how would you like him to behave?
>
> MR. MINNOCCI: I think he's old enough now to talk respectfully to us, instead of yelling and screaming.
>
> MRS. MINNOCCI: I agree.

Exploring the Problem

The physician needs to assess family patterns that may maintain the problem and investigate other family events that may contribute to the dilemma.

1. **Get a detailed understanding of the problem, including onset, duration, and frequency.**

> DR. O: How long have these tantrums been going on?
>
> MRS. MINNOCCI: That's the odd thing. When he was little, he didn't do this. It only started in the beginning of the school year.
>
> DR. O: That would be about five months ago? Was there any- thing else going on at that time?
>
> MR. MINNOCCI: Well, I was working a lot of overtime. You see we had just built a house and moved in.

MRS. MINNOCCI: I started waitressing 3–4 nights a week just before then.
DR. O: It sounds like you all were going through a lot of changes. Do you
    remember anything else Mark?
MARK: I don't know. Just the work.

Here Dr. O learns that the tantrums usually occur after school on days when Mark's mother has to work. Mark usually asks for something when his mother is busy getting ready for work. When she cannot respond immediately, he yells at her and throws things. Typically father is not home yet. Mother ends up in tears and Mark ends up in his room. Dr. O recognizes the link between Mark's behavior, his father's absence, and his mother's preparation for work.

2. **Find out what advice parents have received from significant others**. This helps the physician understand who is important to the family, how they may be a resource to the parents, and how the parents may be pulled in different directions by the advice they have received.

DR. O: Because you've both been so concerned, I'm sure you've talked to
    other people about this. What advice have you received?
MRS. MINNOCCI: My mother says I'm too hard on Mark, but I don't think I am.
    She thinks I ought to quit my job and stay home all day like she did.
MR. MINNOCCI: Mark's teacher feels we need to structure him more. She
    talked to us about behavior charts.

3. **Explore the impact of the problem on all family members.**

DR. O: It sounds to me like this has had an impact on everyone. Could each
    of you tell me how it has affected you?
MR. MINNOCCI: I think it has led to some tension between my wife and me.
MRS. MINNOCCI: I agree. We don't seem to think about anything else. We're
    yelling a lot.
DR. O: What about you, Mark?
MARK: Everyone is always mad at me.

By exploring how the child's behavior problem affects others, the physician broadens his or her understanding of the issue to include all family members.

4. **Find out what other stressors may be affecting the family.** It is not unusual for child behavior problems to emerge at times when the family is experiencing other difficulties.

DR. O: Earlier you mentioned that some other changes have taken place—a
    new house, Mr. Minnocci working overtime, and Mrs. Minnocci starting a
    new job. How has that been for the family?
MR. MINNOCCI: What does this have to do with my son's behavior?
MRS. MINNOCCI: If he would only straighten up, none of the rest of this would
    be as upsetting.
DR. O: It is hard to say if these changes have anything to do with Mark's
    behavior. Sometimes kids begin to act up at times when lots of changes

are occurring. And when lots of changes are occurring, it can be doubly hard for parents to deal with a misbehaving child.

MR. MINNOCCI: There's no excuse for the way he treats his mother.

DR. O: I agree.

MRS. MINNOCCI: Since I started working I've been exhausted all the time, and, of course, that's when Mark gets on me. (To Mr. Minnocci) And when you get home you don't seem to care.

MR. MINNOCCI: I've got a million things on my mind!

Focusing on Solutions

The physician should engage the parents in developing solutions that are clear and specific. This involves supporting the parents' use of their own resources to solve the problem and providing ideas and suggestions to undergird their efforts.

1. Discuss what the parents have tried in order to solve the problem.

DR. O: What have you tried so far?

MR. MINNOCCI: Well, I haven't been as directly involved. I usually get home during the aftermath.

MRS. MINNOCCI: I've tried everything. I've told him to go to his room; I've threatened to take the TV away. Everything! He just won't listen.

MR. MINNOCCI: But you never follow through. That's the problem.

Dr. O learns that Mr. and Mrs. Minnocci have not been able to work together on discipline. Mrs. Minnocci usually has full responsibility for disciplining Mark and finds it to be a distasteful task. Dr. O learns that Mr. Minnocci has much less responsibility but often criticizes his wife for not doing a better job.

2. Find out if there are times when the problem does not occur.

DR. O: Are there ever times when this problem with Mark does not occur, times that are pretty good?

MRS. MINNOCCI: Actually things go pretty smoothly on the weekends.

MR. MINNOCCI: The pace is a lot slower. Everyone is at home.

Mark: We do things together.

Dr. O learns that when Mr. and Mrs. Minnocci work together and are doing activities with Mark, then family life goes much better. He beings to wonder if a similar approach could be used to solve Mark's behavior problems.

3. Ask the family what they feel their strengths are. Parents facing child-rearing problems often feel they have failed in some way. By helping them discuss family strengths, the physician shifts the family's focus from deficits to assets. The family can then use those strengths to make constructive changes.

Dr. O: One of your family's strengths seems to be knowing how to have fun together.

Mr. Minnocci: I don't know if that's strength or not. It's been awhile since we've had much fun.

Dr. O: It sounds like you want to regain some of that.

Mr. Minnocci: What I want is a son who listens.

Dr. O: And if you had that it might be more enjoyable to be together.

Mr. Minnocci: Yes, it would. We used to have lots of good times.

Dr. O: What would you say are the strengths of your family?

Mr. Minnocci: I don't know.

Mrs. Minnocci: Well, we work hard, and we worry a lot about our son, if that's a strength.

Mr. Minnocci: That's for sure.

Dr. O: You worry a lot, even get angry because you want him to head in the right direction.

Mr. Minnocci: That's right.

Dr. O: Is there any area in which you feel he's heading in the right direction?

Mr. Minnocci: His teacher says he's doing well in school.

Dr. O: That's an area in which the two of you have Mark right on track.

Having the parents begin to think about family strengths enables Dr. O to comment on Mr. and Mrs. Minnocci's success as parents.

4. Engage the parents in developing a plan of action for solving the problem.

Dr. O: Mr. and Mrs. Minnocci, what do you think could be done, a first step, that would make things a little bit better at home?

Mr. Minnocci: (to Mrs. Minnocci) I think if you'd just follow through things would work out.

Mrs. Minnocci: (to Mr. Minnocci) That's easy for you to say. You're not there.

Dr. O: One of the things that strikes me is that when the two of you are working together as parents, like you do on the weekends, things go very well.

Mrs. Minnocci: That's true.

Mr. Minnocci: I agree.

Dr. O: How could you make that happen at other times?

Mr. Minnocci: If I knew that, I wouldn't be here. I thought you could tell us.

Dr. O: You were hoping I could give you an answer.

Mr. Minnocci: Yes, I was.

Dr. O: All I know is that two parents working together are stronger than any one child. I think your son's behavior is so difficult that it's going to take both of you to make a difference.

Mrs. Minnocci: I don't know what could make a difference. But I know I would feel much better if we could talk once in a while about what to do with Mark. (To Mr. Minnocci) I always feel like I'm making decisions you don't agree with.

Mr. Minnocci: Well, usually I don't agree with them.

Dr. O: It sounds like both of you have your own ideas on how to deal with Mark's behavior, but being so busy there is seldom time to plan together what to do.

MR. MINNOCCI: That's true.

DR. O: You've helped him be successful in school, and when you are home together on the weekends, he behaves better. I think when you work together things go more smoothly. What would help make that happen at other times?

MRS. MINNOCCI: (to Mr. Minnocci) What do you think?

MR. MINNOCCI: I don't know exactly.

MRS. MINNOCCI: Maybe if we set some time aside after he goes to bed, we could talk about . . . . I don't know.

MR. MINNOCCI: Talk about what?

MRS. MINNOCCI: What we want from Mark.

MR. MINNOCCI: You mean how Mark should behave . . .

Dr. O intervenes by suggesting that when the parents work together they are successful. With Dr. O's support the Minnocci's decide to talk together more about Mark. Over the next few months Mr. Minnocci increases his support of Mrs. Minnocci's efforts with Mark. Mr. Minnocci also takes a more active role in disciplining his son. Mark's behavior improves markedly.

When Parents Are Stuck

Often times parents are ready to work on more effective discipline but do not know where to begin. The physician can help such parents by providing several basic guidelines for parents to consider:

1. **It is important for both parents to agree about the plan for discipline.** Parents who cannot work together on a parenting plan will have greater difficulty following through. Lack of cooperation between parents also makes it easier for the child to split the parents. Parent cooperation on discipline is equally important in families of separation and divorce.

2. **The discipline should be clear and concrete.** Grounding a child for "the rest of his life" is often a parental threat but never an effective plan. Telling Suzie she will have to go to her room for 20 minutes if she yells or throws anything is clear and specific enough for everyone to understand.

3. **The discipline should be something the parents can monitor and the child can do.** Billy is much more likely to do his after school chores if a parent is available to monitor the task. All discipline requires parental supervision. Discipline should also be clear, concrete, and behaviorally oriented. For example, it is very difficult for a child to know what to do when a parent says "Change your attitude." However, identifying swearing as a behavior to change, and having the child substitute "I am angry because . . ." instead of swearing, helps to change his attitude and has a better chance of being effective.

4. **The discipline should be time-limited.** Open ended discipline ("You can't watch TV until you've shown us you've changed") often leads to ongoing additional battles between parents and children over the fairness of the punishment. Knowing when a punishment is going to end adds to the likelihood that a child will comply.

5. **Once a plan is developed by the parents they should share it with the child and be sure it is understood.** Parents can share the plan with their child and then have the child verbally repeat the plan. Another approach involves making a brief written "contract" that outlines the details of the punishment.

6. **The parents should also be encouraged to increase positive parent–child interaction.** For some families with child behavior probems, it may seem like parenting is reduced to constant disciplining. Conflict becomes the rule rather than the exception between parents and children. Without some opportunity for fun, enjoyment, or just time together, parents and children can find themselves at odds a great deal of the time. Since children often express their need for parent attention by misbehaving, giving attention when a child is not misbehaving can interrupt the pattern and bring parent and child closer together. In the busy lives of most families such time together does not always happen spontaneously, but needs to be planned. Parents with children having behavior problems should plan brief, regular, even daily, time with their child in order to talk, play a game, or do some other activity. This plan should also be communicated to the child so that the child will know that he or she will have time with both parents on a regular basis. This can make it less necessary for the child to get attention from his or her parents in other, more problematic ways. Dr. F illustrates some of the guidelines for working with parents who feel stuck when needing to discipline their child.

> Dr. F met with Ms. O'Brien, who was a single parent, and her mother regarding Ms. O'Brien's 10-year-old daughter, Melinda. Ms. O'Brien lived with her mother who helped raise Melinda and Melinda's 15-year-old sister. Melinda had been caught several times stealing money from her mother and grandmother. When the corner grocer reported to Grandma O'Brien that the girl had stolen some candy, Ms. O'Brien became so upset that she almost hit Melinda. When asked about any recent changes in the family, Ms. O'Brien indicated that her mother had been ill with pneumonia. Grandma O'Brien said it had taken two months for her to recover.
>
> Dr. F helped Ms. O'Brien and her mother explore Melinda's problem around stealing and plan an appropriate punishment. They decided Melinda would have no TV in the evening for the remainder of the week and no play time with friends on Saturday. Dr. F also asked Ms. O'Brien how it had been for her during her mother's illness. Ms. O'Brien said she worried "day and night" and even took time off to care for her mother. Melinda had also been

very upset by her grandmother's illness, but Ms. O'Brien had had little time to talk with her about it. It was during this time that Melinda had begun to have trouble with her school work. In a family discussion with Dr. F, Ms. O'Brien talked further about how scary it was to see her mother become ill at her age. Since Grandpa O'Brien's death two years ago, the family was more sensitive to loss and death. Discussing these feelings enabled the family to share in a grieving process. As a result of this conversation, Ms. O'Brien wondered if both she and Melinda might benefit from more special time together. Everyone agreed. Dr. F helped them all plan an outing for Sunday and a weekly time that Ms. O'Brien and her mother would spend alone together. Grandma O'Brien planned to help Melinda with her school work in the afternoons and take a snack break on a daily basis.

When to Refer

A physician cannot be expected to treat every child behavior problem. At times the physician's most important function is to identify situations that call for a referral to an appropriate mental health professional and then guide the family through the referral process. A physician may want to consider a referral when:

- The parents cannot agree on a plan.
- There is evidence of long-term marital discord.
- The child's problem has been going on for more than a year.
- There is family violence, substance abuse, sexual or physical abuse, suicidal intent, an eating disorder, or evidence of psychosis in the family.
- The physician does not feel he or she has the time or training to address the matter adequately (7–9).

In any of these situations the physician can encourage the parents to see a mental health professional with a family orientation. (See the Protocol at the end of this chapter, as well as Chapter 22, for a discussion of making referrals.)

Managing Child Behavior Problems During an Office Visit

One of the most difficult situations for a physician is dealing with disruptive patient behavior during an office visit. Typical responses range from taking over the parenting role with a misbehaving child to ignoring the problem behavior. These situations can provide an opportunity for the physician to intervene in a way that supports and empowers the parent and allows the parent to learn how to manage effectively their child's behavior problem in other settings. In this section we will outline ways to work with both passive and aggressive parental responses to child misbehavior during an office visit.

When a Parent's Response Is Overly Passive

Mrs. Spencer brought her son Eddie, age 7, for a routine checkup for school. As Mrs. Spencer and Dr. D talked, Eddie became louder and louder. Then he opened a drawer of the examining table and began to play with the medical instruments. Mrs. Spencer seemed to ignore her son's behavior.

1. **Clarify that you are in charge of the office, its contents, and what transpires during the visit** (10).

> Dr. D: I should have mentioned at the beginning that there are some things I do not want children to do in the office. These include not playing with the instruments or the contents of the drawers, and not making so much noise that it is difficult for me to talk with parents.

2. **Help the parent be in charge of the child's behavior** (10).

> Dr. D: Would you have Eddie quiet down and also put the tongue blades back in the drawer?
> Mrs. Spencer: He doesn't listen to me.
> Dr. D: I think it's important that he listen to you so why don't you give it a try?
> Mrs. Spencer: Come on now, Eddie. (Eddie continues the same behavior.)
> Dr. D: What else could you try?
> Mrs. Spencer: I don't know. Maybe you could get him to settle down. Maybe he would listen to you.
> Dr. D: I think it's much more important that Eddie listen to you. And I know it can be hard, especially when you have a high-spirited boy like Eddie. Is there anything else you could do?
> Mrs. Spencer: I can't think of anything.
> Dr. D: Maybe you could tell him what you would like him to do.
> Mrs. Spencer: Eddie, stop playing with those things and sit down. (Eddie listens, but continues his behavior.)
> Dr. D: Maybe for today you may need to hold him on your lap. Please do whatever you need to do and if I can help, let me know.

Mrs. Spencer gets up, draws Eddie to her and holds him as he stands beside her. Eddie resists at first but then begins to settle down. Dr. D acknowledges how difficult this is for Mrs. Spencer and congratulates her for doing such an effective job.

3. **Plan with the parent how to approach the next visit.**

> Dr. D: You handled things well today, Mrs. Spencer. What do you think would make it easier, next time?
> Mrs. Spencer: Maybe if I bring some toys or something to draw with. He likes that.
> Dr. D: Good idea. Sometimes I also encourage parents to bring a family member or friend to help out.

MRS. SPENCER: My husband works and there's really no one else.

DR. D: Okay. Maybe your husband could come for a visit in the future. Is there anything else that would help?

MRS. SPENCER: I guess I'll just have to keep him right by my side until he can behave better.

When a Parent's Response is Overly Aggressive

Mrs. Hurt brought her daughter Jayne, age 5, to see Dr. L for an immunization. During the visit Jayne started singing and would not stop even when her mother asked. Mrs. Hurt then yelled at her daughter and struck her on the shoulder twice.

1. Explore the parent's feelings of frustration.

DR. L: Boy, it must be hard being a mother at times.

MRS. HURT: Yes, sometimes I get very frustrated. She just won't listen.

2. Discuss the frequency of the child's behavior and the parent's response.

DR. L: Do you have problems with Jayne very often?

MRS. HURT: Yea, a couple of times a week, a couple times a day on a bad day.

DR. L: It must be pretty hard on you.

MRS. HURT: I take care of it.

3. Ask how the other parent responds to similar situations.

DR. L: How does your husband deal with this?

MRS. HURT: He's more patient. He says I shouldn't hit, but he's not home all day, every day.

4. Find out if the parent was treated in the same way as a child.

DR. L: How did your parents discipline you?

MRS. HURT: What do you mean?

DR. L: Did they hit you at times?

MRS. HURT: Sure they did; ten times more than I hit Jayne.

DR. L: How was that for you?

MRS. HURT: I didn't much like it but I guess they thought I had it coming.

5. Explore other ways the parent could respond.

MRS. HURT: Don't get me wrong, I love Jayne, but when she gets on my nerves there's only one way to get her to stop.

DR. L: Nothing else seems to work?

MRS. HURT: Huh uh.

DR. L: And I'll bet you've tried a lot of different things.

MRS. HURT: Have I ever! I've tried groundings and time-outs and they don't last five minutes. I threaten her but she doesn't seem to care. She gets so defiant. Often times, she's made me so mad that the only thing I feel I can do is spank her. Usually I don't, but sometimes I have to.

DR. L: You don't like it when she makes you that mad.

MRS. HURT: No I don't. My fuse can get pretty short when she doesn't listen.

DR. L: I'm sure it does. Would it be easier to deal with Jayne if she didn't make you angry so quickly?

MRS. HURT: What do you mean?

DR. L: Well, is there any way to make the fuse a little longer?

MRS. HURT: If there is, I haven't found it yet.

It took Dr. L several visits over the next year to help Mrs. Hurt find different ways to manage Jayne's behavior. Mr. Hurt was only willing to come with Mrs. Hurt to see Dr. L once during this time, but Mrs. Hurt reported that her husband was a little more supportive. Mrs. Hurt succeeded in "lengthening her fuse" and, while she still got very angry at Jayne, was able to discipline her without hitting.

A parent who acts aggressively with a child in the office may be asking for help. It is important to respond to the parent's signal. Dr. L will set up a follow-up visit or phone contact to see how Mrs. Hurt is doing. This physician may want to invite both parents in to discuss the situation further if problems continue.

Jayne did not appear to be at risk for physical injury. She had no visible bruises, and there had been no complaints at school about unexplainable injuries. Dr. L would have been legally bound to report the situation to the area child protective agency if he felt Jayne was at risk of physical abuse. (See Chapter 19 on physical and sexual abuse.)

In this chapter we have emphasized that when dealing with more serious child behavior problems the physician needs to intervene in an active, authoritative manner. Nevertheless, the primary goal is still to support the parents in taking charge of the child and his or her behavior. The picture changes again when the child becomes an adolescent and the family enters a new stage. The next chapter will discuss how the physician's role changes to accommodate this individual and family transition.

References

1. Clarke-Stewart KA: Popular primers for parents. *Amer Psychologist* 1987;**33**:359–369.
2. Gabel S (ed.): *Behavior Problems in Childhood: A Primary Care Approach.* New York, Grune and Stratton, 1981.
3. Chamberlain RW: Prevention of behavioral problems in young children. *Ped Clin North Am* 1982;**29**(2):239–247.
4. Ahrons CR, Perlmutter MS: The relationship between former spouses: A fundamental subsystem in the remarriage family, in Jansen JE (ed.), Messinger L (vol. ed.): *Therapy With Remarriage Families.* Rockville, MD, Aspen Publication, 1982, pp. 31–46.
5. Grief JB: The father-child relationship subsequent to divorce, in Hansen JE (ed.), Messinger L (vol. ed.): *Therapy With Remarriage Families.* Rockville MD, Aspen Publication, 1982, pp 47–48.

6. Friedman HJ: The father's parenting experience in divorce. *Am J Psychiatry* 1980;**137**(10):1177–1182.

7. Frenck N: A time-conserving protocol for pediatric behavioral problems. *Fam Syst Med* 1984;**2**(2):146–149.

8. Johnson SB: Guidelines for short-term counseling, in Gabel S (ed.): *Behavioral Problems in Childhood: A Primary Care Approach.* New York, Grune and Stratton, Inc., 1981, pp. 67–80.

9. Chamberlain RW: Management of preschool behavior problems. *Ped Clin North Amer* 1974;**21**(1):33–47.

10. Doherty WJ, Baird MA: *Family Therapy and Family Medicine.* New York, Guilford Press, 1983.

PROTOCOL
Working with Parents on Child Behavior Problems

Getting Started

1. Meet with the parents, the child or children, and other primary child caretakers.
2. Clarify what the parents would like to change.

Exploring the Problem

1. Get a detailed understanding of the problem, including onset, duration, and frequency.
2. Find out what advice parents have received from significant others.
3 Explore the impact of the problem on all family members.
4. Find out what other stressors may be affecting the family.

Focusing on Solutions

1. Discuss what the parents have tried in order to solve the problem.
2. Find out if there are times when the problem does not occur.
3. Ask the family what they feel are their strengths.
4. Engage the parents in developing a plan of action for solving the problem.

When Parents Are Stuck Regarding Discipline

1. It is important for both parents to agree about the plan.
2. The discipline should be clear and concrete.
3. The discipline should be something the parents can monitor and the child can do.
4. The discipline should be time-limited.
5. Once a plan is developed by the parents they should share it with the child and be sure it is understood.
6. The parents should also be encouraged to increase positive parent–child interaction.

A Referral Should Be Made When

1. The parents cannot agree on a plan.
2. There is evidence of long-term marital discord.

3. The child's problem has been going on for more than a year.
4. There is family violence, substance abuse, sexual or physical abuse, suicidal intent, an eating disorder, or evidence of psychosis in the family.
5. The physician does not feel he or she has the time or training to address the matter adequately.

Managing Behavior Problems during an Office Visit

1. When a parent's response is overly passive:
   a. Clarify that you are in charge of the office, its contents, and what transpires during the visit.
   b. Ask the parent to be in charge of the child's behavior.
   c. Plan with the parent how to approach the next visit.
2. When a parent's response is overly aggressive:
   a. Explore the parent's feelings of frustration.
   b. Discuss the frequency of the parent's behavior.
   c. Ask how the other parent responds to similar situations.
   d. Find out if the parent was treated in the same way as a child.
   e. Explore other ways the parent could respond.
   f. Evaluate the child's risk for physical injury. If the risk is high, refer to a child protective agency.

CHAPTER 11

Balancing Alliances
Family-Oriented Care of Adolescents

The family-oriented physician cares for the adolescent best by respecting both the adolescent's growing autonomy and the parents' vital role in the adolescent's overall health and development. The adolescent's need to individuate, to develop a sense of identity and independence, has been established as important in adolescent health care (1–4). Unlike child health care, the physician often sees the adolescent alone and deals with many medical, developmental, and other issues with the confidentiality afforded adult patients. It has been suggested that the absence of the parent is essential to developing a trusting relationship between the physician and the adolescent, and that the physician can play a role in "accelerating the process of children becoming independent patients"(4).

While we agree with the importance of a one-to-one relationship between the adolescent and his or her physician, we believe that the physician must also consider the context that shapes the adolescent's development most—the family. Studies of adolescents indicate that parents have the greatest influence on the development of adolescent values and that, even with their need to rebel, adolescents derive much of their self-esteem from their parents' approval and support (5–7). This is not to suggest that adolescence is conflict free. At times adolescents must challenge their parents and other adult authorities in order to establish their own autonomy. Parents sometimes must stand firm, so that their adolescent offspring are safe and secure. While the relationship between the adolescent and parents may be qualitatively different than when the adolescent was a child, it is still just as important. The family-oriented physician treats the adolescent with the family in mind, collaborating with the adolescent and the parents in order to provide the best health care possible. This chapter will discuss how to work with adolescents and their parents in a balanced and effective way.

Primary Care of Adolescents: Guidelines for Office Visits

Appointments for adolescents can be made by parents or by adolescents themselves and can range from a sports physical to a request for an abortion. No matter what the concern or who makes the request, the office visit should be adolescent-focused with a family orientation. This perspective puts the physician in the best position to care for the adolescent, utilize parent resources, and not be pulled into unhealthy coalitions with either the adolescent or the parents.

Adolescence begins with the onset of puberty, as early as age 10, and ends in the early twenties. During this period the individual faces dramatic physical, emotional, and relational changes. The adolescent begins to address many important issues at this time (3,8–10):

• Discovering more about his or her body and learning about sexuality.
• Beginning to explore and develop new and intimate peer relationships.
• Starting to establish a sense of personal identity and values.
• Making a first step into the world of work.
• Beginning to establish independence from his or her parents.

Adolescent development does not take place in a vacuum but is part of a larger transition for the family as a whole. Combrinck-Graham (11) describes this as a centrifugal period in the family life cycle in that the normal processes of family development during this time pull family members in different directions. Not only is the adolescent trying to establish an identity, but his or her parents may be reassessing their own identities as well. Parents may be experiencing a "midlife crisis" as they question career choices, directions for the future, and even their marriage. Furthermore, grandparents also may be reviewing their lives as they approach retirement and/or face the declining capacities that are associated with normal aging. Along with the issues associated with adolescent development, some teenagers may also have to deal with their parent's separation and divorce, living in a single-parent household, and coping with the death of grandparents.

Ideally, during this period of family transition, parents make adjustments in their parenting as they recognize that adolescents are no longer children and not yet adults. Parents protect their adolescent offspring even as they try to give their sons and daughters more responsibility. Adolescents continue to count on their parents even as they seek more independence.

Adolescence is a period in which parents and teens fluctuate between closeness and distance, dependence and independence, as they all anticipate the adolescent's eventual leave-taking. Some guidelines for working with adolescents and their parents that reflect these developmental considerations include:

1. Maintain a relationship with both the adolescent and his or her parents. Avoid entering coalitions with either the adolescent or the parents. Siding with the parent against the adolescent or the adolescent against the parent runs the risk of eventually losing the trust of both. The art of being a family-oriented physician involves forming supportive relationships with multiple members of a family. And, the physician is best able to help parents and adolescents work together when there is a problem if the physician is allied with both.

> Mrs. Mendoza, a single parent, called Dr. M to make an appointment for her daughter Melinda, age 16:
> Mrs. Mendoza: Melinda needs a physical, doctor. And there's something else.
> Dr. M: What's that?
> Mrs. Mendoza: I don't want Melinda to hear this, but I'm afraid she may be, you know, messing around with some boys. I accidentally found her diary in her room. It was open and I glanced at it. Well, I saw some pretty shocking things.
> Dr. M: That must have been upsetting to you.
> Mrs. Mendoza: I knew you would understand. I was hoping that, since you're a lady doctor, maybe you could talk some sense into Melinda. Or is there some kind of birth control that I could maybe put in her food so she wouldn't know?
> Dr. M: Does your daughter know you are concerned about this?
> Mrs. Mendoza: No, I'm too embarrassed to bring it up.
> Dr. M: It is clear to me how concerned you are about your daughter's well-being. I think it would be very helpful if you could come to see me with Melinda so we could all talk together about this.
> After several minutes of further discussion, Mrs. Mendoza reluctantly agreed to come with her daughter.

Parents may refuse to come to the office to discuss their concern with the adolescent. When this is the case it is important for the physician to support the parents in their concern, but to also underscore the value of the parents and the adolescent talking together. The physician should not become a go-between for the parents and the adolescent. The physician may offer to meet with the parents once to plan how to talk with the adolescent or to meet with the parents and the adolescent when the parents feel ready to come in to the office.

2. Be sensitive to the emotional issues that can arise for anyone working with adolescents. Many physicians experience a natural pull to either side with parents against teens or with teens against their parents. This side-taking can reflect the physician's own unresolved issues around adolescence. A male physician may see in a 16-year-old male patient his own efforts to work out a relationship with his father. Or the physician who wants to protect her own 15-year-old daughter may strongly identify with the parents of an adolescent female who has come for a confidential pregnancy test. These responses are normal. It is important for the physician to recognize and understand how these responses may influence the health care he or she may give to adolescent patients.

> Dr. M felt angry after Mrs. Mendoza's phone call and did not know why. Perhaps it was just that Dr. M was extremely busy that day and the phone call was just one more intrusion. It was not until the next day that Dr. M realized it was Mrs. Mendoza's "intrusiveness" that bothered her. It reminded Dr. M of times in her own adolescence when her mother wanted to know everything she was doing. Knowing this, Dr. M decided to monitor her reactions to see how much they related to the Mendozas and how much they had to do with Dr. M's relationship with her own mother. By doing so, Dr. M would be less likely to react to the Mendozas in ways that would disrupt the provider–patient relationship.

3. Be aware of how adolescent efforts to individuate play a part in adolescent health care. Individuation is often an underlying issue in adolescent office visits. It can play a part in everything from discussions about who will come into the exam room, to physicals for work, to requests for contraception, to pregnancy tests. The physician is in an excellent position to help parents and adolescents appropriately address issues of independence and autonomy with each other.

> Dr. M saw Melinda alone for the physical exam and talked with her about school friends, and other close relationships. Dr. M learned that Melinda had a boyfriend with whom she was sexually active. When Dr. M asked about contraception, Melinda said she was not using anything but that her boyfriend occasionally used condoms.
>
> After Dr. M completed Melinda's physical, she invited Mrs. Mendoza into the exam room.

DR. M: (to Mrs. Mendoza) As I explained to Melinda, she is in excellent health. Everything is normal.
MRS. MENDOZA: Good.
DR. M: I was wondering if either of you have any other concerns or questions? (silence). Was there anything else that either of you wanted to talk about?
MELINDA: No. (silence)
DR. M: Mrs. Mendoza, do you have any concerns?
MRS. MENDOZA: Not really, just that I worry about her.
DR. M: What do you worry about?
MRS. MENDOZA: She's growing up.
MELINDA: Of course, I'm growing up!
DR. M: What concerns you about that?
MRS. MENDOZA: I worry about her when she's out with all these boys; what's going to happen?
MELINDA: Mom! I can't believe you're bringing this up! It is none of your business! (Melinda begins to cry)

Dr. M encourages Mrs. Mendoza to comfort her daughter. Mrs. Mendoza hands Melinda a tissue. Melinda rejects it.

MRS. MENDOZA: (to Dr. M) I'm afraid she could get pregnant if she doesn't watch out. I told her she couldn't date until she was sixteen which was five months ago. Since then she is out all the time.

MELINDA: What do you mean, "out all the time." I've dated just a few boys, mainly Jack.

MRS. MENDOZA: Have you done anything?

MELINDA: That's none of your business.

DR. M: This is a tough time for both of you. Melinda is growing up and becoming a young woman and you, Mrs. Mendoza, have all the concerns a good mother has for a teenage daughter. (to Melinda) Have you thought about pregnancy?

MELINDA: I don't want to get pregnant.

MRS. MENDOZA: I don't want that either, honey.

DR. M: Have you ever talked about birth control?

MRS. MENDOZA AND MELINDA: No.

DR. M: I would be willing to discuss with you the various methods available, but it may help if you talk about it with each other first.

MELINDA: There's nothing to talk about. (silence)

MRS. MENDOZA: Well, I guess it's really up to her.

DR. M: (to Melinda) If you decide that birth control is necessary, please feel free to make an appointment.

A month later Melinda made an appointment to start on birth control pills.

It is awkward and unnecessary for parents and teens to discuss the details of a teenager's sexual behavior, but it is very helpful to have parent assent to contraception. In this case Mrs. Mendoza's permission made it easier for Melinda to take that step when she was ready.

Structuring the Interview When a Parent Accompanies the Adolescent

It is important to talk with both the adolescent and the parent when a parent accompanies the adolescent on a visit, but it is rarely appropriate for the parent to be involved in the exam itself. The physician needs to structure parent involvement in a way that respects the parent's role, but makes it clear that the adolescent is the patient.

1. Meet with the parent(s) and adolescent together initially. The physician can greet the adolescent first, then the parent, and thank both for coming.

2. Ask how you can help them today. Let the parent and adolescent decide who will respond first. This gives the physician a picture of how the parent and adolescent interact: Does the parent let the adolescent talk? Do the parents and adolescent agree on why they are here? Do either the parent or adolescent have special concerns? This format is also a way for the physician to model his or her expectation that concerns of parents and adolescents should be talked about together.

3. See the adolescent alone for the majority of the visit. Once the purpose of the visit has been clarified, the parent may wait in the waiting room while the physician interviews the adolescent and performs the exam. (The doctor may say to the adolescent's parent: Please wait in the waiting room during Larry's exam and when I'm finished I'd like you to come back in again to discuss the results.)

The physician should ask young adolescents if they would prefer to have their parent with them for the exam. The physician may see older adolescents alone for a majority of the history as well as the exam.

4. Clarify with the adolescent what will be shared with the parent(s). This should be a negotiated process in which the physician specifies what he or she wants to discuss with the parent and the adolescent has the opportunity to agree or disagree. In cases where there is disagreement, unless there is substantial risk to the adolescent's or someone else's life, the adolescent's wishes need to be respected.

5. Meet conjointly with the parent(s) and the adolescent at the end of the visit. Discuss the findings with the parent. Plan together with the parent and adolescent what the treatment plan will be.

In the following case Dr. V discovers a significant concern in a routine office visit with an adolescent and his mother. Because of his work with both the adolescent and the parent, Dr. V is able to help the family address the problem.

> Mrs. Chase brought Howie, 15, to have a physical for a school trip. Dr. V greeted them in the exam room and thanked Mrs. Chase for coming.

> DR. V: I would like to spend a little time with you together before I see Howie alone for the exam. Then we can talk together again at the end. How can I help you today?
> MRS. CHASE: Howie is going on a trip to Washington and the school wants everyone to have a physical ahead of time.
> DR. V: Okay, is there anything else that either of you wanted to bring up today?
> MRS. CHASE: Well, I wasn't going to bring this up, but, well, Howie has been very moody lately and hard to reach.
> DR. V: Hard to reach?
> MRS. CHASE: He just doesn't talk to us. (Howie frowns and sighs.)
> DR. V: Do you understand what your mother is talking about, Howie?
> HOWIE: No.
> DR. V: (to Howie) Is there anything that you are concerned about? (Howie shakes his head "no"). What do you think is going on, Mrs. Chase?
> MRS. CHASE: I don't really know.
> DR. V: Does Mr. Chase have the same concern?
> MRS. CHASE: Oh, yes, he especially doesn't like Howie's new friends.
> HOWIE: Big surprise.

DR. V: What doesn't he like about this?

MRS. CHASE: We don't know them very well and they're older than Howie.

HOWIE: Al is not older.

MRS. CHASE: Well, most of them are. (silence)

DR. V: Well, Mrs. Chase, I'd like to give Howie a chance to change for the exam. You can wait in the waiting room and I'll call you back in after the exam.

Dr. V steps out. When he returns, Dr. V tries to follow up on Mrs. Chase's concern.

DR. V: Your Mom seems pretty concerned. (Howie does not respond.) What do you think about what she was saying?

HOWIE: Nothing.

DR. V: Has it been hard on you at home?

HOWIE: No. (Silence. Dr. V begins the exam.)

DR. V: How is school going?

HOWIE: Lousy.

DR. V: Why is that?

HOWIE: The teachers are all jerks.

DR. V: What do you like to do?

HOWIE: Hang out, you know, spend some time with my friends.

DR. V: What kind of things do you like to do with your friends?

HOWIE: We go out on the weekend, cruise around, get some beer, you know.

DR. V: You and your friends like to drink.

HOWIE: When we can, yeah. Not that much, though.

DR. V: How much would you say you drink on a weekend?

HOWIE: I don't know. Not that much. A couple of six packs.

DR. V: Do you ever get together during the week to drink?

HOWIE: Once or twice, maybe.

DR. V: Is this with the friends your mother was talking about?

HOWIE: Yeah, but they are all great guys. I'm not changing my friends for anyone.

DR. V: Sounds like they are very important to you.

HOWIE: Yeah.

DR. V: How long have you and your friends been drinking together.

HOWIE: About five months or so.

DR. V: Do your parents worry about you drinking?

HOWIE: They asked me about it once.

DR. V: What did you say?

HOWIE: I wasn't gonna tell them anything because they'll never let me see my friends again.

DR. V: Do your parents or relatives drink?

HOWIE: Not much. My Dad ties one on every once in awhile, but it's no big deal.

DR. V: What about relatives?

HOWIE: Well, I've heard my Dad tell some stories about his Dad, but I don't think he drinks much now.

DR. V: What do you enjoy about drinking?

HOWIE: It's just fun.

DR. V: What is most fun?

HOWIE: Just being with my friends and relaxing.

DR. V: Is it hard to relax at times?

HOWIE: No, not really. School is a pain and sometimes my parents get on my nerves.

DR. V: Do you talk to your parents?

HOWIE: No.

DR. V: Would you like to?

HOWIE: Not really, it just leads to an argument.

DR. V: It sounds like being with your friends and drinking is one way you have to relax and get away from things. Whenever I talk with any teenager who drinks from time to time, I'm always concerned that the drinking not become a problem. Do you ever think about that?

HOWIE: Sometimes, but I think I can handle it.

DR. V: One thought I had for making sure it's not becoming a problem is to keep a record of when, what, how much, and how often you drink over the next two weeks. Then we could get together and see how you're doing.

HOWIE: I don't think that's necessary.

DR. V: It may not be, but it may be a good idea to check things out to make sure.

HOWIE: Are you going to tell my parents I drink?

DR. V: No, but I would encourage you to talk to them.

HOWIE: Okay, I guess I'll come back.

Dr. V leaves the room and returns with Mrs. Chase. Dr. V briefly discusses the physical with Howie and Mrs. Chase.

DR. V: I was wondering, Mrs. Chase, if there was anything else you wanted to say about your concern for Howie?

MRS. CHASE: Well, I guess my husband and I both have wondered if Howie was drinking with these boys.

DR. V: Why did you wonder that?

MRS. CHASE: He came home pretty late a few times and we heard him getting sick in the bathroom. He always says he just had too much to eat.

DR. V: But you wonder.

MRS. CHASE: Yes, I suppose, but he has told us he isn't. You aren't drinking are you Howie? (Howie shakes his head "no.")

DR. V: I can see why you would worry about your son drinking. Has anyone in your family ever had problems with drinking?

MRS. CHASE: Well, my father-in-law did years ago but not now.

DR. V: He's recovering.

MRS. CHASE: Yes.

DR. V: That's great. So you have some experience with a family member having drinking problems and what difficulties can arise.

MRS. CHASE: Yes, I do.

DR. V: I think you and your husband have done a good job taking these changes in Howie's behavior seriously. I'd like to suggest that you and Mr.

> Chase watch these behaviors for the next couple of weeks and then all of
> us can get together to see how things are going. Would Mr. Chase come?
> MRS. CHASE: I'm not sure, I think he would.
>
> Three days later Mr. Chase called Dr. V. Howie had come home intoxicated
> the previous night. Mr. Chase didn't know what to do. Dr. V suggested a
> counselor at a local alcohol treatment facility where Howie could go for an
> evaluation. Dr. V contacted the counselor to let her know the Chases would
> be calling that day. Dr. V also suggested that the Chases return for their
> appointment with him to follow up on the steps they were taking for Howie.

In this case, Dr. V maintained an alliance with Howie and his mother.
He used that alliance to help Howie monitor his drinking and to support
Mr. and Mrs. Chase's vigilance regarding their son's behavior. This
helped bring the issue to a head so that the family, with Dr. V's aid, could
get Howie treatment for the problem.

When Adolescents Refuse to Talk

Talking with teenagers can be one of the most challenging aspects of
working with adolescents, especially when they refuse to speak.

> Jordan, age 14, was sent by his mother to see Dr. S for a follow-up visit
> regarding a throat infection. Since Jordan was doing well, Dr. S decided to
> talk with him about some developmental issues of adolescence. Dr. S
> explained that he wanted to get to know Jordan and asked Jordan to "tell me
> about yourself."Jordan looked at Dr. S and shrugged his shoulders. Dr. S tried
> again, "What can you tell me about school and other things you enjoy
> doing?" "Nothing much," Jordan replied. Dr. S asked a few more open-ended
> questions to which Jordan responded with assorted shrugs, grunts, and nods.
> Dr. S, feeling frustrated, told Jordan it would help if Jordan would talk so Dr. S
> could get to know him. Jordan just looked at Dr. S.

Clearly in this situation, Dr. S was becoming angry and frustrated
in a way that potentially could have made it impossible to move forward with the interview. It is not unusual for adolescents to be less
verbal with adults, especially those in authority. Adolescents are self-
conscious about their bodies, as well, and may be embarrassed just sitting
in an exam room, let alone talking with a physician. The physician who
expects or pushes the adolescent to be verbal may endure many silent
visits with teenagers. Here are some suggestions for talking with nonverbal adolescents:

**1. The physician should continue to talk and give the teenager
permission to be silent.** It is important to avoid power struggles with
adolescents over whether or not they are going to talk. Such battles
will usually increase a teenager's reluctance to speak. By giving the
teen permission to be silent, the physician eliminates potential power
struggles and helps make the adolescent more comfortable. For some

adolescents feeling less pressure to speak makes talking easier. The physician needs to be active even when the adolescent refuses to talk.

> Dr. S realized he could not force Jordan to talk. At that point Dr. S said he understood that going to the doctor's could hardly be at the top of Jordan's list of things he'd like to do, and if he did not want to talk, that would be fine. Dr. S explained that there were some things he wanted to talk about and Jordan should feel free to just listen. Dr. S then began to talk in a general way about some of the changes that all adolescents face.

2. Start with close-ended questions and move to open-ended ones. When talking with nonverbal adolescents, it is often more effective to begin with questions that can be answered in monosyllables and then expand to questions that can be answered in phrases and sentences. Factual questions or ones that require "yes" or "no" answers are safest. The adolescent needs to feel comfortable before he or she will open up.

3. Explore areas of possible interest or accomplishment for the adolescent. This approach facilitates the joining process and gives the adolescent an opportunity to talk about areas of personal importance. The physician can explore school, peers and outside interests, such as music and sports.

> Dr. S had another appointment with Jordan 10 months later for a sports physical. Remembering the previous visit, Dr. S decided to approach Jordan differently:
>
> DR. S: Have you had a birthday since I last saw you, Jordan?
> JORDAN: Yeah.
> DR. S: So that makes you how old?
> JORDAN: Fifteen.
> DR. S: What grade would that be?
> JORDAN: Sophomore.
> DR. S: Is tenth grade better than ninth?
> JORDAN: Not much.
> DR. S: My understanding is that you're here today for a physical. Is that right?
> JORDAN: Yeah.
> DR. S: Is it for anything in particular? (Jordan gives Dr. S a form from school)
> DR. S: So this is a physical for sports. What sport are you trying out for?
> JORDAN: Basketball.
> DR. S: I used to play basketball in high school. How long have you been playing?
> JORDAN: About six years.
> DR. S: You must be pretty good by now. Is this JV or Varsity?
> JORDAN: Varsity.
> DR. S: What position do you play?
> JORDAN: Point guard.
> DR. S: That's like being the coach on the floor, isn't it?
> JORDAN: Yeah, you have to know a lot.
> DR. S: I'll bet. You must practice pretty hard.

JORDAN: Yeah, we practice every night except on game days. Those are Tuesdays and Fridays. We practice Saturdays, too.

DR. S: That's a lot of work.

JORDAN: Yeah, coach is pretty tough.

4. Use the physical exam as an opportunity to talk (1). The physical exam is probably the most uncomfortable part of the visit for adolescents. The heightened attention given to the body during a physical can be extremely embarrassing for teens. During the physical the physician can continue to talk and gather psychosocial information about the adolescent. This approach helps reduce the adolescent's anxiety and also gives him or her a chance to talk about personal matters without the parent present.

5. After speaking to the adolescent for some period of time, involve the parent(s) in the interview. If the parent(s) are available, the physician can invite the mother and/or father in for the interview. The physician can explain to the adolescent that it is not necessary for him or her to talk, but that the physician needs to get some information from the parent and would like the teen to be present. Often times, teenagers find it uncomfortable to listen to such a conversation without being an active participant in the discussion. They will frequently talk voluntarily in order to make sure that a balanced view is presented to the physician.

6. When appropriate, facilitate discussion of important adolescent issues. The physician who has developed rapport with the adolescent patient has an opportunity to explore issues related to the adolescent's health and development. Typically these will focus on sexuality, peer conflicts, problems with parents, and the use or nonuse of drugs and alcohol.

> Dr. S saw Jordan two times over the next year for a minor illness and a sports injury. Their conversations revolved around athletics. Usually Dr. S talked more than Jordan, but slowly Jordan began to talk more freely. In particular, he talked about his friends, hinting at some confusion regarding his relationships with them. Dr. S used the discussion about friendships to talk about sexuality. Jordan listened intently as Dr. S described the confusion that all adolescents can experience as they try to sort out their feelings toward females and males. When Dr. S asked if Jordan had thought about these issues much, Jordan said he had, but he did not want to discuss it. Dr. S said that was fine and that he would be glad to talk with Jordan further if he ever wanted to.
>
> Eight months later Dr. S saw Jordan for the flu. During the visit Jordan said he was still having some problems with his friends. When Dr. S invited Jordan to say more, he told the doctor that he had "odd feelings" toward a boy who was his best friend. Dr. S guessed that Jordan wondered if he was gay. Jordan had not had any sexual relations with his friend or anyone else, but was feeling very confused and upset. Dr. S asked if Jordan's parents were aware of his

concern. Jordan said "no," and he wanted to keep it that way. After further discussion Dr. S offered to talk with Jordan on several more occasions to address these concerns. Jordan appreciated the help and accepted Dr. S's offer.

Dr. S saw Jordan six times over the next year. Jordan gradually began to recognize and accept his homosexuality, although he did not want his family to know at this time. As Jordan became sexually active, Dr. S talked openly with him about AIDS and the need for safety in his sexual relations. He also referred Jordan to an area gay support and advocacy group. Although Dr. S continued to encourage Jordan to talk with his parents at some point, Jordan refused.

Two years later, while Jordan, now 20, was home from college for the summer, he decided to tell his parents. Dr. S offered to see Jordan and his parents together, but Jordan wanted to handle it on his own. Dr. S helped Jordan clarify what he wanted to say to his mother and father. Jordan's disclosure to his parents led to a great deal of conflict. Dr. S met with Jordan and his parents once, and recommended they see a family therapist to talk further about their concerns. Dr. S was able to arrange the referral to a local therapist he knew.

In this case, by going slowly with a reluctant adolescent the physician was able to develop a relationship over time which had a significant impact on the adolescent's development. This case also illustrates a common dilemma that physicians who work with adolescent patients can often face: being asked to keep certain information confidential. In the next section we will discuss the issue of confidentiality in adolescent health care.

Confidentiality and Adolescent Health Care: A Family-Oriented Approach

Confidentiality is one of the most important issues in adolescent health care. Supreme Court rulings and state statutes have extended a teenagers' rights to confidential health care in a variety of areas. In 1977 the Supreme Court held that adolescents have a right to privacy regarding the purchase and use of contraceptives (12). The U.S. Department of Health and Human Services' effort to require federally funded programs to notify parents regarding teenage use of contraceptives was found unconstitutional in 1983 (12). In a series of decisions between 1976 and 1983 the Court also declared that state statutes requiring parental consent for abortion were an unconstitutional violation of a girl's right to privacy (12). All states have statutes protecting the adolescent's right to confidential treatment of venereal disease and most have similar statutes regarding drug and alcohol treatment (12).

The traditional age of majority with regard to medical care is 15 (13). Teenagers who have reached majority can consent for treatment if they understand the treatment and its risks, if the treatment risks are not very serious, and if the physician judges them capable of giving the same degree of informed consent as an adult (12). A 15-year-old may be able to give informed consent for treatment of a minor skin condition, but a physician would not consider treating the same adolescent for a malignancy without the family's knowledge.

The law has given adolescents the right to consent to treatment but the responsibility for judging whether or not the adolescent is capable of exercising that right often falls to the physician. It should be noted that, because of economic reasons, the adolescent's right to consent to medical treatment usually only applies to outpatient settings. Few adolescents have insurance to cover inpatient care. It is unlikely that an adolescent would be admitted to a hospital for non-emergency treatment without the hospital contacting the family to establish who would be financially responsible for the medical care (12).

Changes in the law over the past 15 years have clarified the legal rights of adolescents. The law has also introduced a potentially adversarial note into the relationships among the health care provider, the adolescent, and the parents. It is important for family-oriented physicians to have a plan for dealing with confidentiality so that they do not inadvertently enter into coalitions with adolescents or parents that may hinder them from providing the best health care to adolescents. Some guidelines regarding confidentiality include:

1. The physician's main consideration is to provide necessary and adequate health care service for the adolescent. The health care needs of the adolescent should be the first priority in questions of confidentiality. The purpose of confidential treatment is not only to protect the adolescent's right to privacy but to provide health care to adolescents who might not otherwise seek it if parental consent was required. In these cases, such as venereal disease, the physician needs to assure the adolescent that his or her health needs will be addressed confidentially.

2. Blanket confidentiality should not be extended to any patient. Under certain circumstances the physician is legally bound to breech confidentiality in order to keep the patient and others safe. The most common examples are when a patient is suicidal, homicidal, or has a communicable disease. In those situations the physician needs to involve others to help make the patient safe or to warn those who may be endangered by the patient.

> DEBBIE (AGE 15): Doctor, there is something I want to tell you, but you can't tell anyone else, especially my parents.
>
> DR. D: I would be glad to talk with you. It must be very important. But I must tell you that I can't always keep information confidential. For instance, if you told me you were going to hurt yourself or someone else I would have to involve other people. If it is something less than that, I may encourage

you to talk to other people but I myself won't breathe a word of it. I just want that to be clear so there isn't any confusion.

In most cases, adolescents will share their concern even with these constraints on confidentiality. The physician needs to protect his or her range of options for treating the adolescent.

3. Involve parents whenever it is possible and appropriate. Parents should not be contacted when teens are adamantly opposed to parent involvement, or would not seek health care if their parents were notified, or would be at risk for abuse if parents knew about treatment. Parents should be involved in any treatment, though, in which the teen does not object. Since the adolescent's development takes place within the family, involvement of parents can help the physician understand how the adolescent's difficulty will affect and be affected by the larger family context (14). In cases such as pregnancy, abortion, or substance abuse the physician should try to include parents. This involves encouraging teenagers to talk with their parents or getting their permission to contact them yourself.

As an example, national surveys indicate that over half of the teenagers who obtain abortions have told at least one parent about their pregnancy and planned abortion (15). Parent involvement and support can be invaluable to teens who are facing such stressful situations.

4. Assess what role family dynamics may play in the adolescent's request for confidentiality. As we have indicated, confidential medical care is often required in order to provide necessary or desired treatment for adolescent patients. At times, though, the request for confidentiality may be related less to health care issues than to family dynamics. The adolescent may be trying to draw the family physician into a coalition against his or her parents:

> Hector, 14, told Dr. J he was having problems with his parents, especially his father. Hector said his father hassled him "all the time, for no reason." Hector told Dr. J he was so angry at his father that he was going to run away. Hector asked Dr. J not to tell anyone about his plans.
>
> Dr. J asked Hector if he was running away because his parents were hitting him or abusing him in any other way. Hector said no, they just were a "pain." Dr. J then explained he did not feel it would be best for Hector or his parents for Dr. J to keep this information a secret. Dr. J told Hector he wanted to call his parents and would prefer doing it while Hector was there and could hear the conversation. Hector was angry but reluctantly agreed. During the call, Dr. J asked the parents to join him with Hector for a family conference later in the week so they could talk further about these concerns.

Parents may also give the physician information which appears to put him or her in a confidentiality bind.

> Mrs. Demas asked to speak privately with Dr. L before he saw Wendy. Mrs. Demas explained that she and her husband were worried about Wendy. A family friend had seen Wendy using drugs with some friends at a party. Mrs. Demas said that if Wendy found out how they learned of her drinking, she would be furious and might get "violently angry." Mrs. Demas wanted Dr. L to "subtly" question Wendy without letting on he knew anything.
>
> Dr. L said she could understand Mrs. Demas' concern about Wendy, but she did not feel she could act on this information. Dr. L said it would be better if Mrs. Demas could talk directly with Wendy. She offered to help Mrs. Demas do that. Mrs. Demas said she could not risk talking with Wendy. Two weeks later Mrs. Demas called Dr. L saying she had had a fight with Wendy. She asked Dr. L if she could come in to talk. Dr. L suggested that Mr. and Mrs. Demas and Wendy come in together. At that point, Mrs. Demas agreed.

In both cases the main issue is not confidentiality but the patient's and parent's effort to triangulate the physician into a family problem by getting the physician to take sides and keep a secret. This usually reflects patterns of indirect communication that may be typical for these families. The physician needs to avoid such triangles and make every effort to have adolescents and parents communicate more directly with one another.

This chapter has advocated a family-oriented approach to adolescent health care which respects both the teenager's need for increased independence and autonomy and the significant role that the family still plays in his or her life. A physician can play a very important part in the lives of families with adolescents. A structured and planful approach to working with adolescents is not only more efficient and effective, but it can also make the interaction more enjoyable for the physician.

References

1. Gallagher JR: The care of adolescents, in Gallagher JR, Heald FP, Garell D (eds.): *Medical Care of the Adolescent.* New York, Appleton-Century-Crofts, 1976, pp. 57–86.
2. Blaine GB: Common emotional problems, in Gallagher JR, Heald FP, Garell D (eds.): *Medical Care of the Adolescent.* New York, Appleton-Century-Crofts, 1976, pp. 211–219.
3. Felice ME, Friedman SB: Behavioral considerations in the health care of adolescents. *Ped Clin North Am* 1982;**29**(2):399–413.
4. Cogswell BE: Cultivating the trust of adolescent patients. *Fam Med* 1985;**27**(6):254–258.
5. Douvan E, Adelson J: *The Adolescent Experience.* New York, Wiley, 1966.
6. Winch RF, Gordon MT: *Family Structure and Function as Influence.* Lexington, MA, Heath, 1974.

7. Lerner RM, Spanier GB: *Adolescent Development: A Life-Span Perspective.* New York, McGraw-Hill, 1980.
8. Erickson EH: *Identify, Youth and Crisis.* New York, W.W. Norton and Co., Inc. 1968.
9. Lourie RS: Psychology of adolescence, in Gallagher JR, Heald FP, Garell D (eds.): *Medical Care of the Adolescent.* New York, Appleton-Century-Crofts, 1976, pp. 32–41.
10. McAnarney ER: Social maturation: A challenge for handicapped and chronically ill adolescents. *J Adol Health Care* 1985;**6**:90–101.
11. Combrinck-Graham L: A developmental model for family systems. *Fam Proc* 1985;**24**(2):139–150.
12. Holder AR: Minors' rights to consent to medical care. *JAMA* 1987; **257**(24): 3400–3402.
13. Strasburger VC, Eisner JM: Teenagers, physicians, and the law in Connecticut, 1982. *Connect Med* 1982;**46**(2)80–84.
14. Henao S: Evaluating and counseling adolescents, in Henao S, Grose NP (eds.): *Principles of Family Systems in Family Medicine.* New York, Brunner/Mazel, 1985, pp. 150–164.
15. American Civil Liberties Union: Parental notice laws: Their catastrophic impact on teenagers right to abortion. American Civil Liberties Union, 1986.

PROTOCOL

Family-Oriented Care of Adolescents

Guidelines for Office Visits

1. The family in transition – developmental considerations:
   - Maintain a relationship with the adolescent and his or her parents.
   - Be sensitive to the emotional issues that can arise for anyone working with adolescents.
   - Be aware of how adolescent efforts to individuate play a part in adolescent health care.
2. Structuring the interview when a parent accompanies the adolescent:
   - Meet with the parent(s) and adolescent together initially.
   - Ask how you can help them today.
   - See the adolescent alone for a majority of the visit.
   - Clarify with the adolescent what will be shared with the parent(s).
   - Meet conjointly with the parent(s) and the adolescent at the end of the visit.
3. When adolescents refuse to talk:
   - The physician should continue to talk and give the adolescent permission to be silent.
   - Start with close-ended questions and move to open-ended ones.
   - Explore areas of possible interest and accomplishment for the adolescent.
   - Use the physical exam as an opportunity to talk.
   - After speaking to the adolescent for some period of time, involve the parent(s) in the interview.
   - When appropriate, facilitate discussion of important adolescent issues.

A Family-Oriented Approach to Confidentiality

1. The physician's main consideration is to provide necessary and adequate health care service for the adolescent.
2. Blanket confidentiality should not be extended to any patient.
3. Involve parents whenever it is possible and appropriate.
4. Assess what role family dynamics may play in the adolescent's request for confidentiality.

CHAPTER 12

Recognizing the Signs of Strain
Counseling Couples in Primary Care

The problems that couples face in an intimate relationship, especially marriage, are often the underlying reasons for patient visits in a primary care setting. It has been estimated, for example, that over one in ten visits involves a sexual problem (1). The primary care physician is in an excellent position to address a variety of marital difficulties by virtue of his or her relationship with a family over time. From premarital exams, to well-child visits, to acute illnesses, to the experience of loss, the physician has access to a couple throughout the life cycle and can be the one to whom a couple turns when facing problems in their relationship.

Often times, though, only a fraction of these marital problems are identified by health care providers. The reasons for this include:

1. Physicians often see only one person in an office visit. It is very difficult to assess or treat a relationship problem without talking to both partners. Even sexual problems, which are often presented as an individual dilemma, are best thought of as the product of couple interaction (2).

2. Couples do not typically present marital and sexual problems to a physician directly. Often marital problems underlie a patient's presentation of vague physical complaints (2,3–5). Recognizing the link between a patient's somatic symptoms, such as headaches or irritable bowel, and marital discord can be difficult.

3. Physicians may feel uncomfortable asking patients questions that seem "too personal." Questions about a patient's marriage or sex life are sometimes believed to be too intrusive or embarrassing, and indeed they may be uncomfortable for the physician and patient. Nevertheless, a study of patients in a primary care setting found that subjects would be more likely to consult their family physician about sexual problems than any other professional (6). These patients' willingness to consult their family physician depended on whether or not they perceived their physicians as being interested or concerned about sexual matters in general. By physicians simply informing patients of their interest in sexual concerns, patients were more likely to discuss the issue.

Physicians who are attuned to the signs of marital strain and who talk with couples about such difficulties can help couples take the first steps toward resolving their problems. In this chapter we will discuss how to recognize marital difficulties, areas to assess in couple's relationship, and guidelines for primary care couple counseling.

Pursuers and Distancers: Recognizing Common Relationship Patterns in Couples

The following example illustrates a common relationship pattern in marriages that can become problematic, how it may then be presented to the physician, and ways in which the physician can recognize the signs of marital discord.

> Mr. and Mrs. Washington had been married seven years. They had one child, Ron, age 6. From Mrs. Washington's perspective, their marriage had been a stable one until the last several months when there had been considerable conflict. A homemaker and part-time beautician, Mrs. Washington felt her husband was not there for her during this time. If she told him about problems she was having, he was never in the mood to talk. When she asked him why, he never seemed to have an answer. Sometimes Mrs. Washington told herself her husband must not care about her. When Mr. Washington got angry, he rarely spoke and left the house. Mrs. Washington did not understand why, no matter how hard she tried, that her husband would not "open up to her." Why wouldn't he even talk about his day at work, she wondered. Mrs. Washington was becoming more and more convinced that her husband was rejecting her.
>
> From his perspective, Mr. Washington wished his wife would stop nagging him. No matter what he did, she thought it was never right and it was never enough. Didn't she know he had to answer complaints all day long as an apartment building maintenance supervisor? He didn't want to come home and listen to more complaints and problems. Mr. Washington was perplexed and becoming more and more irritated about why his wife doesn't understand that. Doesn't she know he needs time to himself, not more pressure from her?

Fogarty (7) suggests that there are two primary ways people respond to anxiety: one is to pursue; the other is to distance. When stressed, the pursuer tends to move toward other people to get his or her needs met. The pursuer believes in togetherness, unity, and hopes that happiness can be attained through attachments to others. Distancers want relationships, but also see them as dangerous. When distancers are anxious, they withdraw, fall silent, and shoulder their difficulties alone. Distancers try to be rational and objective and are confused by the emotionality of pursuers.

Pursuing and distancing are styles of relating that can characterize people in marital relationships, work relationships, doctor–patient relationships, and other important relationships. Everyone is a mix of pursuer and distancer. In fact, over some issues (like sex) a person may pursue, while over other issues (like expressing feelings) the same person may distance. Everyone uses pursuing and distancing responses, but most people tend toward one primary style much of the time. Fogarty believes the majority of women tend to be emotional pursuers (and sexual distancers) and the majority of men tend to be emotional distancers (and sexual pursuers). While differential socialization may support these sex-role stereotypes, many exceptions prevent them from being universally applicable.

Interestingly, pursuers and distancers are typically attracted to each other and often marry (8). Their differences can be a resource for a relationship as long as there is enough flexibility in the marriage for both partners to pursue or distance when either feels it necessary. In this way a healthy balance of togetherness and separateness, of intimacy and privacy can be maintained. Whenever one person only pursues and the other only distances, then the couple may enter a seemingly endless vicious cycle which is rigid, exhausting, and unrewarding for both. The more the distancer withdraws to refuel, the more the pursuer feels anxious and unloved and looks to the distancer for acceptance, making the distancer feel anxious and intruded upon, leading to further withdrawal by the distancer which results in more pursuit by the pursuer. (See Fig. 12.1.)

> Mr. and Mrs. Washington are caught in just such a cycle. Mrs. Washington pursues her husband in hopes of getting the closeness that will make her feel complete.
>
> Mr. Washington distances from his wife fearing such closeness will swallow him up. Both want to be understood and cared for. Mrs. Washington feels she can only get what she wants by trying harder to achieve intimacy with her husband. Mr. Washington feels he must stay beyond her reach or there will be no way to preserve his identify and independence.
>
> Mr. Washington found himself leaving for work earlier in the morning and staying later in the evening. Mrs. Washington began to have trouble sleeping. She felt exhausted and often had headaches. When Mrs. Washington developed stomach pains, she decided to see Dr. R.
>
> Mrs. Washington reported her symptoms to Dr. R, saying she had had them "off and on" for a few weeks. Dr. R's examination revealed nothing remarkable. Mrs. Washington was relieved and began to tell Dr. R about the pressure she was under trying to raise her son, keep the house, and work part time. Dr. R listened and was supportive. When Mrs. Washington asked if Dr. R had any

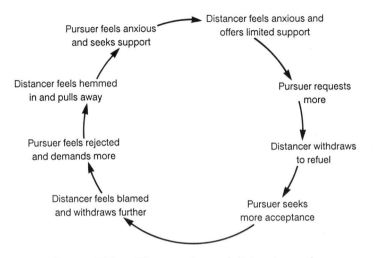

FIGURE 12.1.   The pursuing and distancing cycle.

"tricks" for reducing stress, Dr. R suggested a breathing exercise for her to try. He also suggested she make a return appointment for three weeks to follow up on her progress.

Mrs. Washington felt good when she left Dr. R's office. Dr. R was glad he had helped Mrs. Washington, but felt slightly perturbed when he realized he was fifteen minutes late for his next appointment.

Pursuers are more likely than distancers to seek help from a professional, such as a physician. Distancers may withdraw into their work, as does Mr. Washington, drink more, or have extramarital affairs which can provide gratification without the risks of genuine intimacy. If Mrs. Washington's emotional needs are met by the attention the physician gives to her somatic complaints, she may pursue him further and become an even more regular visitor in his office. **The first signal that the patient may have underlying marital problems is the physician's mixed reaction to her visit.** Dr. R felt glad to be a help to Mrs. Washington, but at the same time feels uncomfortable with her neediness.

Mrs. Washington was very pleased by her visit with Dr. R. She talked to her husband about how "lousy" she had been feeling. Mr. Washington felt his wife was overly sensitive to aches and pains. Mrs. Washington said the doctor believed she was under too much stress. Mr. Washington wondered if this comment was a criticism of him. He told his wife he didn't want to talk about it; he had "enough on his mind."

Two days later, Mrs. Washington again experienced stomach pain and developed diarrhea. She called Dr. R at home, upset that she was not feeling better. Dr. R spoke to her for fifteen minutes and succeeded in soothing her.

He offered her an appointment for the following day. When he hung up the phone, Dr. R was angry at Mrs. Washington for calling him at home and realized he didn't want to see her the next day.

What happened to Dr. R and Mrs. Washington is not unusual, and is not limited to marital problems. Physicians often find themselves in pursuer–distancer relationships with certain patients. With noncompliant patients, like noncompliant diabetics or hypertensives, the physician is often the pursuer, trying everything possible to get the patient to cooperate in treatment (e.g., increasing the frequency of visits), while the patient appears to be doing everything possible to sabotage treatment (e.g., "forgetting" to take medication). With other patients, physicians may feel pursued and find themselves distancing in response (e.g., taking greater time to return these patients' frequent phone calls).

Steps can be taken to both protect the physician from unproductive interactions with patients and also identify any marital problems that may underlie a patient's office visit.

1. The physician should use his or her reactions to a patient as a diagnostic tool. When a physician finds him- or herself consistently pursuing or distancing from a patient, it is a signal that a problem exists. The solution begins with the recognition that the physician can alter his or her behavior with the patient. Distancing encourages the patient to pursue and pursuing encourages the patient to distance. With difficult cases, it may be helpful for the physician to consult with a colleague in order to develop a more balanced approach to the patient. For example, with patients who pursue it is important to set appropriate limits. Those may include: no phone calls at home, regularly scheduled visits, and prescribed phone contact between visits. In this way the patient has access to the physician, but the physician has set limits on their contacts. With distancing patients different approaches that emphasize patient autonomy may be needed. For example, the physician may need to put the patient in charge of the frequency of their contact, while alerting the patient and the family to the risks of not complying with treatment.

Recognition of a pursuer–distancer pattern helps the physician understand the nature of the patient's relationships with significant others. Patients who pursue physicians, for instance, in all likelihood pursue those closest to them as well. Patients who pursue physicians excessively are often not getting their needs met in their closest relationships. Physicians may not see distancers in their office as frequently. These people may be less revealing or expressive with their families as well. Problematic interactions between the physician and patient can parallel problems in the patient's marriage and can be a sign to the physician to assess the patient's marital situation.

2. Be aware of the psychosocial dimension of each patient encounter. This is not to suggest that every patient has an underlying emotional or relational problem or that every patient's marriage must be fully assessed during each visit. It is important, though, to recognize that most marital and sexual problems come to the physician's attention as somatic complaints first. Lower back pain, abdominal pain, pain in the thighs, and urinary frequency are often association with sexual problems among women (3). In men sexual problems are often presented as nonspecific rectal or urinary difficulties (2). Vague somatic complaints, fatigue, headaches, weight loss are often associated with the stress that occurs in conflictual marriages.

3. Make psychosocial questions a routine part of your interview. In order to avoid the "my-doctor-thinks-it-is-all-in-my-head" trap, psychosocial questions should be interspersed with biomedical questions and be symptom focused:

• When you are feeling ill or in pain, who do you turn to for support?
• Have you discussed your symptoms with your spouse?
• What does he or she think is the cause of this problem?
• Has your spouse suggested anything for you to do about your symptoms?
• What is it like for you at home when you are feeling ill?

Questions such as these help the physician explore relationship issues in a safe way while remaining focused on the patient's symptoms. If there appears to be marital discord, it is often easier for the physician to invite a partner to a follow-up session to help with the patient's symptoms and treatment rather than to discuss "marital problems."

> Dr. R recognized that his strong reaction to Mrs. Washington's neediness may have been a sign that there were other issues contributing to her request for medical care. He decided to explore Mrs. Washington's psychosocial situation further.
>
> Mrs. Washington (as Dr. enters the room): I thought those exercises would work, but I just feel worse everyday. The headaches are stronger. They go down the back of my neck. . . .
> Dr. R: It sounds like you've been in a lot of discomfort.
> Mrs. Washington: . . .and I've had stomach pains and even diarrhea. I can't get any rest. I've got to keep working. Sometimes I have to get up at night two or three times.
> Dr. R: With the headaches?
> Mrs. Washington: No, to go to the bathroom.
> Dr. R: So all of these symptoms have been pretty constant since you were here a few days ago?
> Mrs. Washington: Yes, I've felt awful.

DR. R: I'm sure you have. Have you talked with your husband at all about your illness?

MRS. WASHINGTON: Yes, a little.

DR. R: So, he's aware of how sick you've felt.

MRS. WASHINGTON: I would think anyone would notice.

DR. R: Does he get up with you when you are sick at night?

MRS. WASHINGTON: No.

DR. R: When you get up, have you had any vomiting?

MRS. WASHINGTON: No, just diarrhea.

DR. R: Have you had a fever with this?

MRS. WASHINGTON: No, it's been normal.

DR. R: This must be very uncomfortable and exhausting for you. What does your husband say about it?

MRS. WASHINGTON: Well, I think he thinks it's all in my head. But he's around so little, how would he know. . . .

Mrs. Washington went on to talk about some of the conflict that had occurred in the marriage.

DR. R: It sounds like this has been a hard time for both of you. Your husband is working a lot of hours. You have been working hard too, at home and on your job; and both of you are trying to be good parents. At times you haven't felt as close as you'd like. To top it off, you've been feeling pretty sick.

MRS. WASHINGTON: That about sums it up.

DR. R: This is what I would suggest at this point. I would like to invite your husband in to get some of his thoughts about how you are feeling and how things are going in general.

MRS. WASHINGTON: Well, if you think it's necessary. I don't know if he'd come. He can't get off work very easily.

DR. R: Would you mind if I give him a call to invite him in?

MRS. WASHINGTON: No, that's okay. I'll give you his number.

Dr. R remains sensitive to Mrs. Washington's physical problems while gaining valuable psychosocial information. By inviting the husband to the next appointment, Dr. R interrupts the pursuer–distancer cycle that had begun between himself and Mrs. Washington. It also gives him the opportunity to assess the role that marital discord may play in Mrs. Washington's complaints.

Assessing Couples' Relationship Problems

Mr. Washington came with his wife for the next appointment with Dr. R. In talking with Mr. Washington, Dr. R learned that it was unclear to him how sick his wife "really" was and that Mr. Washington seldom knew how to help her. Mrs. Washington became angry with her husband, feeling he never tried to understand. Dr. R discussed how difficult this situation was for both of them. The Washingtons agreed that things had not been good between them for months. Dr. R offered to meet with the Washingtons for a longer visit to discuss the difficulties they were having and to follow up on Mrs. Washington's symptoms. Mrs. Washington was willing to return, but her husband was skeptical about the value of "just talking more" and wanted time to think about it. Dr. R agreed that this was an important decision that they both should think over. Dr. R suggested the Washingtons call in a week to let him know their decision.

Two weeks later Mrs. Washington called. Things had gotten worse and Mr. and Mrs. Washington wanted to talk with Dr. R about it.

By reading the signs correctly, Dr. R recognized the existence of a problem and succeeded in stimulating the couple's willingness to discuss their marital difficulties. In the next visit Dr. R assessed the Washington's relationship. There are several purposes of an assessment session: (1) to gain additional information about the couple and their problems; (2) to help the couple clarify their concerns and wishes for their relationship; and (3) to assist the physician and couple in deciding what the next step should be. The following are areas of a couple's relationship that are important for the physician to assess: family background, the nature of the problem and attempted solutions, strengths of the marriage, sexual intimacy, and the couple's motivation to change.

Family Background

If the physician does not already have a genogram of the couple, it is helpful to develop one early in the assessment interview. This can be done informally as part of the joining process. Oftentimes marital problems reflect unresolved issues related to each partner's family of origin or difficulty blending the different relationship styles of two families. Having information about the families can be useful when discussing other areas of assessment. Some possible questions include:

• Do your parents and family live in this area?
• Are both of your parents living?
• How many brothers and sisters do you have?
• Where are you in the birth order?
• How often do you have contact with your parents and family?
• Do your parents know about the difficulties you are having?

Nature of the Problem and Attempted Solutions

Having the couple discuss their problems and how they have tried to resolve them not only gives the physician important information but also the opportunity to observe how the couple interacts. How do they communicate verbally and nonverbally? Does one partner intellectualize while the other is emotional? Who pursues and who distances? In what areas are their interactions similar to that of a parent and child at times? Does one blame while the other accepts guilt? While observing the couple's style of interaction, the physician's questions to each partner should help to discover whether the problem is chronic or situational, severe or mild.

• What do you feel is the problem?
• How long has the problem been going on?
• What changes have occurred in your life during this time?
• How do you think these changes have affected your relationship?
• What do you think is the cause of the problem?
• How have you tried to solve the problem in the past? Any previous counseling? What has worked? What has not worked?
• What have family and friends said to you about your problems?
• Has anyone else in either of your families had similar problems?

> Mr. Washington was an only child who grew up in what he described as a strict household where emotions were seldom expressed openly. His parents were loving but not demonstrative. Mrs. Washington was the oldest of five. She reported that her family showed a lot of emotion, fighting often, but always making up. The differences in their family backgrounds were reflected in Mr. and Mrs. Washington's descriptions of their problems.
>
> Mr. Washington felt his wife was always upset about something. Nothing he did for her was right. Mrs. Washington was angry that her husband was "never affectionate" and did not listen to her. She said her husband had always been quiet but that things had been much worse in the last five months. Mr. Washington had not noticed a problem until several weeks ago, although he acknowledged that something was up over the last few months.
>
> In talking about their son it was apparent to Dr. R how much both parents loved him. Ron had been very ill with pneumonia seven months ago and Mrs. Washington had taken time off work to care for him. Mrs. Washington said it was very stressful for her, especially since her husband had to work a lot of overtime during the illness. Mr. Washington reported that he worried about his son all the time. The couple reported arguing several times during their son's illness. Since that time the Washingtons had not been able to resolve the tensions between them. Now they report to fighting "at the drop of a hat."

Strengths of the Relationship

It is just as important to understand the strengths of a committed relationship as it is to understand its problems. Couples usually find it easier to discuss problems than strengths when they are angry or disappointed. Those couples who are able to identify strengths are usually more flexible, and open in how they view a marriage and, consequently, more hopeful about change. Couples who are rigidly problem-focused about their marriage tend to be more stuck and less hopeful about change. Questions which focus on the couple's strengths include:

- Are there times when there are few problems in your relationship?
- What do you do differently during those times that makes them better?
- What do you feel are the strengths of your marriage?
- When was the best time in your relationship?
- What made it good?

> The Washingtons smiled when Dr. R asked them about the good times in their relationship. They talked humorously about their ill-fated honeymoon camping trip during which it rained for five days, and the excitement and closeness they felt when their son was born. Those were times in which they talked more and felt they were headed in the same direction.
>
> Mr. Washington felt the greatest strength they had was their "willingness to keep trying." Mrs. Washington said that their greatest strength was their commitment to each other and to their son, although she worried whether or not these commitments would endure. Dr. R said he was impressed that even with the difficulties they were having, their marriage obviously had clear strengths that they could draw on to try and solve their current problems.

Sexual Intimacy

Assessment of sexual problems depends in large part on the initiative of the physician. Patients who present with low back pain, abdominal pain, urinary difficulties, and a host of other somatic complaints may have underlying sexual problems that they are hesitant to discuss. It is not unusual for somaticizing patients or any patient who has experienced a lifetime of physical discomfort to also have sexual problems which may never be discussed with a physician.

Masters and Johnson (9) have estimated that 50% of all marriages experience sexual problems at some time. Studies indicate that physicians who do not inquire about a couple's sexual relationship will only learn about problems 10% of the time, but physicians who routinely inquire identify sexual problems 50–100% of the time (10).

It is important to assess sexual difficulties from a biopsychosocial perspective. Problems with sexual functioning may arise because of organic factors that then affect the marital relationship or because of general difficulties with intimacy that then affect the physiology of sexual functioning. Because they are intertwined, it is best to assess both the biomedical and psychosocial dimensions of all sexual problems.

Among men the most common sexual problems are premature ejaculation and impotence (3,9,11–13). The most frequent difficulties faced by women include anorgasmia, vaginismus, dyspareunia, and low sexual desire (3,11–13). The causes of sexual problems can range from marital discord, to performance anxiety, to lack of sexual knowledge, to the side effects of medication or organic problems (2).

Organic causes of sexual problems, such as disease (diabetes, circulation problems, endocrine problems, depressed liver function, multiple sclerosis) or the use of a medication or drugs that affect sexual functioning (alcohol, antidepressants, antihypertensives) make up a small percentage of sexual problems (3,12,13). If a sexual problem is situational, it is less likely to be primarily organic in nature. Sexual problems that are chronic and occur under all circumstances have a greater likelihood of having primarily organic causes (12).

The process of assessment should clarify both the nature of the problem and its possible causes. Some evaluation questions include (12,14):

• Are you satisfied with your sex life?
• If not, what difficulties are you having?
• Do these difficulties occur all the time or only in certain circumstances?
• (To men) Do you have problems obtaining or maintaining an erection? Do you have problems controlling ejaculation?
• (To women) Do you have difficulty becoming sexually aroused? Do you ever have pain during intercourse or difficulty achieving an orgasm?
• What do you feel is the reason for these difficulties?
• How would you like your sexual relationship to be?
• Have either of you been ill recently? Are you on medication?
• Do you drink or use any other drugs?

> Dr. R asked the Washingtons if the difficulties they were having affected their sexual relationship. At first they both said everything was "okay," but when Dr. R asked if they were satisfied with their sex life, Mrs. Washington said she was not. She felt they should be closer. When asked what she meant by "closer," Mrs. Washington said she wished they could have sex more often. Dr. R learned that the Washingtons were having sex approximately once every six weeks. Mr. Washington acknowledged that this was less than it had been, but said he often felt too tired at night. And, he said, when he wasn't tired, his wife was angry. Dr. R asked if they were able to have intercourse satisfactorily when they had tried. Both said that several times Mr. Washington had not been able to get an erection. Dr. R explored this further and learned that Mr. Washington had erections at other times, as well as nocturnal emissions. Mrs. Washington had not had problems of any kind until a month ago when she reported pain during intercourse so they stopped. They had not attempted intercourse since.

Motivation to Change

It is important to establish how much both partners want to change the relationship; it is a mistake to assume that a couple wants to change their situation without first asking them. For some change may involve improving the relationship, but for others it may mean ending it. Some couples are not happy with their marriage but are not ready to make changes. This can be for a variety of reasons including anxiety about giving in to a spouse or fear that discussing problems openly may make things worse. If the couple's desire to change is not clarified or if the physician appears more motivated than the couple, then the prospects for effective counseling are greatly diminished. Questions that help clarify each partner's motivation to change include:

• Do you want your relationship to continue?
• Do you feel your relationship can change?
• If your relationship does not change, what do you think will happen to it?
• Do you want to continue to work on the relationship in counseling?

> Dr. R asked whether or not the Washingtons felt their relationship could change. Mrs. Washington said they could probably try harder to get along. Mr. Washington did not know what they could do, but felt things had to get better, so maybe they could "do things differently." When asked if they wanted to work further on changing their relationship, both said "yes," although Mr. Washington made it clear that he didn't want to go off to see some "shrink" for an extended period of time.

Primary Care Couples Counseling

The physician's decision to enter into primary care counseling with a couple can be a difficult one. One partner may be very eager while the other is reticent. The goals for counseling may be vague, but the couple may be motivated. The physician may want to help but not feel his or her skills will be effective. A concern that a couple presents as related to a recent crisis may upon closer examination reveal more difficult problems of longer duration. "Lack of communication" may be related to physical violence or substance abuse. Because of these complicating factors, most couples with marital difficulties will need to be referred to a marriage therapist. But under certain circumstances the physician can provide effective, brief counseling to help troubled couples.

Indications for Primary Care Couples Counseling

1. The problem is situational and has a recent onset. These problems include facing difficulties that have arisen within the previous six months related to life cycle changes or specific crises of limited duration. The birth of a child, a death in the family, recent illness, and job change or loss are among the issues that may create problems of this nature.

2. The problem is specific rather than general. Couples seeking to improve their ability to argue productively, for example, are more likely to make changes because they have clearly defined the problem. Couples who have "communication problems" or who want to "make the marriage better" have a less well-defined focus for counseling. This may be because the problems are multiple and long term.

3. The couple has a history of a good relationship. Couples who report a stable, close relationship prior to the onset of the problem have a good foundation to build on in counseling. Couples who have "always fought" or have "never gotten along" in all likelihood need to be referred.

4. The couple is motivated to change. Both partners need to express a desire to change the relationship for primary care couples counseling to be effective. If one or both partners are not clearly motivated, it is less likely that counseling will be effective.

5. The physician has the time and the skills to work with the couple. If a physician is concerned about the amount of time or the skills necessary for couples counseling, then he or she should refer the case to a marital therapist.

If it is clear from the assessment that these indications for primary care couples counseling are met, then the physician can negotiate the structure of the counseling with the couple.

Guidelines for Primary Care Couples Counseling

The following are suggestions for counseling couples in primary care (13,14):

1. Involve both partners in counseling. It is important not to fall into the pattern of seeing one spouse because the other one is reportedly motivated but unavailable or is not interested. Marital counseling with only one partner may increase the problems that the couple is facing (15). It also encourages the participating partner to depend on the physician inappropriately.

2. Primary care couples counseling should be short term. This is best accomplished by establishing a clear format for the counseling process which includes:

• number of counseling visits (4–6)
• frequency of visits (weekly, monthly, etc.)
• length of each visit (25–45 minutes)
• clarifying what other contacts between the couple and the physician are acceptable (none, 1 phone call between visits, no phone calls at home, etc.)
• assessing the couple's progress on or before the final contract visit

3. Problem solving should be the focus of counseling. The physician should help the couple:

• clarify the changes they want to make
• discuss what each would have to do for the changes to occur

• make a clear plan for implementing the desired new behaviors
• carry out appropriate tasks between counseling visits
• give feedback to each other on progress made

The use of "quid pro quo" techniques can be an effective approach (16–18). In this process, the couple identifies the behaviors they would like each other to change. Each partner then agrees to try a new behavior in exchange for a new behavior that the other partner will try. In this way the couple builds trust and begins to get their needs met (e.g., a wife agrees not to "nag" her husband about jobs around the house and the husband agrees to talk more to his wife).

It can also be useful for the physician to discuss pursuer–distancer patterns in the couple's relationship. Such a discussion can be a springboard from which the couple can negotiate changing their pursuing and distancing behaviors. Whatever approach is taken, it is important to focus on the couple's ability to bring about changes in their behavior.

4. Couples who are not making progress in primary care counseling should be referred. The physician and couple can assess whether or not the couple's goals are being met on the final contract visit or before. It is unwise to recontract for additional visits if change is not occurring with the hope that more sessions will be the solution. It is better to focus on what progress has occurred and how a referral may be the next step in the process of change. (See Chapter 22 for a discussion of referrals.)

> Dr. R and the Washingtons agreed to meet four times over two months and then assess the couple's progress. During their first session both partners discussed wanting to get closer. Dr. R encouraged them to be more specific. After talking further the Washingtons decided they needed to spend more time together and talk more. Both felt this would be difficult due to their busy schedules but wanted to try. Nevertheless, with Dr. R's encouragement the Washingtons planned an evening out together. Since Mrs. Washington was usually in charge of planning such outings, it was decided that Mr. Washington would handle the arrangements. Mrs. Washington agreed to remind her husband about the details of their date only once. The Washingtons chose a day for their date and set up an appointment with Dr. R to discuss the outcome.
>
> At the second session the Washingtons were very pleased with their success. They had gone out twice and enjoyed themselves both times. Dr. R encouraged them to share with each other what made it enjoyable to be together. They said they were beginning to talk together for the first time in months. Mrs. Washington felt her husband was more available and Mr. Washington felt less pressured by his wife. For the next visit they decided to go out again and also make a list of what they most wanted from each other.
>
> At the third visit the Washingtons were very subdued. They had not made their lists although they had gone on another date. Mr. Washington felt things were "not working out." He was not able to explain why. Finally Mrs. Washington became angry and told Dr. R that things had gone well until they

had tried to make love. She felt her husband had rejected her while Mr. Washington insisted he was just too tired from a long day at work. Dr. R learned that the Washingtons had had sexual problems since the time of their son's birth. In the beginning Mrs. Washington was so involved with a new-born that she seldom felt like making love. And when they did she felt her husband was not "tender" with her. Mr. Washington felt his wife criticized how he made love and gradually his interest decreased. Several times he had been unable to maintain an erection. Eventually the Washingtons stopped talking about sex at all, and made love infrequently.

Dr. R emphasized the progress the Washingtons had made on their original goal of increasing their time together and talking more. He suggested that perhaps they were trying to make changes in their sexual relationship prema-turely and needed more time to "get to know each other again." Dr. R sug-gested that the Washington's not have sex before the next appointment. He explained that sexual intimacy may be the next step but for now the Washing-tons needed more time just being together. The Washingtons planned a project to do together and decided to talk together once about how they would like their sexual relationship to be.

Dr. R learned that the Washington's problem was of longer duration than he had assumed. He saw that the pursuing and distancing process in their marriage may have protected them from the hurt or risks of get-ting too close and being disappointed. Dr. R's ban on intercourse is an attempt to slow the couple down and help solidify some of the gains they have made.

Restraining the couple from further attempts at sexual intimacy is an approach that is common in sex therapy (9,12,19). The most familiar treatment approach developed by Masters and Johnson involves work on a couple's communication, the prohibition of sexual intercourse, and the use of sensate focus exercises. Through sensate focus exercises the couple learns to give and receive pleasure by touching and caressing. The couple begins with nongenital touching, graduates to genital pleas-uring, and eventually is encouraged to have intercourse.

Dr. R has focused on the beginning steps in this process by encourag-ing further communication and removing the pressure to perform sexu-ally. In the fourth session Dr. R and the Washingtons assessed their progress and decided on future directions.

The Washingtons did well on their project, which was papering the bedroom. They report, though, that they never had a discussion about sex. Mrs. Washington blamed her husband for this since he had been "too busy" to talk. Mr. Washington admitted that sometimes he is too angry to talk to his wife. The Washingtons felt frustrated. They wanted to be more intimate but felt stuck. Dr. R helped the Washingtons summarize the progress they had made in a short time. Mr. and Mrs. Washington felt they were closer than they had been. They had made strides with their goals of talking more and spend-ing more time together. But both partners felt the relationship had not changed enough.

Dr. R emphasized that couples who are making progress often realize how much more they want from their relationship. The Washingtons wanted to work more on their marriage. Dr. R responded: "I am glad to hear that you want to continue because you've showed that you can make changes. At this point I would recommend that you continue counseling with a marriage counselor that I often work with. He is well trained to deal with sexual difficulties that couples are trying to resolve."

The Washingtons agreed to the referral, although Mrs. Washington was concerned that she would no longer be able to see Dr. R. Dr. R clarified that he would continue to see either of them for her medical concerns and would be in communication with their counselor.

In this case Dr. R engaged the Washingtons in effective, brief primary care counseling which helped the couple begin to make progress and prepared them for an appropriate referral.

Recognizing that relationship problems may be a significant factor in a patient's somatic complaints is one of the most important tasks of the physician when working with patients who are in a committed relationship. Early recognition helps the physician avoid developing a relationship with the patient that may only replicate problem patterns in the patient's marriage. The physician who recognizes the importance of marital dynamics to patient health can either help couples use their strengths to make changes or, as in most cases, refer couples to a marital or family therapist. Of all the professionals who are routinely a part of a couple's life, no one is more advantageously positioned to recognize problems and help couples who are experiencing distress than their primary physician.

References

1. Lanier DC, Graveson RG: Detection of sexual problems by family medicine residents: Effects of a sex education program. *J Sex Educ and Ther* 1982;**8**:21–24.
2. Doherty WJ, Baird MA: *Family Therapy and Family Medicine*. New York, Guilford Press, 1983.
3. Medalie J (ed.): *Family Medicine Principles and Applications*. Baltimore, Williams and Wilkin, 1978.
4. Briggs GW, Banahan BF: A model for marriage counseling in family medicine. *Contin Educ Fam Physicians* Oct.1980:83–85.
5. Waring EM: Marital intimacy and medical practice. *Inter J Psychiatry Med* 1982;**12**(1):59–66.
6. Nease DE, Liese BS: Perceptions and treatment of sexual problems. *Fam Med* 1987;**19**(6):468–470.
7. Fogarty TF: The distancer and the pursuer. *The Family* 1976;**7**(1):11–16.
8. Lerner H: *The Dance of Anger*. New York, Harper Row, 1985.
9. Master WM, Johnson VE: *Human Sexual Inadequacy*. Boston, Little, Brown and Co., 1970.

10. Pauly TB: Human sexuality in medical education and practice. *J Psychiatry* (Australia/New England) 1971;**5**:204–208.
11. Masters WH, Johnson VE: *Human Sexual Response.* Boston, Little, Brown and Co., 1966.
12. Kaplan HS: *The New Sex Therapy.* New York, Brunner/Mazel, 1974.
13. Steinert Y: Working with couples: Sexual problems, in Christie-Seely J (ed.): *Working with the Family in Primary Care: A Systems Approach to Health and Illness.* New York, Praeger, 1984.
14. Kolodny RC, Masters WH, Johnson VE: *Textbook of Sexual Medicine.* Boston, Little, Brown and Co., 1979.
15. Gurman AS, Kniskern D (eds.): *Handbook of Family Therapy.* New York, Brunner/Mazel, 1981.
16. Lederer WJ, Jackson DD: *The Mirages of Marriage.* New York, W.W. Norton, 1968.
17. Stuart RB: An operant interpersonal program for couples, in Olson DH (ed.): *Treating Relationships.* Lake Mills, IA, Graphic Publishing, 1976.
18. Steinert Y: Working with couples: Marital problems, in Christie-Seely J (ed.): *Working With the Family in Primary Care: A Systems Approach to Health and Illness.* New York, Praeger, 1984.
19. Hoeck BJ, Cole C, Rosenfeld BL: A systemic approach to sexual dysfunctions, in Henao S and Grose NP (eds.): *Principles of Family Systems in Family Medicine.* New York, Brunner/Mazel, 1985.

PROTOCOL

Counseling Couples in Primary Care

Recognizing the Signs of Relationship Discord

1. The physician uses his or her reactions to a patient as a diagnostic tool.
   - Consistent pursuing or distancing between the physician and patient may be a sign that the patient's primary relationship has problems.
2. Be aware of the psychosocial dimension of each patient encounter.
   - Most marital and sexual problems first come to the physician's attention as somatic complaints.
3. Make psychosocial questions a routine part of your interview.
   - When you are feeling ill or in pain, who do you turn to for support?
   - Have you discussed your symptoms with your spouse?
   - What does he or she think is the cause of this problem?
   - Has your spouse suggested anything for you to do about your symptoms?
   - What is it like for you at home when you are feeling ill?

Assessing Couples' Relationship Problems

1. Family background
   - Do your parents and family live in this area?
   - Are both of your parents living?
   - Where are you in the birth order?
   - How often do you have contact with your parents and family?
   - Do your parents know about the difficulties you are having?
2. Nature of the problem and attempted solutions
   - What do you feel is the problem?
   - How long has the problem been going on?
   - What changes have occurred in your life during this time?
   - How do you think these changes have affected your relationship?
   - What do you think is the cause of the problem?
   - How have you tried to solve the problem in the past (including previous counseling)? What has worked?
   - What have family and friends said to you about your problems?
   - Has anyone else in either of your families had similar problems?
3. Strengths of the relationship
   - Are there times when there are few or no problems in your relationship?

- What do you do differently during those times that makes them better?
- What do you feel are the strengths of your marriage?
- When was the best time in your relationship?
- What made it good?

4. Sexual intimacy
   - Are you satisfied with your sex life?
   - If not, what difficulties are you having?
   - Do these difficulties occur all the time or only in certain circumstances?
   - (To men) Do you have problems obtaining or maintaining an erection? Do you have problems controlling ejaculation?
   - (To women) Do you have difficulty becoming sexually aroused? Do you ever have pain during intercourse or difficulty achieving an orgasm?
   - What do you feel is the reason for these difficulties?
   - How would you like your sexual relationship to be?
   - Have either of you been ill recently? Are you on medications?
   - Do you drink or use any other drugs?

5. Motivation to change
   - Do you want your relationship to continue?
   - Do you feel your relationship can change?
   - If your relationship does not change, what do you think will happen to it?
   - Do you want to continue to work on the relationship in counseling?

Indications Favoring Primary Care Couples Counseling

1. The problem is situational with a recent onset.
2. The problem is specific rather than general.
3. The couple has a history of a good relationship.
4. The couple is motivated to change.
5. The physician has time and the skills to work with the couple.

Guidelines for Primary Care Couples Counseling

1. Involve both partners in counseling.
2. Primary care couples counseling should be short term. Establish a clear format:
   - number of counseling visits (4–6)
   - frequency of visits (weekly, monthly, etc.)
   - length of each visit (25–45 minutes)

- clarify what contacts between the couple and the physician are acceptable (none, one phone call between visits, no phone calls at home, etc.)
- assess the couple's progress on or before the final contract visit.

3. Problem solving should be the focus of counseling. The physician should help the couple.
   - clarify the changes they want to make
   - discuss what each would have to do for the changes to occur
   - make a clear plan for implementing the desired new behaviors
   - carry out appropriate tasks between counseling visits
   - give feedback to each other on progress made

4. Couples not making progress in primary care counseling should be referred.

CHAPTER 13

Anticipating Loss

Health Care for the Elderly and Their Family Caregivers

In Collaboration with Bernard Shore*

The elderly are living longer and are increasing in numbers. The average life expectancy is now 74 years, 20 years more than it was at the turn of the century. Five percentage of the population is over 75, and this is the fastest growing segment of the population (1). Primary care geriatrics offers the physician the rewards of working with people with long and interesting life histories. And it offers a special poignancy in the opportunity to help patients and families resolve important issues before death.

Extending the length of an individual's life has also extended the joys, the pains, and the responsibility of family life. Three or four generations surviving in one family is now commonplace. Marriages can last longer; over half of the nation's population over 65 are married. For those over 80, the large majority of men are married while only 21% of women this age are married, primarily because their spouses have died earlier (2).

Most of the elderly live with or rely on family members. Of those over 65, more than 50% live with a spouse, 25% live alone, and about 18% live with adult children or other relatives, leaving only 5% in nursing homes or institutions (3). The majority live near at least one of their children and visit them often (2). The popular modern myth of families abandoning their elderly parents has been shown to be just that: a myth (4,5).

After the relative independence of the empty-nest period, the importance of family connections increases with aging. Physical deterioration and social and financial changes often push people back to their families so that many elderly come to depend heavily on their offspring and other family members. As the physical realities of aging increase dependency between the elderly and their caregivers, the specter of death

---

*Bernard Shore, M.D., is Medical Director of the Jewish Home of Rochester, New York.

hangs as a backdrop to this life stage and makes the emotional process between the elderly and their families intense and sometimes difficult. More and more, the young old (ages 65–80) are caring for their old old (those over 80) parents (6). Because of their age, the caregivers may have medical disabilities of their own. The overwhelming majority of these caregivers are relatives, and most are women (7). Regardless of who provides the care, decision-making regarding the medical care and placement of the elderly is often a highly emotional process that highlights old family dynamics, unresolved conflicts, loyalties, obligations, and responsibilities. For these reasons, primary care of the elderly needs to be consciously family-oriented. In this chapter we will focus on a range of issues relevant to medical care of the elderly, beginning with a discussion of the role of the physician, then specifics about interviewing the elderly and their families and evaluating the patient's relationships with family caregivers, and finally a discussion of issues around nursing home placement.

The Role of the Physician

For most patients and their families, the role of the physician at this phase of the life cycle is a powerful one; he or she is seen as an important supporter, advisor, and healer. For the isolated, the physician can mean a social contact; for the frail, the physician can seem to be a lifeline to living, an advocate and a guide for the patient and his or her family.

For the physician's part, he or she must be able to consider and evaluate multiple systems and use them to the patient's advantage. The biopsychosocial model is very important for integrating the complexity of issues involved in providing comprehensive care for the elderly. Providers must have a sound practical base in primary care geriatrics, distinguishing disease from normal aging. More important, they must relate any problems to the level of the older person's functioning, then weigh the benefits of any diagnostic or treatment procedures against the effect these procedures would have on the person. Physicians should be able to effectively connect the older person with other needed health care and social services, while coordinating the work of these various professionals to the patient's benefit.

To work constructively with the elderly, physicians should be aware of their own attitudes and biases toward the aged, the chronically ill, and the disabled. These attitudes are influenced by society's myths about aging, the physician's experience with his or her own aging family members, and the physician's personal reaction to becoming older. Prejudices toward the elderly can be quite subtle, but powerfully affect their medical care. These may include equating aging with senility, assuming that the elderly have (or should have) no sexual life, or thinking that the aged cannot care for themselves. Because the elderly have longer and more varied life experiences than most physicians, they are likely to have different beliefs and attitudes toward health and medical care. For example, the elderly person may be more concerned about maintaining their level of functioning and quality of life, than in prolonging their life. Family-oriented care of the elderly involves many of the same principles as care at other ages; however, we would like to emphasize several functions of the physician that are particularly important at this stage of the life cycle:

- **Guiding** patients through the intricacies of the health care delivery system, translating medical language, and educating patients and families about the meaning and appropriateness of various technological procedures.

  > For example, Mr. Long commonly "no showed" for his doctor visits after losing his driver's license due to failing vision. When Dr. U discovered the problem, he was able to inform Mr. Long that his medical insurance covered transportation for doctor visits. Failed visits were no longer a problem for this patient.

- **Coordinating** care for the patient, coordinating the efforts of the multidiscipinary team, professional consultants, community agencies, family and support networks.

  > Mrs. Bonner was found on the floor of her apartment 36 hours after her fall. She had pneumonia, congestive heart failure, and a hip fracture. It was only through longstanding knowledge of the patient and the family that Dr. Z was able to advise the emergency room staff about the appropriateness of a Swan-Ganz catheter and ICU care. Much to the family's relief, she was able to relay the DNR order, carefully worked out over months of discussion. When the surgeons began considering treatment options for the hip fracture, she made certain they recognized the patient's goal of independent ambulation in her own apartment. Applications for a short-term rehabilitation stay, with supporting paperwork, were made soon after the successful surgical repair.

- **Advocating** for the patient and family members, especially in preserving autonomy and choice regarding medical care.

  > Mrs. Dorr was a delightful strong-willed 93-year-old woman. Despite several transient ischemic attacks, she made clear her wish to forego diagnostic evaluation and possible carotid artery surgery. Dr. E received a flurry of anxious calls from family members urging him to "do something." Dr. E supported Mrs. Dorr's right to decide and suggested a family conference to discuss the patient's decision and questions the family might have regarding her medical status and her care.

- **Consulting** to the patient and family in their decision-making processes, whether about diagnostic testing or treatment, resuscitation status, or changes in living arrangements.

Mr. Jones was concerned about his elderly mother who lives alone in another state and had become quite confused over the past several months. He was thinking of bringing her back to live with him, but wanted his physician's advice. Dr. M suggested that he go see his mother and accompany her to an appointment with her physician. He could then find out her physician's assessment of the situation, whether she had received an adequate medical evaluation to date, and what services could be provided in her own community.

• **Collaborating** with the family caregivers, gathering information from the caregivers about the patient's status, educating them about the care of their loved one, assessing the abilities and capacities of the caregivers and trying to prevent them from reaching a point of burnout.

It took several phone calls and an office visit to plan the interim care for Mr. White when his caregiver son, with great hesitation, took his first vacation in over five years. Both father and son were quite pleased with themselves when the son returned home, and both agreed to make this an annual event.

• **Supporting** of the patient and the family caregivers, especially in situations where the caregiving is labor-intensive and demanding.

When Dr. O learned that Mrs. Yabinowitz had discovered another way to lay out her father's clothes so he was able to continue dressing himself, he told Mrs. Yabinowitz how surprised and impressed he was by her inventiveness and her devotion. She clearly was buoyed by the doctor's recognition and support.

Interviewing the Elderly and Their Families

1. **Be prepared to pace the interview more slowly** than with younger patients. Sensory deficits that are often present in older patients necessitate that more time be taken with them. Evaluate and explicitly ask about communication problems, such as hearing, speech, vision, memory, and other aspects of mental status. Direct communication about these issues has a modeling effect and allows patients and family members to explore present or future dysfunctions. Accommodate to any deficits and other physical limitations as necessary. [See Santora (8) for specific suggestions.] Some patients may require or benefit from a home visit. Working with the elderly requires careful attention to communication. However, realizing that communication deficits are common among older patients, be flexible enough to recognize the older person who neither needs nor wants special accommodations.

2. **Address the patient first.** It can be tempting with elderly patients to find the person in the family who is easiest to communicate with and speak primarily to that person, to the exclusion of the patient

or other involved family members who may be more difficult to deal with. Communicating with one person may be efficient in the short term, but can result in hard feelings and even noncompliance from the patient in the long term. Some older people already feel their family is ganging up on them to take away their autonomy. It can be difficult to balance the issues of safety and autonomy, as in the case below. It may be helpful to first interview the patient alone, then invite the family member in to find out how both patient and caregiver are doing. It is important for the physician to be supportive to both the patient and the caregivers.

> MRS. FEISTER: Doctor, you have to help us. My mother, as you know, is not capable of driving safely. We have not allowed her to renew her driver's license and we have sold her car. But she has twice called car dealerships and had them send out new models to her house so she would have a car. We've talked to her about our worries until we're blue in the face.
>
> DR. M: I can see you're concerned and frustrated. Mrs. Toms, can you tell me what your concerns are?
>
> MRS. TOMS: I just need to be able to get around, Doc. I'm not in my grave yet, in spite of what my children think. How do they expect me to go to the store, or visit my friends? Am I supposed to just wait until it's convenient for them to cart me around? I know I can't see well enough to drive any more, but my children are busy people with families of their own to take care of.
>
> DR. M: Mobility seems very important to your mother, Mrs. Feister. Do you have any ideas?
>
> MRS. FEISTER: Well, my brother and I would gladly pay for her to take a cab when she wants to go, if she'd stop calling the car dealerships and trying to buy cars.
>
> DR. M: That seems like a solution that really might work. It would allow you to leave home at your discretion, Mrs. Toms. You wouldn't have to rely on your children or friends to drive you. Would this be an acceptable compromise to you?
>
> MRS. TOMS: Yes, I suppose so.

3. **Involve caregivers and family members early** in the patient's care. In the end, this is a time-saver. Family members can provide important information the patient may not be able to provide.

> Dr. T enters the office to greet a smiling elderly woman, a new patient, still in her coat.
>
> DR. T: Hello, how are you?
>
> MRS. PARRISH: (smiles and nods briefly)
>
> DR. T: What brings you to the office today?
>
> MRS. PARRISH: (pauses for a moment, then notices the doctor is waiting) Oh, I'm not feeling too badly. It's just these legs. I live with my daughter and she's been on me to see somebody about these legs. They don't hurt at all, mind you, they just swell up a bit at night. I don't think it's very serious.
>
> DR. T: Hmm, and how long have you . . . (The door opens and a younger woman peers in, sees her mother and says:)

MRS. VITALE: Oh, Ma. Sorry to interrupt. I just wanted to bring you your pad and marker. Excuse me, Doctor, it's just that she's deaf and her vision has been blurred a bit lately so we use this big magic marker to write our notes to her. I thought this might help you both.

Early involvement of family or other knowledgeable people allows the physician to know about any problems or deficits that are relevant to medical care, deficits about which the patient may be sensitive and trying to compensate. This kind of problem can be particularly acute with a demented patient.

4. **Recognize the emotional concerns** underneath the explicit requests. Many patients and caregivers are fearful about the possibility of the patient's functional deterioration, or death, but may not make these concerns explicit to the physician. Making explicit the emotional concerns underneath the stated requests can allow these concerns to be aired, addressed, and sometimes resolved. For example, Mrs. Parrish in the preceding example did not draw the physician's attention to her visual and hearing deficits and minimized the meaning of her newest symptoms, swelling in her legs. Mrs. Toms, in the earlier example, obviously did not want to accept the lack of autonomy that went with not driving a car (especially with her children wanting to control this part of her life). It should be noted, however, that sometimes the elderly patient accepts the reality of disability better than his or her spouse or children.

5. Do not make significant changes in a treatment plan based solely on the family's report without **evaluating the elderly patient directly.** While family members provide invaluable information about an elderly person, they should not be relied upon exclusively. Family concerns can reflect changes in the patient's condition, an increase in family distress, or both. When receiving a call regarding a change, assess the level of distress in the caregiver as well as any changes in the patient. In this way, the actual problem can be addressed by the treatment plan, whether it be a change in the patient's medication, placement for the patient, or respite care to prevent caregiver burnout.

Dr. V received a call saying his patient, Mrs. Brown, was deteriorating at home and needed to be hospitalized. Mrs. Pale, Mrs. Brown's daughter, spoke urgently, saying she had flown in from out of town, had not seen her mother in five months, and was worried that her mother was "at death's door." Dr. V asked to speak to Mrs. Brown and the patient repeated the complaints she had had since her stroke three months ago. Dr. V told Mrs. Brown and Mrs. Pale he would make a home visit to try and evaluate Mrs. Brown's condition. When he arrived, he found Mrs. Brown to be in stable condition, much as she had been in recent months. He discussed her condition with the patient and her daughter and reassured both that the current treatment plan was appropriate. Mrs. Pale spoke about how much the stroke had affected her mother, how difficult it was to see her deteriorate, and her own determination to visit her mother more frequently. Dr. V invited Mrs. Pale to call him with any concerns she might have about her mother.

Evaluating the Patient's Relationships with Family Caregivers

Care of the elderly, especially as their physical or mental health begins to deteriorate, can be a challenge to the healthiest and most resourceful of families. Two or three times as many housebound and bedridden elderly live at home as live in an institution (7). These patients require responsible, attentive care from family members and from community supports. The balance between the patient's and family caregivers' needs can be difficult to achieve successfully. The following example is, unfortunately, not so rare.

> Mrs. Houser told Dr. P she did not know what to do. Her mother had managed her father's blindness and other health needs with seeming ease, by solely devoting herself to him. But, since her mother's death and her father's moving in to their home, Mrs. Houser's life had been a shambles. Her volunteer work at the museum had been the first to go, then she had had to get neighbors to take the children to their piano lessons. There was no time for friends and less and less socializing for the Housers as a couple. Her father, on the other hand, seemed pleased with the arrangement. He did not seem to notice his son-in-law's irritation when he visited with him while the younger man worked at his hobby of woodworking. Today, Mrs. Houser reported, her husband had said: "That's it. This can't go on. Either he goes or I do." Dr. P suggested Mr. and Mrs. Houser and her father come in together to discuss the current living arrangement, and each person's satisfactions and dissatisfactions with it.

Clearly, family caregivers are essential members of the health care team. They provide clinical observation, direct care, case management, and a range of other services (9,10). In chronic illnesses, such as Alzheimer's Disease, these caregivers may devote years of their own lives to caring for a loved one. Unfortunately, our current health care system offers little in the way of institutional support for families who are burdened with caregiving (11). Home services are not well-coordinated. Physicians are not adequately reimbursed for home visits nor for what can be the very time-consuming task of coordinating services. Insufficient respite care is available for those families who need a break from caregiving. The lack of respite care can encourage an all-or-nothing mentality for families taking care of their sick loved ones, so that the family may push themselves to exhaustion and then demand placement for the patient. The patient's status may not have changed, but the caregiver clearly says, "I can't take it any more." It is important that physicians provide emotional support and connect the family with any available home services and community support groups to help prevent caregiver burn-out.

Family-oriented physicians need to monitor patients and their care-givers to assess and reduce the burden of caregiving. Caregivers them-selves need to be evaluated for symptoms of depression, fatigue, somatization, and illness, especially those with heavy responsibilities for patients that require long-term care. The possibility of elder abuse by caregivers or other family members should also be considered; this may be a result of burnout or of longstanding conflictual relations. Houlihan, in his review of the literature, found several common predictors of severe caregiver burden. He found that, on the whole, caring for demented rela-tives is more burdensome than caring for the physically impaired. He found that female caregivers feel more burdened in general than male caregivers, and spouses of the patient feel more burdened than adult chil-dren. And, he found that families with community resources for the patient and the caregiver feel less burdened than those without (10). The physician can help the patient and family assess the adequacy and the burden of caretaking by evaluating the relationships between the patient and the caregivers along several important dimensions:

1. **Nature of the illness.** Does the disease process result in physical limitations or in cognitive impairment? Is the caregiving likely to be long-term, over a 10-year period as with Alzheimer's, or short-term, as with some metastatic cancers?

2. **Trust and dependability.** Can the patient trust the caregivers? Are the caregivers able to handle the patient's deficits?

3. **Availability.** Do the caregivers have the resources, both finan-cially and emotionally, to manage the tasks of caring for their sick rela-tive? What kind of back-ups exist, should the caregiver become ill or wish to take a vacation? Will they be able to pay for respite care if it is not, as is typical, covered adequately by insurance?

4. **History of the relationship and current family dynamics.** In families there is a history of obligations, debts, and loyalties that often emerges in bold relief around questions of how to care for a loved one. This history must be balanced with present day demands and a realistic assessment of available resources. Given this history and the current family dynamics, can the patient and caregiver work together success-fully to meet the needs of the patient and at least sustain the needs of the caregiver?

5. **Support network.** Does the family and patient have adequate support for this venture? Can the physician help to strengthen the sup-port network to improve caregiving? What community resources are available: case managers, geriatric assessment units, family therapists familiar with elderly issues, respite home care programs, day services, support groups, rehabilitation services, psychoeducation programs for the caregivers? (See the protocol at the end of this chapter for more on evaluating caregiver burden.)

Many of the issues around family caregiving are evident and can be explored during routine primary care before an acute health event makes them of crucial importance. For example, knowing a patient's or family's financial status, their ability to afford medications and food, may help in planning for care after a hospital stay. Knowing who helps an older patient with shopping or who brings them to the doctor in the winter may help in knowing who might be available if a patient breaks a hip. Knowing family dynamics may also help when a family is struggling to accept their mother's dementia.

> Mrs. Towner came for her first visit with Dr. U accompanied by her youngest daughter, Miss Green. The daughter related the following story: Mrs. Towner, twice a widow, had worked for 25 years as a legal secretary in a prestigious law firm. She had always been bright, witty, practical, and much respected by her five children. Over the last 3 years her behavior had become more erratic; her work performance began to fall off noticeably, so that while she was kept on at the firm, no important matters were entrusted to her anymore. Several oblique comments were made to family members by her employers, but last week the senior partner had called Miss Green and insisted that her mother must see a doctor or face outright dismissal.
>
> A full evaluation strongly suggested Alzheimer's Disease. Dr. U convened a family meeting including Mrs. Towner and the 5 children. It seemed clear that all lived busy, demanding lives, and all were fiercely independent. The children's questions were many and pointed: Is there a test for Alzheimer's? Are you a neurologist? What are our legal obligations as far as our taking care of her? How do we get a second opinion? Dr. U answered these, then asked: "How do you think we should best proceed?" Many alternative options were offered by the children, with the eldest strongly urging a thorough evaluation at Johns Hopkins. Dr. U then asked Mrs. Towner what she thought about all this: "Do you see a problem? What do you feel would be best?" Mrs. Towner, who had remained silent through most of the meeting, smiled blandly for a moment, then said: "Well, my memory's just no good anymore. I think they should just take me out and shoot me." After a wave of reassurance and genuine avowals of her importance to them, the eldest exchanged pointed glances with her youngest sister and said: "Well, we'll never put her in a nursing home no matter what you say she has."

In this case, the patient's feeling of being abandoned, the family's spontaneous denial of her diagnosis, and the daughters' potential disagreement over placement are indicators that working out caregiving for this patient is likely to be problematic. Intensive support and intervention may be required with this family before a successful plan is achieved.

Working with the Elderly and Their Families Around Nursing Home Placement

In spite of widespread guilt and ambivalence about nursing home placement in our culture, nursing homes can be a solution for some serious health problems. Placement can result in positive consequences for both the patient and the patient's family (12). Although only a small proportion of all elderly live in institutions at any given time, this option can be an important one for patients with serious impairments and for families who are not able to provide care for their loved one. Even so, the decision to make such a placement is often fraught with emotions–guilt, anger, rejection, depression–for both the patient and responsible family members. Many nursing home residents are 85 years or older, so often these decisions are made by the old old and their aging children.

In 1973, Williams found that the decision for placement was most often made at "a time of desperation, exhaustion, and with too little participation by the patient." In his study, institutionalization often occurred with a lack of thorough and current medical or nursing evaluation of the patient (13). This and previous studies suggested that more than half of all persons in long-term care facilities were at an inappropriate level of care. Not studied, but implied, was the fact that other-than-medical factors, such as depletion of caregiving resources, could be precipitating these inappropriate referrals. With current stricter regulations, placement is more likely to be at the appropriate level of care; however, caregiver resources remain a factor in determining the timing and pressure for placement.

The **decision for placement** of an elderly person in an institution should be made by reviewing **the fit between the family's health care and personal needs, and the family's resources and desires.** Patients and families should make these decisions, balancing the needs of the patient and the family, in consultation with their primary care physician. Multiple options are available: the elder may live alone and receive home services ranging from public health nurse visits to a live-in home health aide; the elder may receive these services while living with a family member; or the elder may need institutionalization. The level of care at this last institutional level can range from little in an adult care facility to a high level of care in skilled nursing facilities at nursing homes. (See Fig. 13.1.) Different levels of care match different family and patient needs. When assessing the level of care needed, the question is: **How can the patient and family needs be met in the most effective way by the available institutional supports?**

Assessing the Need for Placement

Given the problems regarding determination of placement, Herr and Weakland suggest the primary care physician ask the following questions before making any recommendations:

• **Who says the elder needs to move? And why?**
• **When an elder requests information about alternative living arrangements:**

Institution	▲	Skilled nursing facilities
		Health–related facilities
		Institutional respite care
		Rehabilitation care
		Adult home/Domiciliary facilities
Community		Enriched/supervised/shared housing
		Hospice
		Foster care
		Adult day care
		Coordinated home care
		• Nursing services
		• Personal care attendant
		• Homemaker/Housekeeper
		• Nutrition/"Meals on Wheels"
		• Rehabilitation services
Home	▼	• In-home respite care

FIGURE 13.1.   Range of services for the elderly.

Why is the elder *presently* concerned about alternative housing?
What are the elder's expectations for the alternative housing?
What needs would be met that cannot be met by the current arrangements?
Is the elder moving to meet his or her needs or some other presumed needs of the family system?
• **When family members request information about alternative living arrangements:**
Who has decided something must be done? Why?
How was the spokesperson "elected"?
What are the pressures being experienced by the family? (14)

It is important for primary care physicians to discuss issues around long-term care with their older patients, long before the need arises. One such question might be: "What are your plans for the future should you become sick and need help, or possibly not be able to care for yourself?" Like discussions around DNR policies, it is important for patients and families to first discuss these issues while they are healthy and able to consider the range of alternatives. These early discussions are, in themselves, diagnostic: some families will discuss the issue and implement their decision should the need arise, others may be unwilling to consider the possibility or may make an entirely different decision when faced with the reality of ill health. Certainly when an elderly person starts to have functional difficulties, it is important to discuss the possibility of increased care needs in the future.

Patients and families vary in their decisions regarding the level of care they desire. Some families jump to nursing home placement early in an illness; others go to great lengths to keep their loved one in a family home. Many families use a range of caregiving services. To return to the example of Mrs. Towner:

As Mrs. Towner and her family began to absorb the fact that Mrs. Towner's symptoms were strongly suggestive of Alzheimer's, they began to plan for her caretaking. They were able to begin with a low level of care, that of increasing family support, given their resources and the status of her illness at that time.

Mrs. Towner's Alzheimer's Disease became progressively worse over the next year. After numerous problems and complaints by her employers at the law firm, she resigned from her job. Her family became increasingly concerned that she was unsafe living alone, that she might leave the gas on or have some other accident. After several months of discussion, the oldest daughter, Mrs. Centre, asked her mother to move into her family home with her husband and two children.

After a year, Mrs. Towner had deteriorated, requiring Dr. U and the family to consider increasing the level of care given to her. At that time, Dr. U met with Mrs. Towner and Mrs. Centre and verified that Mrs. Towner's condition had further deteriorated. Mrs. Centre now worried about leaving her children alone with her mother for fear her mother would lose track of important information. Mrs. Centre also made some comments about her husband "not realizing what he was in for." Dr. U suggested Mrs. Centre arrange for a home health care aide to come in three times a week to help Mrs. Towner with some of her daily activities. Mrs. Towner protested that she was capable of taking care of her grandchildren, but agreed to accept the help from the home health care aide.

Because of the stress and strain on the family and Mrs. Towner's further deterioration, the Towner family found it necessary to consider increasing her care to include services outside the home over the next 6 month period. During this time period, Dr. U saw Mrs. Centre twice for what seemed to be stress-related headaches. After the second visit, he asked how she was handling her mother's illness. Mrs. Centre became teary and said she either had to devote herself to her mother or to her husband and children. Currently she felt she was no good to either. She said her sister had been pushing the idea of a nursing home "for everyone's good." Mrs. Centre said she had told herself she would never do such a thing to her mother. Dr. U suggested Mrs. Centre and her husband and children come in with Mrs. Towner for a family conference to discuss how Mrs. Towner was doing.

At this conference, Dr. U saw that Mrs. Towner had further deteriorated, that Mr. Centre was quite perturbed by her frequent lapses of memory, and that Mrs. Centre felt stuck in the middle. With a knowledgeable social worker present, he discussed the possibility of a day treatment program, something he said would give Mrs. Towner the daily activities she had enjoyed when she was a busy person living on her own. The social worker also informed the family of a support group composed of other families going through similar experiences with their loved ones with Alzheimer's. Everyone seemed

pleased with the arrangement for day treatment. Mrs. Towner looked forward
to having "something to do," and the strain eased on Mrs. Centre's face.

   Mrs. Towner did well in the day program for about a year. At the end of that
time her continuing deterioration and other family concerns led to the
Towners considering placement. At that time, Mrs. Centre called Dr. U about
her mother becoming more irritable and combative, and wandering in the
middle of the night. She said if something was not done, she was afraid her
mother and her husband were going to come to blows. After examining and
talking with Mrs. Towner, Dr. U called another family conference, this time
with Mrs. Towner, the Centre family, all Mrs. Towner's other children and her
social worker. At that time, the group discussed the alternatives, including
home nursing service and placement in a nursing home. Mr. Centre and Miss
Green favored placement. Mrs. Centre seemed to favor placement as well, but
all she could say was that she was worried about how all this was affecting
the children. Mrs. Towner's sons suggested that they go out and canvas the
nursing homes to see the possibilities first hand. Mrs. Towner would not agree
or disagree to accompany them during the meeting. Within 3 months, Mrs.
Towner was placed in a local nursing home. Dr. U helped her and the family
adjust to the changes the placement brought. After an initial depressive
period, Mrs. Towner adjusted well to the social life at the nursing home and
did well there until the last 6 months of her life when she became bedridden,
unresponsive, and finally died.

As with the Towner family, a family conference is a useful format for
discussing the advantages and disadvantages of placement with many
patients and their families. (See Chapter 6 for the specifics of conducting a family conference.) Once the patient, family, and physician agree
that placement is desirable, the physician can help provide access to
information so the family can choose the best possible nursing home to
meet their needs (15). Facilitating an assessment of the patient's financial resources is an important step in the process. Financial considerations have become such a complex, often overwhelming burden that
usually a referral to a social worker and/or financial counselor skilled in
this area is required.

Dr. U was able to help the Towner family make decisions along the
way about increasing Mrs. Towner's care through family conferences
and some primary care counseling. Some families with more serious
difficulties warrant a meeting with a family therapist for either consultation or referral. (See Chapter 22 on referral to a family therapist.) As
with other situations, the physician needs to be alert to signs of serious
family stress or dysfunction around questions of caregiving or placement for the elder. Signs of stress include people refusing to speak to one
another, refusing to allow the elder access to certain family or friends,
the existence of family secrets, a series of important losses, overinvolvement or threats of abandonment directed at the elder, or overutilizing
medical services by any member of the family.

Postplacement

Once a reasonable plan has been established regarding placement, and the patient has been accepted by a nursing home, the primary care physician can provide continuity of care by following the patient in the nursing home. Some large nursing homes have their own medical staff, so that a decision needs to be made about which physician will retain primary responsibility for the patient. Whether the physician retains responsibility for the patient's medical care or not, it is useful to define what one's role will be to the patient and the family postplacement, recognizing the family's ongoing need for support and trying to diminish any sense of abandonment felt by the patient. It is important at this point to be specific in explaining the extent and limits of your care, as well as what can realistically be expected from long-term care. Lack of timely communication about these issues can foster unrealistic expectations.

The early period of adjustment to a nursing home placement can be difficult for both the patient and the family. The family will often need extra attention as they work to support the patient in a new environment. The highest period of morbidity and mortality for patients in a nursing home occurs in the first 3–6 months after placement (16), so closer attention from family and health-care staff is warranted at this time. Problems occur even for the majority of patients who do make the transition successfully; it is useful to normalize this for the patient and family. It is helpful to let family members know that although there are problems early on, it does not mean that the placement will not eventually work well.

Even for the physician who turns over the patient's care to the nursing home medical staff, he or she often continues to take care of the elderly person's family members. In this capacity the primary care physician may play an important role in supporting and advising the family to remain active participants in their relative's life postplacement. The family is an important source of support in helping the patient make the early adjustment to placement. Reisman talks about the importance of families reassuring their loved ones during the stressful adjustment period, helping with logistical problems such as locating important rooms on the floor, reading the signs, and learning the routines, as well as facilitating relationships between the patient and the staff and other residents (17). The family can usefully become involved in the policies and procedures of the nursing home by joining and being active in the family organization that is a part of some nursing homes. Finally, family members may need consultation on issues related to medical care, such as the patient's code status. The primary care physician can provide information, support, and, when necessary, redirect the family to bring up questions or problems with nursing home staff. Nursing home placement is a situation in which the primary care physician can be an advocate for both the patient and the family in helping all parties to adjust to a new stage of life.

> Mr. Yalom had gradually developed severe Parkinsonism with associated dementia, often tinged with paranoid ideation and hallucinations. This was very difficult for his wife and son, especially, to accept. Mr. Yalom had, with little formal education, risen high in his engineering firm. He had always maintained a very close relationship with his son. This family had proved to be a "model family" in weathering some life-threatening complications of his psychiatric problems and was well-liked by staff and other families. However, a series of problems—conflict with a roommate, some delay in a needed surgical procedure, and finally a deferred consultation—produced an eruption of anger from the 33-year-old son. He had left a job opportunity out of state to return home to "supervise" his father's care. He refused to look for another job for many months because "things weren't right with Dad." A simmering conflict with his mother increased. And, during this period, Mr. Yalom began to have increased Parkinsonian symptoms, including anorexia, serious weight loss, and more paranoid thinking.
>
> A family meeting was held, with Mr. Yalom present. The physician reviewed recent events and after asking for other views, began addressing Mr. Yalom. The physician noted that the family was very worried about Mr. Yalom and he sensed that everyone was being affected by the situation. What could be done to help them? Much of Mr. Yalom's reply was confused and circumstantial, but amidst this was a clear message to his son to "get a job." He said knowing his son was set would be a relief when so much else "didn't work right." Both son and mother began to cry together, their first mutual support in months, but Mr. Yalom remained calm. It was helpful to all the family to acknowledge Mr. Yalom's losses and their own losses as well as his continuing strength and love.

In this final example, the physician was able to use the opportunity to help the Yalom family deal with their unresolved family issues prior to Mr. Yalom's death. This family conference facilitated Mr. Yalom's nursing home adjustment and increased the family's ability to cope. Successful adjustment to either nursing home or home care during the period of illness and physical deterioration may help all parties in facing the next stage, that of death of the patient and grieving for the family.

References

1. U.S. Senate Special Committee on Aging: *Aging American—Trends and Projections, 1985*–86. Prepared by the U.S. Senate Special Committee on Aging in conjunction with American Association of Retired Persons, the Federal Council on Aging, and the Administration on Aging.
2. Zopf PE: *American's Older Population*. Houston, Cap and Gown Press, 1986.
3. Smallegan M: There was nothing else to do: Needs for care before nursing home admission. *Gerontologist* 1985;**25**(4):364–369.

4. Brody E: "Women in the middle" and family help to older people. *Gerontologist* 1981;**21**:471–480.

5. Brody E: Parent care as a normative family stress. *Gerontologist* 1985;**26**: 19–29.

6. Brody E: Families: Aging and changing. House Select Committee on Aging. June 4, 1980, p. 56.

7. Goldstein V, Regenery G, Wellin E: Caretaker role fatigue. *Nursing Outlook* 1981;**29**:24–30.

8. Santora G: Communicating better with the elderly. *Nursing Life* 1986;**6**: 24–27.

9. Maletta G, Hepburn K: Helping families cope with Alzheimer's: The physician's role. *Geriatrics* 1986;**41**(11):81–88.

10. Houlihan JP: Families caring for frail and demented elderly: A review of selected findings. *Fam Syst Med* 1987;**5**:344–356.

11. Koren MJ: Home care–who cares? *New Engl J Med* 1986;**314**:917–920.

12. Smith KF, Bengtson VL: Positive consequences of institutionalization: Solidarity between elderly parents and their middle-aged children. *Gerontologist* 1979;**19**:438–447.

13. Williams TF, Hall JG, Fairbank C: Appropriate placement of the chronically ill and aged. *JAMA* 1973;**226**:1332–1335.

14. Herr JJ, Weakland JH: Alternative living arrangements, in *Counseling Elders and Their Families: Practical Techniques for Applied Gerontology.* New York, Springer Publishers, 1979.

15. MacLean H: *Caring for Your Parents: A Sourcebook of Options and Solutions for Both Generations.* New York, Doubleday and Co., 1987.

16. Sekscenski ES: Discharges from nursing homes: Preliminary data from the 1985 National Nursing Home Survey, Advance data from Vital and Health Statistics of the National Center for Health Statistics 1987;**142**:1–15.

17. Reisman B: Adjusting to a residential facility for older persons: A child's perspective. *J Gerontolog Social Work.* 1985;**9**:91–100.

PROTOCOL

Evaluating Burden in Caregivers of the Elderly

The degree of burden and reward in any caregiving situation is determined by factors specific and individual to each patient and their caregivers. What is perceived by one caregiver as overwhelming may be seen as a doable challenge by another. Keeping this in mind, the following is an adaptation and extension of the factors found by researchers to increase caregiver burden, as reviewed by Houlihan (10). This checklist with two columns of positive and negative predictors of caregiver burden, actually represents a continuum from manageable or positive caregiving situations to those that most often result in severe burden or dysfunction for the caregiver and difficulty or deterioration for the patient. This checklist may be used by the primary-care physician as clinical tool in evaluating or monitoring a patient and his or her caregivers. No one factor should be seen necessarily as determining an unmanageable situation, but taken together the factors may be able to assess or predict degree of burden.

Predictors of positive caregiving relationships	Predictors of burdensome caregiving relationships
The caregiver's relationship to the patient	
• the caregiver is able to express anger with the patient when appropriate	• the caregiver feels guilty over anger and resentment of the patient
• the caregiver is concerned for the patient but does not feel solely responsible	• the caregiver has a high sense of responsibility for the family and for the patient
• the previous relationship between the patient and caregiver was positive	• the previous relationship between the patient and caregiver was highly ambivalent or conflictual
The patient's condition	
• the patient has mild to moderate physical impairments	• the patient is demented
• the patient's behavior is positive	• the patient's behavior is disruptive
• the family accepts the patient's diagnosis	• the family denies the patient's diagnosis

Predictors of positive caregiving relationships	Predictors of burdensome caregiving relationships
• the family accepts the reality of the patient's future deterioration	• the family is very fearful of the patient's future deterioration
• the patient does what he or she can independently	• the patient is highly dependent on the caregiver
• the caregiver is knowledgeable about the patient's disease or condition	• the caregiver does not understand much about the patient's problems

The caregiver's condition

• the caregiver is physically strong, healthy, and has stamina	• the caregiver is physically ill or disabled
• the caregiver's mood is positive most of the time	• the caregiver is depressed
• the caregiver has a good support network	• the caregiver is isolated and lonely
• the caregiver has personal time away from caregiving responsibilities	• the caregiver has little or no personal time away from caregiving
• the caregiver basically feels confident in caregiving	• the caregiver feels inadequate for the job
• the caregiver has a reasonable number of responsibilities	• the caregiver experiences role overload
• the caregiver is able to delegate responsibilities to other family members	• the caregiver has negative relationships with other family who do not help
• the caregiver is realistic about the responsibility and monitors self for physical or emotional symptoms	• the caregiver overfunctions denies the reality of the caregiving burden

Family resources

• the family is able to afford the caregiving	• the caregiving represents an economic hardship for the family
• the family is able to cope with the patient's safety needs	• the family has great difficulty keeping the patient safe
• the family is basically happy	• the family is in conflict
• the caregiver and the family have maintained some degree of social activity	• the level of social activity for the caregiver and family has decreased markedly

Predictors of positive caregiving relationships	Predictors of burdensome caregiving relationships

Family resources *(continued)*

• the caregiving family is able to maintain a future perspective and make future plans	• the caregiver and family are steeped in the problems of the present and are unable to make future plans

Community services

• a day care program is available for the patient	• a day care program is unavailable for the patient
• psychoeducation and/or a support group is available for the caregiver	• psychoeducation and/or a support group is unavailable for the caregiver
• good rehabilitation services are available for the patient	• no rehabilitation services are offered
• day respite care is available for the family	• day respite care is not available for the family
• overnight respite care is available for the family	• overnight respite care is not available for the family
• psychological and family therapy services are available for the patient and family	• psychological and family therapy services are not available for the patient and family
• the caregiver has good relations with the medical and support staff	• the caregiver has conflictual relations with the medical and support staff

Looking Death in the Eye
Death, Grieving, and Families

The death of a patient presents the physician with one of the most challenging situations in the practice of primary care medicine. Negotiating the process of dying can also be one of the most rewarding parts of practice as it brings about an emotional intensity for the patient, the family, and other caregivers that can be moving and healing for all who participate. The knowledge of impending death can facilitate resolution of personal and interpersonal conflicts rooted in previous life cycle stages. Of course, that same emotional intensity can also prove traumatic or bring about long-lasting dysfunction for those families who are unable to resolve the challenges raised by the loss of one of their members.

Our society is only beginning to provide institutional support for patients and families facing these changes. On the whole, we are a culture that denies the reality of death (1). In the health care community, death is an event to be prevented, not accepted, and providers often seek emotional distance from the dying patient and the patient's family. Overtly or covertly, the death of a patient is often seen as a failure of the provider's skills. This aspect of our professional socialization makes it difficult for us to facilitate a healthy dying process for our patients or encourage constructive grieving for their families, and for ourselves. In this chapter we will challenge our culture's tendency to deny death by providing a model for constructive interaction between the medical system, the dying patient, and the family. We begin by making practical suggestions about communicating a terminal diagnosis to a patient and family, then turn to treatment planning and making any decisions to limit treatment, notifying a family of a death, counseling around primary care grief issues, and recognizing unresolved grief reactions.

"I believe you may die from this illness"

Communicating the diagnosis of a terminal illness to a patient and family ideally involves clear, direct statements transmitted with a minimum of anxiety. While sometimes a terminal diagnosis is provided by a specialist, the primary care physician is uniquely qualified to communicate this information because of his or her long-standing relationship with the patient and understanding of the family's issues and needs. Several **guidelines for clear communication of a terminal illness** include:

- Communicate directly to the patient about the diagnosis, the treatment, and the prognosis of the illness. ("We don't believe your disease is curable.")
- Use clear, simple language. Avoid overmedicalizing or intellectualizing the information.
- Be honest and straightforward about the information as you know it, acknowledging areas of medical uncertainty. ("Most people with this illness survive 6–18 months.") Avoid giving an overly optimistic or overly pessimistic prognosis.
- Look the patient in the eye and speak calmly. Repeat the message several times.
- Avoid arguments over the diagnosis, or other diversions from the message itself.
- Set up another appointment to answer questions that will inevitably arise when the initial reaction wears off.
- Repeat this process with the family present. Create a safe atmosphere during the family conference for people to express their feelings honestly and directly if they so desire.
- Allow people their sadness or anger rather than trying to reassure them or brighten their mood. In this situation, depression can signal healthy anticipatory grieving, a process that needs encouragement rather than suppression.
- Allow patients some hope. Be humble about predicting how long a patient may survive.
- Meet regularly with the patient and family to discuss medical care, prognosis, and individuals' emotional reactions, even when the medical care is being managed by a specialist. Encourage children in the family to be involved in at least some of these meetings.

Dying patients force us to face our own mortality and that of those we love. Facing these personal issues can help us be calm and straightforward when communicating a terminal diagnosis to a patient, or accept a family member's anger on hearing about the death of a loved one (2). With very difficult or upsetting cases, discussion with a trusted colleague can be invaluable, both for the medical consultation and for the emotional support (3).

After hearing about a terminal diagnosis, the families of dying patients experience a period of high stress. Holmes and Rahe found the death of a spouse to be the single most stressful life event an individual encounters. Death of some other family member ranked 4th, after divorce and separation (4). Primary care physicians can do much in the way of prevention by spending a relatively brief amount of time attending to family members' reactions and functioning during the terminal illness phase. Fuller and Geis recommend a "health check" for the spouse or other significant family members of a dying patient (5). This appointment allows the physician to address this person's physical and emotional concerns and to raise questions about sensitive areas such as sexuality and finances. Many of these issues may be best discussed with the couple together.

Often the medical care of terminally ill patients is shared among a number of specialists. The primary care physician is well positioned to be a case manager and coordinate the medical care of the patient among the specialists and between the medical system and the family. Communicating regularly with the specialists involved can avoid the fragmentation of medical care that is so common with complex or terminal cases. Without someone coordinating services, families can receive differing or contradictory messages about a terminal illness.

> Dr. E had taken care of the Termillo family for over 20 years. Mr. Termillo, the patriarch of the family, had always been in relatively good health, though neither Dr. E nor his family had ever been successful in getting him to stop smoking. Recently, Mr. Termillo was found to have a lung mass on a chest X-ray done during a physical exam. A chest surgeon biopsied the mass, which proved to be malignant. After this diagnosis, Mr. Termillo began to see an oncologist and the surgeon on a regular basis, rarely seeing Dr. E. Both specialists confirmed a diagnosis of lung cancer, but were vague to the patient and the family about prognosis. While Dr. E thought of Mr. Termillo often, he was actually relieved during this difficult period to be able to distance from this man who reminded him of a favorite uncle.
>
> When Dr. E received the specialists' reports on Mr. Termillo, he found the surgeon and oncologist presented very different prognoses for this patient. Soon after reading these reports, Dr. E received a call from one of Mr. Termillo's adult children pleading with him to make sense out of what the doctors were telling her stepmother about the prognosis. Dr. E suggested that the daughter convene a family conference at his office in the next week, allowing him time to communicate directly with the specialists involved in Mr. Termillo's care. When he did so, he found that the surgeon's view was that Mr. Termillo had several months to live, if that long, while the oncologist was not yet ready to label the patient terminal, saying "There's always hope." Dr. E told the specialists of the family's request for more specific information and

his own suggestion for a family conference. He invited the specialists to attend. When both declined, he asked them if they had any special message they would like transmitted to the patient or family. Both reiterated the prognosis as they saw it. Dr. E promised to present both points of view to the family.

Mr. and Mrs. Termillo and three of four of Mr. Termillo's adult children attended the family conference. Mrs. Termillo said she was relieved to be meeting with Dr. E, whom she trusted and had known for a long time. Mr. Termillo's daughter who had requested the meeting appeared nervous and quickly got to her point: "We're having trouble with the specialists because they won't tell us what's *really* going on with our father." Dr. E asked for others' understanding of Mr. Termillo's prognosis. Mrs. Termillo said she understood her husband was going to die but she did not know how soon. The other adult children split on whether they believed there was any hope. One in particular said she was "not going to sit there and just let him die." Mr. Termillo sat through the meeting passively. When asked his own feeling about his prognosis, he said "I don't know."

Dr. E spent the rest of the conference reviewing the reports from both specialists, presenting their differing points of view as well as the available statistics for the particular stage of Mr. Termillo's cancer. As everyone was encouraged to air their feelings, it became more clear that much of the pent-up frustration and anger about Mr. Termillo's illness was being directed at the medical system. At this point, Mr. Termillo asked, "Dr. E, do you think I will die from this?" Dr. E said, "Given the reports from the specialists and the statistics from others with your disease, in all likelihood I believe you will. Whether that will be in 6 months or in several years, we do not know right now."

Dr. E then talked about the difficulty of dealing with an uncertain prognosis and how important it was for the family to continue to support and communicate with each other during this time. Dr. E offered to more actively coordinate Mr. Termillo's care, and rescheduled a follow-up appointment for Mr. and Mrs. Termillo for the next month. Mrs. Termillo agreed to be the primary person to dispense information coming from Dr. E. However, it was clear that the adult children did not entirely trust their stepmother to communicate all the information to them. Dr. E encouraged all the conference participants to communicate directly with him if they had questions that went unanswered. Dr. E said another family conference might be useful sometime in the future, and suggested that anyone at this conference could call and request it. Mr. Termillo appeared visibly relieved and thanked Dr. E for meeting with his family as he left the office.

Ongoing family dynamics and important unresolved issues are frequently highlighted around a terminal diagnosis. Having a shortage of time with a loved one can result in people wanting some resolution to long-term feelings or problems. As a primary care physician, facilitating this kind of resolution can be very meaningful for the patient and the family. For example, in the follow-up session with Dr. E, Mrs. Termillo complained that her husband would not talk with her about his feelings. It turned out that this was a longstanding complaint of Mrs. Termillo's, and one she felt desperate to change in their final months together. By providing some support and communication guidelines, Dr. E was able to help the Termillos talk with each other about Mr. Termillo's illness. The couple then reported feeling closer to each other than they had in years. This was a case where primary care counseling was appropriate and effective. When the conflict is more severe and/or jeopardizes the medical treatment of the patient, a referral to a family therapist may be necessary. In these more severe cases, the goal may be to help the family pull together enough to work through the issues around the dying person.

"It would help me to discuss what kind of medical care you would like should you become extremely ill"

Treatment planning with patients and families around a terminal illness allows everyone to confront the reality of an impending death and to participate in and feel some control over the medical care process. Issues range from whether patients prefer another round of chemotherapy or surgery, to questions of hospice care or whether they wish to be resuscitated if they arrest in the hospital. Most often decisions made to limit medical treatment occur because further treatment is viewed as futile. These decisions can involve weighing the risk of premature death against the risk of prolonged, painful life without dignity. Often these choices should be understood as more ethical than medical (6), and should be made by the patient in consultation with family members.

Negotiations around treatment planning are easiest to accomplish when the physician has had a previous relationship with the patient and family. These discussions tend to be sensitive and emotionally charged. The physician can be most effective when he or she can draw on knowledge of the patient and family's history prior to any crisis. Ideally, prior to any serious illness the physician has discussed with the patient his or her wishes regarding medical care should a catastrophic accident or illness occur (6,7). While these discussions are useful with any patient, they are especially important with elderly patients, patients with chronic illness, or patients facing serious surgery. From an ethical perspective, any decision to limit treatment is best made by the patient, rather than the family or the physician, hence the value of the patient having a "living will." In spite of the compelling reasons to have such discussions with healthy patients, it is rarely done, perhaps because of time constraints in a busy practice, because of the physician's own denial and avoidance of death, out of fear of causing depression or anxiety in patients, or for lack of interactional skills or experience (7). It is possible that having such a discussion will result in the patient becoming depressed, anxious, or resistant, so sensitivity, timing, and support are crucial to a successful interaction of this sort. The following are suggestions to facilitate the **discussion of terminal treatment guidelines in the ambulatory setting:**

1. While taking a routine genogram, ask **"Who in your family do you turn to for support?"** Follow up by asking, "Should you become seriously ill or injured, would that be the person you would like me to consult regarding treatment decisions?" (8).

2. At that point, or at a later session, ask about the patient's own wishes for treatment: "Although you are healthy now and we do not expect anything to happen, **it would be helpful to know what your wishes are about your medical care should something catastrophic happen** and you were unable to tell me what your wishes were at that time."

3. **Be as specific as possible:** "If your lung disease worsened so that I thought that you would never be able to breathe on your own again, would you want to be on a respirator?" "If your heart stopped beating or you stopped breathing, would you want us to start your heart again or put you on a machine to breathe for you?"

4. **Emphasize that the patient's input is helpful to you** and allows you to be the best doctor you can be for him or her.

5. **Encourage the patient to discuss his or her wishes with family members and other loved ones.** "As difficult as it might be, it also might be useful to discuss these issues with your family while you are healthy and well."

6. **Introduce the idea of a "living will."** "Some people feel so strongly about what they do and do not want done for them in the event that they cannot make decisions, they have written living wills. Do you feel strongly about this?" If so, suggest a written living will, which should:

   a. be as specific as possible regarding such possibilities as respiratory support, nutritional support, antibiotics, and resuscitation
   b. name a surrogate or proxy who can have final authority, in consultation with other family members, to make unforeseen treatment decisions
   c. contain the signatures of two witnesses
   d. be updated yearly and/or prior to any hospitalization
   e. be copied and given to family members and the primary care physician (9)

Knowing a patient's preferences is in everyone's best interest. One study asked healthy elderly people whether they wished their preferences about terminal medical care (maximal vs. comfort care) to be recorded in their charts. The researchers found that while not all patients could render a decision, the majority did have a preference they wished to be recorded (10). Most terminal patients, whether young or old, want to participate in treatment planning.

> Mr. Rione was a 36-year-old man with a homosexual lifestyle who had been diagnosed HIV positive. With some difficulty, Mr. Rione decided to inform his family of his health status in the interest of trying to bridge some hard feelings that had arisen when he had revealed his sexual preference some ten years before. Mr. Rione used his primary care physician, Dr. Z, as a support and a sounding board during this period of time. As part of the process of discussing the uncertain course of this potential illness, Dr. Z also discussed how Mr. Rione, his lover, and his family could participate in treatment planning should he become symptomatic or seriously ill. Dr. Z described some of the potential treatments that are available for people who develop HIV syndromes, and solicited Mr. Rione's questions or concerns. She also emphasized that Mr. Rione was currently not symptomatic, may remain well indefinitely, and that research is very active in this area so that new treatments are likely to develop that are unknown now.

Once a patient becomes terminally ill, the hypothetical issues about treatment guidelines become a reality that must be faced. Hopefully, a family conference can be held to discuss these issues while the patient is still competent. The following are **guidelines for a family conference focused on terminal treatment planning:**

1. After a preliminary discussion with the patient, invite all family members the patient wishes to attend. Ask the family if they want to include their priest, minister, or rabbi in these discussions.

2. Join with all the participants. Then begin the conference by asking about less difficult issues, such as the current medical treatment, and move on to more highly charged issues, such as new prognostic information or questions about life-prolonging care.

3. Address the relevant medical issues, such as
   • What are the treatment options?
   • What does the treatment offer the patient?
   • What are the probabilities of success and failure?
   • Will the treatment cause additional illness?(11)

4. Solicit questions to help decide how much and what kind of medical information the patient and family want. It is easy to present medical information in a way that heavily influences the outcome of a patient or family's treatment decisions, so be as straightforward as possible and acknowledge personal biases that may affect the way the information is given. Be careful not to medicalize what are actually ethical issues.

5. Help the patient and/or family weigh potentially good outcomes against potentially undesirable ones.

6. Help both patient and family stay focused on the patient's personal goals as primary in this process.

7. Work on being as nonanxious as possible in the room. These discussions are most frequently highly emotional for the participants, and benefit from facilitation by someone who is clear and calm.

8. Use clear, jargon-free language. Be a supportive, active listener. Track others' communications and clarify confusing statements made by any participant. Care needs to be taken to attend to communication issues in general because the likelihood of someone misinterpreting another's statements or intentions in this emotionally charged situation is high.

9. Model an ability to tolerate the ambiguity and uncertainty that accompanies all these decisions.

10. Communicate a willingness to sustain contact with the patient and the family regardless of their treatment decisions.

Many people are reluctant to limit medical therapy because they equate it with limiting care for the patient. Assure the patient and the family that all supportive care by the staff will be appropriately aggressive, including providing adequate pain control, attending to bladder and bowel functions, discontinuing unnecessary treatments, allowing lengthy or unlimited visiting hours, providing opportunities for the patient to talk (or be silent), and generally showing a high level of patient care (7). Miles suggests that patients or families that respond to discussions around treatment planning with "Do everything!" should be understood as saying "Slow down, give us more time to understand what you are saying" or "Show us that you care and won't abandon us at this time when our options are so profoundly limited" (11). Regardless of the decisions that are made concerning treatment, it is important to let the family know that their physician will stand by them and will not withdraw during their difficult time.

Dr. D requested a family conference after Mr. Mount's discharge from his third hospitalization for chronic obstructive pulmonary disease. The Mount family included the elderly Mr. and Mrs. Mount and their single adult daughter who lived with them. The family had a history of difficult medical and psychiatric problems: Mrs. Mount had cardiac arrhythmias and mild congestive heart failure. The daughter, Nadine, had perplexing neurologic symptoms as well as severe bulimia. The family was known for their resistance to medical intervention and their devotion to each other. In arranging the conference, Dr. D suggested the family bring the home health aide whom they had come to accept and trust. Dr. D invited the psychological consultant who had attended previous family conferences around other important family decisions.

The family arrived nervous but talkative with Mr. Mount in his wheelchair. Dr. D reviewed how Mr. Mount was doing at home. The patient reported that he was doing fine, only worried about the health of his wife and his daughter.

Mrs. Mount complained that her husband was too dependent and would not try any small task without help. The daughter and the home health aide agreed. The consultant talked this over with Mr. Mount and discovered that he rarely even tried to walk because he was certain of failure, he feared being a burden to his family, and he felt to ask for help ahead of time was "unmanly." The family agreed with the consultant that Mr. Mount was a very proud man. They worked out some signals for him to acknowledge he needed their help early in a task so that he could "be less of a burden to the family in the end."

Following this problem-solving discussion, Dr. D asked Mr. Mount and the family for help in planning treatment guidelines for the next time he needed to go into the hospital. She asked Mr. Mount if he wished to go on a respirator if that was warranted. Mr. Mount was evasive and ambiguous in his answer, saying he did not think this would happen and if it did, his family could decide. Nadine left the room at this point, saying she had to go to the bathroom to vomit. Mrs. Mount refused to comment. With support from the consultant, she said she did not want to be responsible for her husband's treatment decisions because she had been the responsible party when her sister was critically ill and incompetent and it had been a very difficult role for her. Dr. D said this was why it was important to discuss these issues now. Mr. Mount agreed this experience had been difficult for his wife. With a lot of support and information, he was able to decide he would like to go on a respirator should he have respiratory failure, but that he did not want to have cardiac resuscitation should he arrest in the hospital. The daughter returned to the room during this discussion, and both she and her mother agreed to support Mr. Mount's decisions.

To summarize, the best situation occurs when a patient, in conjunction with family members, is able to express his or her preferences regarding treatment decisions. If the patient is unable to communicate and has not previously made his or her wishes known, the burden of responsibility falls almost completely to the family members. In one recent study 86% of families of incompetent patients made these decisions (12). Treatment decisions can be difficult for families to negotiate without considerable support and information from the medical staff. The physician may wish to keep in mind the following **principles that guide a family conference for terminal treatment planning in which a patient is unable to participate:**

1. Keep the care, comfort, and concern for the patient primary.
2. Include all available family members in the conference.
3. Hold the conference at the patient's bedside. Even if the patient is comatose, having the discussion with the patient there makes the decisions more real and diminishes family members' sense of guilt about having to decide about their loved one's treatment.
4. Recognize the family's pain, and acknowledge the difficulty of the process.

Patients and families can respond to these discussions about limiting treatment in one of several ways. Bedell et al. found that families were most likely to choose to limit treatment, especially to write a Do Not Resuscitate order, under the following conditions: when the patient was in a coma or brain dead, when physicians and staff supported and reassured them that this was the appropriate decision, when they were assured that the staff would maintain the patient's medical care and comfort, when the patient had expressed a previous wish to the family regarding care, and when they were told the orders could be changed (12). The age of the patient, severity of the illness, and degree of patient suffering did not predict these family members' decisions.

Some family members clearly and unambivalently want "everything" done to keep their loved one alive. Others appear ambivalent, but unable to decide to limit treatment as they seem to view any restriction as abandonment or even murder. These family members may try very hard to get the medical staff to make these decisions for them or they may demand aggressive treatment because of their own feelings of sadness, denial, fear, anger, guilt, or abandonment. Many of these reactions change over time with a focus on making the patient's needs primary, so it is important to have discussions periodically both to update family members on any new medical information and to allow people to express changes that have occurred in their own thinking.

> Mrs. Katz had been hospitalized for 10 days, but her fevers were still uncontrolled. This was her fourth hospitalization in the last six months. With dementia and Parkinsonism, complete incontinence, recurrent infections and deep decubiti ulcers unsuccessfully treated with surgery, death seemed inevitable to her physician and hospital staff. Dr. S initiated a discussion of limiting treatment with the patients' two daughters at their mother's bedside. Adele, the younger daughter, had been unusually attentive and involved. She was always available, left two or three phone numbers, visited daily, and made lists of questions and suggestions about her mother's treatment. Observing this painful daily decline, she reluctantly came to accept her mother's impending death as a certainty and favored writing Do Not Resuscitate orders. Her sister, Robin, was a much less frequent visitor and was often unreachable because of her long and unpredictable work hours. Her ideas were relayed to Dr. S by Adele, accompanied by barely disguised anger, as Robin maintained that she could not "give up on Mom."
>
> When Dr. S finally met with Robin and Adele, Robin expressed bitter frustration at a previous physician's lack of consideration in never consulting her about her father's care the previous year, when he was "allowed to just die." Until Dr. S could have a family conference and meet with these daughters together, he was unable to resolve the issues around treatment planning for their mother. By encouraging them to talk together about what their mother would have wanted and what was in her best interest, Robin slowly agreed that limiting treatment was the best option available. Dr. S encouraged both daughters to visit their mother frequently and reassured them she would get the best available care from the staff.

"I need to inform you that your loved one has died"

Notifying family members about the death of a loved one is a difficult, stressful task. Direct, sensitive communication makes it more likely family members will hear the message clearly. Prior discussions with a family about an expected death make this situation generally easier to deal with than that of an unexpected death. The following are **suggestions for notifying the family about a death:**

1. Encourage the family to be present at the time of death if at all possible. One study demonstrated that a majority of family members were grateful to be present during a resuscitation attempt for their relative (13). Any action that helps family members participate in and acknowledge their loved one's death may be useful.

2. When the family is expecting the death of one of its members, ask how they would prefer to be notified if they are not present.

3. Notify the family immediately at the time of death.
   a. With an expected death, call on the family as previously agreed upon.
   b. With an unexpected death, ask the family as a whole to come to the hospital and discuss the events leading up to the death.

4. While being sympathetic and sensitive, avoid euphemisms. Use the words "death, dying, and dead" rather than "passed away" or other colloquial sayings.

5. Say "You have my sympathy" rather than "I am sorry," which could be construed as an apology.

6. Give the family the opportunity to view the body and say their good-byes.
   a. Arrange for the viewing to occur in a private room.
   b. Make sure the body has been cleaned and prepared, so that wounds have been dressed, blood stains removed, and the body draped and placed in an appropriate position.
   c. Offer to have a member of the health care team stay with the family, especially if only one member is present.
   d. Allow them to remain with the deceased as long as they wish (14,15).

7. Meet with the family.
   a. This may occur before or after the viewing. Either way, it is an important step in showing concern and facilitating a healthy early grieving process.
   b. Provide information about the cause of death. Solicit and answer any questions.
   c. Make any requests for autopsy or organ donations at this time. Clarify the reasons for the request, particularly when there is uncertainty about the diagnosis.

    d. Use active listening skills. Expect and tolerate expressions of intense emotions, especially with a family who learns of an unexpected death. Do not exclude family members who become very upset or emotional. Avoid psychotropic medications in this situation.

    e. Make yourself available as a support for the family. Suggest a follow-up meeting to discuss autopsy results or questions about the deceased that are likely to arise in the future.

    f. Remind the family to call their funeral director.

    g. Encourage the family to include children, especially those over 5 years old, in the funeral and other family gatherings.

8. Send a sympathy card to the family, or attend the wake or funeral.

9. Telephone the family 1–2 weeks after the death to inquire about them, answer any questions, and schedule a follow-up appointment.

"What did I do wrong?"

One of the most difficult aspects of dealing with a patient's death is the physician's own feelings. Though in a different and much less intimate role than that of a family member, the health care provider may also experience feelings of sadness, loss, anger, or guilt. In addition to facilitating the grief process for the family, the provider also needs to attend to his or her own grief and acknowledge his or her own feelings. Rituals such as saying good-bye to the deceased and attending the funeral when possible (16) allow for the emotional side of being a doctor to be nourished and utilized.

Especially with an unexpected death, or the death of a young person, the physician usually examines the patient's history and course of treatment to determine any professional failures on his or her part. This process can be important and useful if it is seen as an opportunity to learn from the careful examination of a case rather than to perpetuate perfectionist, superhuman standards for providing medical care. At those times when mistakes have been made, it is important to face them squarely and create opportunities for confession and forgiveness (17). Discussing the case with trusted colleagues can be both educational and cathartic, especially if uncertainty and guilt remain prominent feelings over a period of time after a patient death (3).

"To feel pain and sadness at this time is a normal, healthy response"

Primary care grief counseling offers significant opportunities for medical providers to encourage healthy grieving and prevent pathological or unresolved grief reactions. In the event of sudden, unexpected death, the supportive role of the primary care physician can be especially important (18). Even in these cases, the usual grief response is time-limited and somewhat predictable in its phases. Normal grieving is characterized by intellectual and emotional awareness of the loss and feelings of guilt, stress, pain, anger, and hostility (19). Grief is typically a cyclical process in which all these feelings may be present at any time, but certain feelings may dominate at different points in the cycle. The acute phase begins with the notification of death and is characterized by emotional shock. This phase typically lasts for up to two weeks. Depression and somatic symptoms are common and persist into the second phase, characterized by rumination over memories of the deceased. During this phase, people may withdraw and become introverted as they examine what the recent death means for their own life. This process typically takes from 3–6 months. The third and final phase is the resolution phase. At this time, somatic symptoms and preoccupation with the deceased lessens. Bereaved family members begin to plan for the future and participate again in activities that were an important part of their lives prior to the death. The resolution phase is punctuated by the anniversary of the loved one's death. After this period, which often involves a temporary increase in grief or symptomatology, most people are able to move on.

The following are **principles for primary care grief counseling:**

1. Schedule an office visit at 6–8 weeks with interested family members to review the death and the autopsy results.

2. Encourage family members to talk about the circumstances surrounding the death, recall memories, and openly discuss feelings of sadness, anger, and guilt. Give them permission to grieve.

3. Inquire about any significant changes in financial status. Settling an estate, the loss of income, and the lack of experience managing money can intensify the grieving process.

4. Normalize signs of grieving, such as crying spells, lack of energy, and preoccupation with the deceased. Tell the family that normal or uncomplicated grief typically takes at least a year for the active phase to resolve.

5. Avoid the use of psychotropic medication, such as sedatives or hypnotics, except in very unusual circumstances. A sedated person at a funeral may not be able to participate or even remember this important time. Starting antidepressant, antianxiety, or antipsychotic medications are rarely indicated during bereavement.

6. Monitor the medical status of the recently bereaved closely as research indicates that the bereaved are at higher risk of serious illness and death. (See Chapter 2.) Encourage family members to come in for a health evaluation at 3 months to assess any increased risk for illness or delayed difficulties with grieving.

7. Refer interested family members to community-based self-help support groups, such as the Widow-to-Widow group, the group for parents of

Table 14.1.   Signs and Symptoms of an Unresolved Grief Reaction

---

1. Prolonged, severe clinical depression (that is, a pervasive sense of worthlessness and self-blame lasting longer than 12–18 months)
2. Prolonged social isolation, withdrawal, or alienation
3. Emotional numbing in which the patient largely denies an emotional reaction to the loss, resulting in a kind of wooden or flat emotional presentation
4. An inability to cry
5. Talking as if the dead person were still alive
6. Persistent compulsive overactivity without a sense of loss
7. Persistence of a variety of physical complaints, such as headaches, fatigue, dizziness or multiple injuries
8. Profound identification with the deceased and prolonged acquisition of symptoms belonging to the illness of that person
9. Extreme, persistent anger (may be directed at the physician)
10. Alcohol or drug abuse, persistent requests for sedative or narcotic medications
11. Marital or family problems (can be especially prominent after the death of a child, but not uncommon after the death of an elderly parent)
12. Work or school problems

SIDS children, or any of the many other illness-focused support groups. Support and information from those who have experienced a similar loss themselves can be extremely helpful to the bereaved.

8. Monitor family members for signs of unresolved grief reaction (19–21). (See Table 14.1.) Refer if necessary.

Prolonged and extreme reactions to grief are themselves dangerous and necessitate referral to a specialist. Such a referral is best made to both the person with the symptoms and that person's family. Referral may be made for evaluation, bereavement counseling, psychiatric treatment, or family therapy, as is appropriate.

The following example describes a close married couple from the time of the acute phase of the husband's illness to the year following his death.

> Mrs. Stowe had cared for her husband for over 20 years. He was blind and suffered from Alzheimer's Disease. Over the previous year he had become increasingly difficult to care for; he became incontinent and began wandering at night. His normally cheerful mood changed gradually as he became more irritable and resisted any assistance. After being struck by him on several occasions, Mrs. Stowe decided she could no longer care for him at home. She had kept him with her in their small apartment with few services long past the point when most families would have institutionalized a demented elderly member. She herself was 84 years old, and the physical and emotional stress of caring for her husband was beginning to affect her health. Her three children had been encouraging her for several years to arrange for placement.
>
> Because the couple had significant savings, Mr. Stowe was placed in a nearby nursing home within a month of Mrs. Stowe's decision. She became quite depressed shortly after he left home. Their family physician, Dr. C,

encouraged her to visit him regularly and ventilate her feelings. She spent most of her day with her husband in the nursing home, but continued to feel that she had betrayed him. Now she felt she had nothing worthwhile to do with herself.

Several months after his admission, he suffered a massive stroke and died within a week. Mrs. Stowe became increasingly depressed over the next 6 months, grieving over his death and feeling that her life, which had been spent caring first for her children and then for her husband, was now worthless. Her family tried to cheer her up, which only made her feel that they did not understand her grief. Efforts to get her involved in social activities in the apartment house where she lived were unsuccessful because she viewed any social activities as "a waste of time."

A month after Mr. Stowe's death, Dr. C met with Mrs. Stowe, her children and several of her grandchildren, who were concerned about Mrs. Stowe's emotional state. Dr. C explained that the intensity of Mrs. Stowe's grief was testimony to what a special relationship the couple had, and that to give up that grief too soon would seem to Mrs. Stowe to be dishonoring her husband. He encouraged Mrs. Stowe's children to share their memories of their father and how much they also missed him with their mother.

Dr. C met with Mrs. Stowe every 3 months for the first year of bereavement. At 6 months, he began to encourage her to get involved in volunteer work where she could help and care for other people. A year after her husband's death, Mrs. Stowe's grief and depression had begun to lift. She was doing some volunteer work at a local hospital and felt she had found some meaning in her life. Her spirits were improved though she continued to miss her husband deeply.

Grief typically sends "shock waves" throughout a family system (22). The goal of primary care management of terminal illness, death, and grieving is to channel these shock waves so they can have a restorative effect, and to monitor their influence to prevent future disruption or symptomatology.

References

1. Becker B: *The Denial of Death*. New York, MacMillan Publishing Co., 1973.
2. Servalli EP: The dying patient, the physician, and the fear of death. *New Eng J Med* 1988;**319**:1728–1730.
3. McDaniel SH, Bank J, Campbell T, Mancini J, Shore B: Using a group as a consultant. In Wynne LC, McDaniel SH, Weber T (eds.): *Systems Consultation*. New York, Guilford Press, 1986.
4. Holmes TH, Rahe RH: The social readjustment scale. *J Psychosom Research* 1967;**11**:213–218.
5. Fuller RL, Geis S: Communicating with the grieving family. *J Fam Pract* 1985;**21**:139–144.
6. Schneiderman LJ, Arias JD: Counseling patients to counsel physicians on future care in the event of patient incompetence. *Ann Intern Med* 1985;**102**:693–698.

7. Lo B, Jonsen AR: Clinical decisions to limit treatment. *Ann Intern Med* 1980;**93**:764–768.

8. Maher E: Establishing treatment guidelines in geriatric patients. Family Medicine Grand Rounds, University of Rochester School of Medicine, Rochester, New York, March 31, 1988.

9. Concern for Dying: *A Living Will*. New York, Concern for Dying, 1983.

10. Snow RM, Atwood K: Probable death: Perspective of the elderly. *South Med J* 1985;**78**:851–853.

11. Miles SH: The limited treatment plan: Part II, planning with patients and their families. *Clin Rep Aging* 1987;**1**:14–16.

12. Bedell SE, Pelle D, Maher PL, Clearly PD: Do-Not-Resuscitate orders for critically ill patients in the hospital: How are they used and what is their impact? *JAMA* 1986;**256**:233–237.

13. Doyle CJ, Post H, Burney RE, Malno J, Keefe M, Rhee KJ: Family participation during resuscitation: An option. *Ann Emerg Med* 1987;**16**:673–675.

14. Tolle S, Elliot D and Girard D: How to manage patient death and care for the bereaved. *Postgrad Med* 1985;**78**(2):87–95.

15. Engel GL: Grief and grieving. In Schwartz LH, Schwartz JL (eds.): *The Psychodynamics of Patient Care*. New York, Prentice Hall, 1972.

16. Irvine P: The attending at the funeral. *New Engl J Med* 1985;**315**(26):120.

17. Hilfiker D: Facing our mistakes. *New Engl J Med* 1984;**310**(2):118–122.

18. Wadland WC, Keller B, Jones W, Chapados J: Sudden, unexpected death and the role of the family physician. *Fam Syst Med* 1988;**6**(2):176–187.

19. Lindemann E: Symptomatology and management of acute grief. *Am J Psychiatry* 1944;**101**:141.

20. Brown JT, Stoudemire GA: Normal and pathological grief. *JAMA* 1983;**250**(3):378–382.

21. Pasnau RO, Fawzy FI, Fawzy N: Role of the physician in bereavement. *Psychiat Clin North Am* 1987;**10**(1):109–120.

22. Bowen M: Family reaction to death, In, P Guerin (ed.): *Family Therapy*. New York, Gardner Press, 1976.

PROTOCOL

Talking to Patients and Families about Terminal Illness, Treatment Planning, and Grief

Communicating a Terminal Diagnosis

1. Communicate directly to the patient about the diagnosis, the care, and the prognosis of the illness.
2. Avoid giving an overly optimistic or overly pessimistic prognosis. Be honest and straightforward about the information as you know it.
3. Look the patient in the eye and speak calmly. Repeat the message several times.
4. Avoid arguments over the diagnosis, or other maneuvers that distract from the message itself.
5. Set up another appointment to answer questions that will inevitably arise when the initial reaction wears off.
6. Repeat this process with the family present.
7. Allow people their depression or anger rather than trying to reassure them or brighten their mood.
8. Meet regularly with the patient and family to discuss care, prognosis, and individual's emotional reactions, even when the medical care is managed by a specialist.

Treatment Planning for a Terminal Illness

A. Discussing terminal treatment guidelines in the ambulatory setting

1. While taking a routine genogram, ask "Who in your family do you turn to for support?" Follow up by asking, "Should you become seriously ill or injured, would that be the person you would like me to consult regarding treatment decisions?"
2. At that point, or at a later session, ask about the patient's own wishes.
3. Be as specific as possible.
4. If your state has a law regulating "Do Not Resuscitate" orders, briefly describe the law to the patient.
5. Emphasize that their input is helpful to you and allows you to be the best doctor you can be for them.
6. Encourage the patient to also discuss their wishes with family members and other loved ones.
7. Discuss the idea of a "living will."

B. Guidelines for terminal treatment planning at a family conference

1. After a preliminary discussion with the patient, invite all family members the patient wishes to attend. Ask the family if they want to include their priest, minister, or rabbi in these discussions.
2. Join with all the participants. Then begin the conference by asking about less difficult issues and move on to more highly charged issues, such as life-prolonging care.
3. Address the relevant medical issues.
4. Solicit questions to help decide how much and what kind of medical information to provide.
5. Help the patient and/or family weigh potentially good outcomes against potentially undesirable ones.
6. Help both patient and family stay focused on the *patient's* personal goals as primary in this process.
7. Work on being a nonanxious presence in the room.
8. Use clear, jargon-free language. Be a supportive, active listener.
9. Model an ability to tolerate the ambiguity and uncertainty that accompanies all these decisions.
10. Communicate a willingness to sustain contact with the patient and the family regardless of their treatment decisions.

C. Principles for terminal treatment planning at a family conference in which a patient is unable to participate

1. Keep the care, comfort, and concern for the patient primary.
2. Include all available family in the conference.
3. Hold the conference at the patient's bedside.
4. Recognize the family's pain, and acknowledge the difficulty of the process.

Notifying the Family about a Death

1. Allow the family to be present at the time of death if at all possible.
2. When the family is expecting the death of one of its members, ask how they would prefer to be notified if they are not present.
3. Notify the family immediately at the time of death.
4. While being sympathetic and sensitive, avoid euphemisms. Use the words "death, dying, and dead."
5. Say "You have my sympathy" rather than "I am sorry," which could be construed as an apology.
6. Give the family the opportunity to view the body and say their good-byes.

7. Meet with the family.
   a. Before or after the viewing, meet with the family to show concern and facilitate a healthy early grieving process.
   b. Provide information about the cause of death. Solicit and answer any questions.
   c. Make any requests for autopsy or organ donations at this time. Clarify the reasons for the request, particularly when there is uncertainty about the diagnosis.
   d. Use active listening skills. Expect expressions of intense emotions.
   e. Make yourself available as a support for the family. Offer to have follow-up meetings, either to discuss autopsy results or questions about the deceased that will likely arise in the future.
   f. Remind the family to call their funeral director.
8. Send a sympathy card to the family, or attend the wake or funeral.
9. Telephone the family 1–2 weeks after the death to inquire about them, answer any questions, and encourage any necessary follow-up.

Primary Care Grief Counseling

1. Schedule an office visit at 6–8 weeks with interested family members to review the autopsy results.
2. Encourage family members to talk about the circumstances surrounding the death, recall memories, and openly discuss feelings of sadness, anger, and guilt.
3. Inquire about any significant changes in financial status.
4. Normalize signs of grieving during the first year, such as crying spells, lack of energy, and preoccupation with the deceased.
5. Avoid the use of psychotropic medication, such as sedatives or hypnotics, except when previously prescribed or in very atypical circumstances.
6. Monitor the medical status of the recently bereaved. Encourage family members to come in for a health evaluation at 3 months to evaluate any increased risk for illness or delayed difficulties with grieving.
7. Refer interested family members to community-based self-help support groups for those who have recently lost a loved one.
8. Monitor family members for signs of unresolved grief reaction. Refer if necessary.

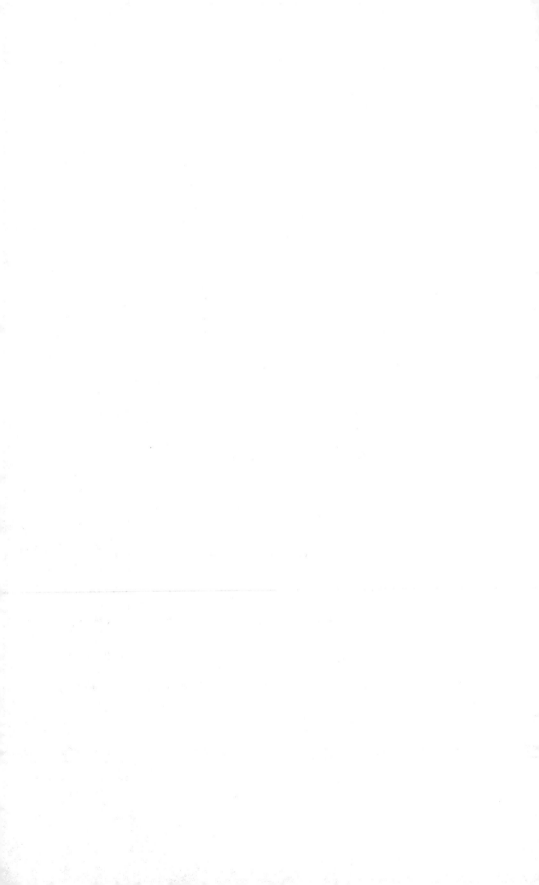

A Family-Oriented Approach to Specific Medical Problems

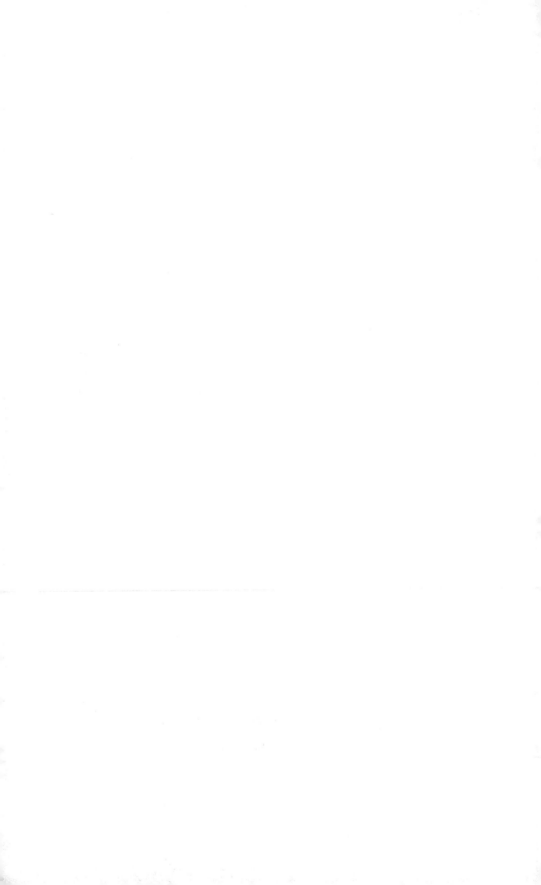

CHAPTER 15

The Developmental Challenges of Chronic Illness

Helping Patients and Families Cope

Most families must face chronic illness in a family member at some time during the life cycle. Chronic illness is increasing in prevalence and has replaced acute illness as the major cause of morbidity and mortality in the United States (1). Half of all people over age 65 and one fourth of those between ages 45 and 65 are limited in their activities by at least one chronic condition (2). As the elderly population grows, this burden of chronic illness increases, and families must play an even greater role in their care. (See Chapter 13 on caring for the elderly.) The experience of chronic illness affects families in profound ways, and how well the family adapts to chronic illness can influence the course of the illness (3). This chapter presents a comprehensive psychoeducational approach to working with families with chronic physical illness, to assess their needs and assist them in coping with illness. (Other chapters deal with family-oriented approach to chronic mental illness including depression, Chapter 17, and alcohol abuse, Chapter 18.)

Families, not health care providers, are the primary caretakers for patients with chronic illness. They are the ones that help most with the physical demands of an illness, ranging from preparing special meals for a family member with heart disease, to assisting with insulin administration for a diabetic, to running a home dialysis machine. In addition families are usually the major source of emotional and social support: someone to share the frustrations, discouragements, and despair of living with chronic illness.

Chronic illness affects all aspects of family life. Old and familiar patterns of family life are changed forever, shared activities are given up, and family roles and responsibilities must often change. Most patients and their families cope well with the stresses and demands of chronic illness, and tend to pull together and become closer (4). Some families may become too close or enmeshed; by assuming too much responsibility and care for an ill member, they may inhibit his or her autonomy and independence. Other families may pull apart under the stress of chronic illness and even disintegrate through divorce (5), institutionalization, or death. The spouses of chronically ill patients often have as much subjective distress as the patients themselves (6). It is easy for health care providers focused on the "patient" to overlook the spouse's distress and not attend to their physical and emotional needs (7). The failure of health professionals to address the needs of family members as well as patients can lead to a downward cycle: the family becomes more distressed and is less able to respond to the needs of the patient, who may then deteriorate physically and emotionally, and put more stress and demands upon the family, leading finally to burnout of the family. By addressing the needs and stresses of the family as well as the patient, the physician can help promote the healthiest functioning of all concerned. This can be best done by establishing a partnership with the families and supporting them as coproviders of care.

Characteristics of Families with Chronic Illness

From their work with families with different chronic illnesses, Steinglass and his colleagues have described four common characteristics of these families (8):

1. The illness and its demands tend to dominate family life, and other family needs are neglected. This response is initially adaptive as the family copes with the crisis, but leads to family disruption over the long term.

2. Family coalitions between the patient and one or more family members develop, or previous coalitions are intensified by the chronic illness. For example, a mother may become overinvolved in the care of her ill child and the father may withdraw or be excluded (9).

3. The family's coping response often becomes rigid, and the family fears that any change may adversely affect the family and their current adjustment.

4. Families tend to isolate themselves in coping with the illness demands.

The primary task for families with chronic illness is to create a balance between the needs of the individual with the illness and those of the rest of the family. The following example illustrates some of the problems and challenges of coping with a serious chronic illness.

Jim Strong had not felt well since he was in his mid-twenties, but it was not until he was 32 and lost part of his vision in one eye, that the diagnosis of multiple sclerosis was made. He had attributed his chronic fatigue and depression to his dissatisfaction and stresses working as a machinist on an assembly line. His primary care physician had initially diagnosed his leg weakness and gait disturbance as a herniated lumbar disc. He and his 30-year-old wife, Harriet, had undergone sex therapy for his impotence. Although therapy helped their sexual relationship, his erections did not return. Their four and six year old boys did not understand what was happening to their father who no longer wrestled with them after work or carried them around on his shoulders. The youngest, Timmy, began having behavior problems at nursery school.

Jim and Harriet's relief at knowing what was "wrong" was balanced by the lack of effective treatment and poor prognosis. Over the next few years, Jim was in and out of the hospital with acute exacerbations of the illness. Initially he recovered from each new neurological deficit, and he and his family maintained hope that he would stabilize. However, gradually he became more disabled and had to quit his job when he could no longer safely work on the assembly line. Harriet returned to work as a librarian, and Jim stayed at home to care for the children after school. With reduced income and the loss of medical insurance from Jim's job, the family was forced to move out of their home and into a smaller apartment.

With time, family life revolved more and more around Jim's illness. There was no longer time or money for going out to movies or restaurants, and many of their friends stopped asking them over for meals. Jim was self-conscious about using a walker in public and stopped going out to the grocery store or to the children's school. Harriet worried constantly about Jim's health and encouraged him to rest as much as possible. At the same time she resented how little housework he did, and felt physically and emotionally burdened by all of her responsibilities. She began developing migraine headaches that occasionally incapacitated her.

This case illustrates many of the challenges of chronic illness and the importance of assessing the patient in the context of the family.

A careful assessment of the patient and the family and their adaptation to the chronic illness is crucial to helping all parties cope with the illness. This assessment occurs over many visits with the patient and family, but usually requires convening the entire family at least once. This family conference is useful at the time of the diagnosis of the illness, or during the initial hospitalization (see Chapter 21). Meeting with the entire family is also helpful early in the chronic phase of the illness, when the initial crisis is over, and the family has settled into the day to day demands of living with chronic illness.

From his work with chronically ill patients and their families, Rolland (10) has developed a clinically useful family systems model of chronic illness. We have organized our assessment of the illness and the family around this model.

Chronic Illness and Its Psychosocial Demands

Physicians are well trained in assessing and managing the biomedical aspects of chronic illness: monitoring blood sugar control, adjusting medication, identifying and treating complications, but are less well prepared to deal with the psychosocial aspects of illness. Each illness is viewed idiosyncratically with different kinds of stresses for each illness. Rolland's psychosocial typology of chronic illness organizes their similarities and allows for important distinctions across illnesses. The typology calls for an assessment of the following areas:

1. Onset: Did the illness begin suddenly or gradually? Illnesses with acute onset such as strokes or spinal cord injuries require rapid mobilization of resources and put enormous acute stress on a family. Illnesses with gradual onset such as lupus or arthritis allow families more time to adapt, but may create great uncertainty and anxiety.

2. Course: Is the illness progressive, constant or relapsing? For slowly progressive diseases such as chronic obstructive pulmonary disease or AIDS, there is a gradual increase in stress on the family with the need for continual adaptation and role changes. With constant course illnesses, such as strokes or amputations, the family attempts to cope with a stable change. Illnesses with relapses such as hemophilia or asthma require that the family shift back and forth from crisis orientation to chronic adaptation. These illnesses demand the most flexibility.

3. Prognosis: Is the illness rapidly fatal, does it shorten life span, or is there a risk of sudden death? Obviously fatal illnesses, such as amyotrophic lateral sclerosis (ALS) or terminal cancer, require that the family cope with impending death. Illnesses where there is a risk of sudden death such as coronary artery disease add an additional stress of unpredictability and constant vigilance.

4. Disability: How severe are the handicaps and incapacitation associated with the illness? The degree to which the disability affects the roles and responsibilities of the patient in the family will influence how the family adapts. A physically disabling illness in a man who works as a laborer will be much more difficult for both the patient and family to cope with than a similar disability in a school teacher. Loss of cognitive abilities (such as in dementia or some strokes) is one of the most difficult burdens for the family (11).

From using this assessment, one can quickly assess the likely stresses and demands that the family faces with a chronic illness. For example, because the onset of multiple sclerosis (MS) is often gradual, there may be confusion, anxiety and sometimes denial initially, and then a paradoxical sense of relief for both patient and family when the diagnosis is finally made. If family members or health care providers have viewed the early symptoms of MS as willful or malingering, they may feel guilty when the diagnosis is made. The most challenging aspect of MS for families is its unpredictability. Patients may do very well for months or years, and then there can be a sudden worsening which will later improve. The stepwise decline that commonly occurs in MS challenges the family over the long haul, and eventually many families become overburdened and cannot care for the patient at home. Other difficult aspects of the disease are the personality changes that occur in some patients. Spouses may describe the patient as "no longer the person I married." This loss of the patient's identity or personality makes coping with all the other demands of the illness particularly difficult.

Assessing Family Functioning and Health Beliefs

This section focuses on those aspects of the family that are particularly important to assess in caring for the chronically ill.

Family Development

1. Where is the family in the family life cycle? The normal developmental tasks of a family will influence and be influenced by chronic illness (12). The impact of serious illness of a parent will be very different depending upon whether the children are very young, adolescent, or adult. Illnesses that are completely unexpected or "out of phase" such as cancer in children or multiple sclerosis in young adult, are usually the most disruptive to normal family development and the most difficult to cope with.

2. How are the developmental tasks that the family is dealing with affecting the chronic illness and vice versa? The direction a family is moving in its life cycle, whether it is pulling together ("centripetal") as during the childbearing years, or pulling apart ("centrifugal"), as when children are leaving home (13), will influence on how it deals with chronic illness. If a chronic illness occurs when a family is in a centripetal phase of development, such as families with a chronically ill child, the additional pull of the illness may lead to enmeshment in which families overreact to each other and discourage personal autonomy (12). Minuchin and colleagues (14) have described psychosomatic families of children with diabetes, asthma and anorexia nervosa, in which an extreme form of this pattern of overinvolvement exacerbates the illness.

When a chronic illness occurs when a family is in a centrifugal period, such as adolescence, the care of the chronic illness can be particularly disruptive and conflict with normal development. The patient may be pushing for autonomy while the illness demands that he or she be closely supervised. Houser (15) has described diabetes, with its demands for strict adherence to diet, exercise and insulin injects, as an "anti-adolescent" illness and has demonstrated how it can impede the adolescent's personal growth and individuation. At the next visit Dr. K explored the impact of Timmy's illness on family developmental issues.

> Dr. K knew the Strong family well from being their family physician for ten years and delivering their two children. He knew that they had developed a strong marital relationship prior to having children, but had initially had some problems parenting their first child. Jim was very strict about discipline, just as his father had been with him, and Harriet tried to compensate by being very lenient. With some brief primary care counseling, they were both able to assume more balanced roles in disciplining.
>
> After the multiple sclerosis was diagnosed, Jim and Harriet became preoccupied with Jim's health, and Timmy, the youngest son, responded by having behavioral problems both at nursery school and at home. Jim again felt that Harriet was too lenient with Timmy and became very strict and authoritarian. Timmy's behavior worsened until they brought him to Dr. K for help. In one session, Dr. K helped the parents find ways to pay special attention to both children in the midst of all the illness-related stresses. This reduced the need for either child to resort to misbehavior to get their parents' attention.

From his work with the Strongs, Dr. K learned how the demands of a chronic illness can compete with the developmental tasks of a healthy family with young children.

Family Strengths and Supports

1. What are the family's strengths and sources of support? Identifying and utilizing the strengths in families, helps the family and the health care provider feel a sense of control in managing the illness. Smilkstein's (16) acronym SCEEM (Social, Cultural, Educational, Economic, Medical) is a helpful way to remember potential sources of support for families.

2. What has helped the family to cope with crises in the past? Reviewing past crises helps identify what kinds of coping strategies have been used before and may be useful dealing with the illness.

3. How adaptable is the family to change? Has the family been able to make the necessary changes in role functioning with this illness? What are the signs of their ability to do so?

4. Does the family accept outsiders, especially health care providers, into the family to help? Some families close ranks around an ill member and are suspicious of health care providers, while other families become excessively dependent upon the health care system. This style may represent the family's way of accepting help or dealing with outsiders, or it may be the result of a previous experience with the health care system that either did not respond to the family's needs or assumed too much responsibility for their problems.

Dr. K met with the Strongs every three or four months to review Jim's medical condition and see how the family was doing. During an early session, Dr. K had the family list and discuss their strengths. These strengths were:

1. a loving and caring marital relationship
2. equal sharing of family responsibilities
3. flexibility in family roles
4. a small group of close friends
5. a supportive extended family, many of whom lived in the area
6. a good working relationship with health care professionals

Dr. K encouraged them to draw upon these strengths and support when they developed difficulties.

Family Health Beliefs

The family's beliefs about the illness, their sense of control over it, and their attitudes toward health professionals will strongly affect how they cope with the illness (17).

1. What does each family member think caused the illness? The family's beliefs about the etiology of the illness can have a powerful effect upon their response to the illness. These health beliefs are usually a combination of the family's medical knowledge about disease (e.g., an understanding of cardiac risk factors), the family's view of health and illness, and their cultural beliefs. Some common beliefs about the etiology of illness include:

• Fate or bad luck
• Blaming the individual who is ill: for not taking care of him or herself, (smoking, lack of exercise) or for misdeeds (an illegitimate birth, divorce).
• Blaming other family members: "Your drinking made me ill." "I get chest pain whenever we fight."
• Genetics: "Cancer runs in our family."
• Religion: "It's God's will."

Health beliefs may be quite idiosyncratic and specific to the disease in question. Thus a woman may believe that illness in general is largely a matter of chance, but that her husband developed heart disease because of stress at work.

2. What do family members believe they or others can do to improve the patient's health? A family's sense of control or mastery of an illness may be quite different than their beliefs about its etiology. A family may believe that the illness is the result of past misdeeds, but that there is nothing they can do to control the illness; or that the disease occurred by chance, but the individual is responsible for maintaining the best health possible. Families will also have different beliefs about how much influence the physician or medicine in general has on the illness. Some families will expect the physician to be responsible for the illness and even blame the physician when the illness is diagnosed or worsens.

> After his diagnosis, Jim read extensively about multiple sclerosis, especially its etiology and treatment. He became especially concerned whether he had been exposed to heavy metals in his job. When a coworker also developed MS, he solicited Dr. K's help in getting an occupational health expert to study the plant he worked in.
>
> Harriet became interested in dietary treatments for MS. For six months, Jim tried a gluten free diet. Although it was time consuming, expensive, and not always very tasty, the couple felt that at least they were doing something to try to get better. Although Dr. K informed them that there was no solid evidence that such a diet would help, he told them it could do no harm and was worth a try.

Multigenerational Patterns of Coping with Illness

How have previous generations responded to serious chronic physical or mental illness? The ways in which individuals and families cope with chronic illness is often passed down from one generation to another. There may be family myths, expectations, or rituals that surround illness and go back many years. An understanding of how previous generations have dealt with illness will help to predict the future adaptations. This information can be elicited by obtaining a family genogram oriented to illness and illness related events and behaviors. Although this can be done with the patient alone, he or she is often unaware of all the multigenerational patterns, so other family members' input can be valuable.

Obtaining an illness oriented genogram can be introduced by saying, "It would help me to learn more about your family history of illness, and how your family has coped with previous illnesses." Ask about all illnesses in the family going back at least three generations: how they were diagnosed, how the family reacted, what happened to the family member and the rest of the family. Look for repeating patterns, such as denial of the illness, over or underfunctioning of the ill person, and family coalitions that develop around the illness.

> The Strongs' genogram revealed that Harriet's maternal grandfather had suffered a severe stroke in his early 30s and had been cared for by her grandmother for over 20 years. She had an excessively close relationship with her daughter, Harriet's mother, who did not leave home and get married until after her father died. Harriet feared that Jim would become similarly dependent upon her, and she did not want to become a martyr as her grandmother had. She also worried about the impact of Jim's illness on their children's development.

Other Stresses and Demands on the Family

What other kinds of stresses or strains is the family dealing with? A chronic illness is a major stress on families, but families commonly face numerous stresses simultaneously. Additional stressful life events will influence the family's ability to cope with the chronic illness. Ask about specific stressors including:

• recent deaths, hospitalizations, other serious illness
• marital distress or recent divorce
• financial or work problems, especially unemployment or the threat of unemployment
• recent moves: change in residence, job, schools

Even positive life events or normal life cycle changes can be quite stressful, such as a new baby, a recent marriage or a job promotion.

> Shortly before Jim's MS was diagnosed, he was promoted at work to a supervisor on the assembly line. Although the job provided more income, it involved more responsibilities and required that he walk up and down the line, trouble shooting any problems that arose. As his illness progressed and he became more disabled, the job got more stressful and exhausting, until he could no longer safely do his work. Unfortunately, there were no sedentary jobs he could transfer to, so he was considered disabled and laid off.

Helping Families Cope with Chronic Illness: A Psychoeducational Approach

We base our family-oriented approach to chronic illness on the psychoeducational model (18). This approach assumes that patients and their families do their best to cope with the demands of chronic illness and have many, perhaps untapped, resources. It emphasizes these strengths rather than the deficits of families, and tries to use them to help chronically ill patients and their families. Families are viewed as partners in the treatment process.

The two key elements of this approach are education and psychological support. The education involves providing information about the illness and teaching specific skills in dealing with a chronic illness. The psychological support involves providing empathy, an opportunity to share feelings, and an assessment of how the family is coping, including referrals of families that are having serious difficulties to mental health professionals.

Families with chronic illness often feel blamed by themselves, friends and neighbors, or health professionals for the difficulties that they experience. Thus they often resent any intervention which suggests

that they have a problem or are in need of therapy (8). With the psychoeducational approach, families are considered part of the solution,
rather than part of the problem.

This family-oriented psychoeducational approach to chronic illness
can be implemented in a meeting with the entire family present. In
addition, this approach can be incorporated into routine visits with the
patient, especially when important family members or caregivers are
invited to these visits.

To implement this family-oriented psychoeducational approach to caring for chronic illness, the provider should:

**1. Provide information and education to the patient and family
about the specific illness.** The physician should help patients and
their families become experts on the illness, and partners in the treatment process. Studies have shown that family members want more
information about illness in their family (19) and that having knowledge and information about an illness gives patients and families a better sense of control and mastery of an illness. It can help them to shift
from a passive to a more active stance in dealing with the illness. For
some illnesses, the physician may not have the time or the knowledge to
educate families fully about the illness.

However, the primary care physician has the responsibility to be sure
that the patient and family have access to and receive comprehensive
and reliable information about the chronic illness. This may involve
recommending books or classes and referring to specialists or self-help
groups with which the physician is familiar. All family members, not
just the patient should be encouraged to become educated about the illness. A patient and his or her family can learn about coronary heart
disease by reading books, attending classes, or joining a cardiac rehabilitation group, but the primary physician must also provide specific
information about the patient's heart disease, especially the prognosis
and recommended treatments. This information is best given in the context of what the patient and family already know and their specific
health beliefs. Therefore, it is useful to elicit what the family already
knows, before providing further information. In this way, specific information can be reinforced, modified or corrected.

> Dr. K learned that Jim and Harriet had read extensively about multiple sclero-
> sis and were quite knowledgeable about the illness. In addition to answering
> their questions, he referred them to the local MS association. There they
> joined a monthly support group and met other couples and families who
> were dealing with different stages of the illness. They were able to share their
> frustrations and sorrow and learn very specific and practical coping skills.
> From other patients with MS, they learned that Jim's difficulty concentrating
> and his sensitivity to temperature changes were common in the illness.

**2. Help the family become effective advocates for the patient and
themselves in dealing with the health care system and utilizing**

community resources. Most serious chronic illnesses involved extended and repeated contact with multiple medical specialists and community agencies. The primary care physician can help the family work effectively within the health care system and become empowered and assertive, without being overly aggressive and demanding or alienating providers. When the patient or family encounter roadblocks or problems in getting information or appropriate medical care, it is most helpful for the primary care physician to suggest ways that the family can proceed rather than directly intervening to solve the problem. If the family is able to solve the problem, their self confidence will increase and they will be able to deal more effectively with similar problems in the future. For example, if the family does not feel they have received sufficient information from a surgeon about a planned operation, the primary care physician should remain in contact with the surgeon and encourage the family to call the surgeon and explain that they need this information before proceeding further. This will be more helpful than the primary care physician obtaining the information directly from the surgeon and becoming the go-between with the specialist and the family.

For most chronic illnesses, there are organizations that provide services for patients and their families (e.g., American Cancer Society, American Heart Association). Some of them are primarily self-help groups that run support groups. Others provide specific services such as transportation for the disabled or informational classes on the specific illnesses. Unfortunately, only a few specifically address the needs of family members (e.g., Alzheimer's Disease and Related Disorders Association). The family-oriented physician should be familiar with these organizations and encourage the patient and family to contact them and become involved. Roback (20) has described many of the functions that groups for patients and family can provide.

> Through the MS Association, the Strongs learned of an experimental treatment for MS being studied at a medical center 150 miles from their town. They sent for information on the treatment and reviewed it with Dr. K. They visited the medical center and learned the details of the study from the investigators. Finally, Jim decided not to enter the study because the treatment seemed too risky, without enough promise for success, and it required frequent trips to the medical center.

3. Encourage the family to openly discuss the illness and their emotional responses to it. Most families do not often talk about the chronic illness, except the most pragmatic aspects of day to day coping (8). It is common for families to feel overwhelmed, angry, and depressed about the illness, but be reluctant to share those feelings, fearing that it will put more burdens on the patient. Yet they may be aware of negative feelings they have about the patient and his or her illness, such as disappointment, anger, and guilt, but believe these feelings are unacceptable in light of the patient's suffering. Encouraging the honest discussion of feelings at a family conference can have a very powerful and therapeutic effect upon the patient and family.

Sometimes a single experience of sharing feelings in a safe environment allows families to open up and communicate emotional reactions that have been suppressed for years. Families who are either over or under-reactive to these feelings may need to be referred for family therapy.

When meeting with the family, the physician can encourage open communication about their experience of living with chronic illness. Some ways to facilitate this communication include:

a. **Ask directly about their experience.** "What has it been like for all of you to deal with your mother's illness day after day and week after week?"
b. **Elicit and empathize with feelings associated with the family's specific problems concerning the illness.** When a family member describes a problem, ask "That sounds pretty tough, how do you feel about having to face that every day?"
c. **Normalize feelings of anger, guilt, and depression.** "Dealing with a chronic illness like this can be very difficult. Most families I have cared for feel a great deal of frustration and sadness about what's happened. What's it been like in your family?"
d. **Inquire about common emotional responses.** "Jim, do you ever get angry at Harriet for being healthy and able to do the things you cannot?" or "Harriet, how often do you feel guilty about being healthy when your husband has been so ill?"
e. **Ask the patient or a family member what kind of feelings they have seen in other family members.** "Jim, how has Harriet dealt with your illness?" "Who in this family is the most upset about Jim's illness?"
f. **Do not try to "cheer up" the patient or other family members; help family members accept the patient's feelings and share their own experiences.**

> Jim: I am so discouraged! None of these treatments seem to help at all, and I keep getting weaker and weaker. Sometimes I just want to give up and stop everything.
> Harriet: Don't say that, Jim. You haven't had as many relapses since you've been on Cytoxan, and your vision seems a bit better.
> Dr. K: Harriet, it sounds like it's difficult for you to hear how discouraged Jim is at times about his illness.

Attempts to cheer up someone who is discouraged or depressed can make that person feel misunderstood and more alone and depressed. Families who are able to share their emotional responses to an illness are more likely to give and receive emotional support from each other. With encouragement the family may be able to share feelings for the first time within a family conference. This can have a powerful therapeutic effect and may stimulate the family to be more open at home.

Patients and family members go through stages of dealing with chronic illness that are often similar to those dealing with death: shock, denial, anger, bargaining, grief, and acceptance. However, each family member may be at different stages in dealing with or accepting the illness. Some may deny aspects of the illness or be angry while others are grieving, and a family member may go back and forth between stages. Because of the personal demands of illness, the patient is often ahead of the rest of the family in dealing with the illness, and this can create conflicts. For the Strongs, Harriet's efforts to get Jim to look at the bright side of this illness were partly because she was still trying to deny the seriousness of the illness, while Jim was grieving the loss of his health. The physician can help the family by normalizing these different responses to the illness.

4. Facilitate the family's involvement in the care of the patient through negotiations with the patient. Most families would like to assist the patient in the care of his or her illness, but sometimes have difficulty negotiating an optimal plan. Physicians may recognize the family has become either over or underinvolved in the patient's care.

a. **Encourage all appropriate family members to learn specific skills involved in the care of the patient.** It may be particularly useful to have the patient teach his or her family how to do certain tasks such as having a spouse draw up the insulin syringes and learn to give injections if the patient is sick or begins to lose vision. Even when the family members do not take over a task, teaching them about specific procedures provides a way to educate them and communicate about the illness. For example, having a colostomy patient demonstrate how to change the colostomy bag can help to normalize the disability.

b. **Have the patient tell other family members how they can help.** Except when he or she is incompetent, the patient should remain in charge of the illness. Problems arise when family members try to decide what is best for the patient or try to help in ways that feel intrusive to the patient. Negotiating how the family can help can be done in a family meeting or in a routine visit when another family member is present.

> DR. K: Jim, it sounds like getting dressed in the morning can be quite difficult. Would you like Harriet's help with any of it?
>
> JIM: Yeah, I guess so.
>
> DR. K: Harriet, would you be willing to help Jim in the morning when he gets dressed?
>
> HARRIET: Of course, I offer to help him every morning but he just snaps at me.
>
> JIM: Well, I'm not an invalid!

DR. K: Jim, what kind of things would you want Harriet to help you with?

JIM: She could start by not treating me like I'm an invalid . . . .

DR. K: Let's start with things she can do to help.

JIM: The one thing I have trouble with is putting on my ankle brace.

DR. K: Would you like Harriet to help you with this?

JIM: Sure.

DR. K: Harriet would you be willing to help with this?

HARRIET: Of course.

DR. K: Is there anything else you'd like her to help with?

JIM: No, I can handle the rest.

DR. K: Are there things you would prefer that Harriet not do for you?

JIM: Yes, I don't like her hovering around me asking if she can help me get dressed.

DR. K: Harriet, would you be willing just to help Jim with his brace and let him dress the rest of himself, no matter how long it takes him, and only give additional help if he asks for it.

HARRIET: If that's what he wants.

JIM: That's what I want.

DR. K: It is important for Jim to remain as independent as possible. You may help him the most by letting him ask for help when he needs it and not offering it at other times.

5. Help the family to develop an appropriate balance between the demands of the ill member and the need for further growth and development for the patient and other family members. Encourage the family to normalize family life as much as possible and only change those aspects of family life that must be altered. This can help to minimize the impact of the illness. For example, it is usually better to maintain family routines and rituals, such as mealtimes, birthdays, and holidays. Family members should be encouraged to pay attention to their own needs. Often family members will view this as being selfish ("How can I think about myself when he/she is so sick?"). It can be explained that taking care of one's own needs is necessary in order to be able to care for the ill family member. Sometimes patients will encourage other family members to do things for themselves.

DR. K: Jim, in the process of helping you with your illness, do you think Harriet is taking good care of herself?

JIM: No, and I worry about that. She used to have lunch with her friends every Wednesday, and now she comes home to check on me. I wish she wouldn't sacrifice those lunches.

The challenge for the family is to find an appropriate balance between caring for the ill member and caring for the family and to put the illness in its appropriate place in the family's life. Families need to continually reassess this balance.

6. Identify families in trouble and refer them for family therapy. Because of the enormous disruptions involved, most families dealing with serious chronic illness would benefit from supportive family counseling, and the physician should offer this to all such families. However, some families develop serious difficulties and family dysfunction. These families should be identified and referred for more intensive therapy. (Details for how to refer for family counseling are discussed in Chapter 22.) Common warning signs are listed below.

Warning Signs of Patient Dysfunction

1. Poor management or complications of the illness. This is often a result of poor compliance with the medical regimen and may result from lack of support or assistance from the family or may be a form of resistance to family overinvolvement.

2. Poor Coping. Poor coping with the illness can result in underfunctioning, such as exaggerating the disability, not participating in rehabilitation (e.g., the cardiac patient who won't do anything that "stresses" his heart) or reporting an increase in symptoms. Poor coping can also result in over functioning, such as denial of symptoms or illness, overdoing the rehabilitation (e.g., the cardiac patient who runs a marathon). The development of any serious psychiatric disorder, such as severe anxiety, depression, suicidal thinking, eating disorders (anorexia or bulimia) is an indication for referral.

Warning Signs of Dysfunction in Family Members

1. Illness or symptoms in other family members. These symptoms result from the stress of caring for an ill family member or be a way of competing for attention and care via health problems. The symptoms may be functional (e.g., tension headaches) or represent serious organic illness (e.g., development of angina).

2. Emotional disturbance in other family members. In addition to psychiatric problems such as depression and anxiety, these signs of poor coping may include school or work problems or chronic insomnia.

3. Family, marital, or sexual problems. Superficially these problems may appear unrelated to the chronic illness (e.g., sexual dysfunction in the parents of a diabetic child), but the illness often plays an important role.

> As Jim's illness worsened, the stress on the couple and their relationship worsened. Jim became withdrawn and depressed, and Harriet's migraine headaches became incapacitating. Despite Dr. K's counseling during office visits, the couple fought more about Harriet's attempts to help Jim. Dr. K suggested that they might benefit from seeing a counselor on a more regular basis to deal with the tremendous stresses related to the illness. The couple agreed.

Chronic illness is a nearly universal part of the life course of families. It is often a crisis that severely stresses families and threatens to disrupt them. The shared experience of coping with chronic illness is also an opportunity for growth; to become closer and develop new and healthier patterns of interaction. Physicians have a unique opportunity to work with patients and families over the long course of chronic illness. Through careful assessment and planned intervention, the family-oriented physician can help families cope in healthy ways to chronic illness.

References

1. Dever GEA: *Community Health Analysis: A Holistic Approach.* Germantown, MD, Aspen, 1980.
2. U.S. Department of Commerce: *Statistical Abstracts of the United States* (101s.d.1S.P.-25,N.802,888), Washington, DC, Government Printing Office, 1980.
3. Doherty WA, Campbell TL: *Families and Health.* Beverly Hills, CA, Sage Publications, 1988.
4. Steinglass P, Temple S, Lisman S, Reiss D: Coping with spinal cord injury: The family perspective. *Gen Hosp Psychiatry* 1982;**4**:259–264.
5. Sabbeth B, Leventhal JM: Marital adjustment to chronic childhood illness: A critique of the literature. *Pediatrics* 1984;**73**:762–768.
6. Klein RF, Dean A, Bogdonaoff MD: The impact of illness on the spouse. *J Chronic Dis* 1967;**20**:241–248.
7. Strong M: Mainstay: *For the Well Spouse of the Chronically Ill.* Boston, MA, Little, Brown & Co., 1988.
8. Gonzales S, Steinglass P, Reiss D: Family-centered interventions for people with chronic physical disabilities: The eight-session multiple family discussion group program. Washington, DC, Center for Family Research, Department of Psychiatry and Behavioral Science, George Washington University Medical Center, 1988.
9. Penn P: Coalitions and binding interactions in families with chronic illness. *Fam Syst Med* 1983;**1**:16–25.
10. Rolland JS: Psychosocial typology of chronic and life threatening illness. *Fam Syst Med* 1984;**2**:245–262.
11. Houlihan JP: Families caring for frail and demented elderly: A review of selected findings. *Fam Syst Med* 1987;**5**:344–356.
12. Rolland JS: Chronic illness and the life cycle: A conceptual framework. *Fam Proc* 1987;**26**:203–221.
13. Combrinck-Graham L: A developmental model for family systems. *Fam Proc* 1985;**24**:139–150.
14. Minuchin S, Rosman BL, Baker L: *Psychosomatic Families: Anorexia Nervosa in Context.* Cambridge, MA, Harvard University Press, 1978.
15. Houser S: Personal communication, Hilton Head, 1988.
16. Smilkstein G: The cycle of family function: A conceptual model for family medicine. *J Fam Pract* 1980;**11**:223–232.
17. Rolland JS: Family illness paradigm: Evolution and significance. *Fam Syst Med* 1987;**5**:482–503.

18. Anderson CM, Reiss DJ, Hogarty G: *Schizophrenia and the Family.* New York, Guilford Press, 1986.
19. Morisky DE, Levine DM, Green LW et al.: Five year blood pressure control and mortality following health education for hypertensive patients. *Am J Public Health* 1983;**73**:153–162.
20. Robach HB (ed.): *Helping Patients and their Families Cope with Medical Problems.* San Francisco, CA, Jossey-Bass, 1984.

PROTOCOL

Assessing a Family's Coping with Chronic Illness

Instructions: Give the family a global score on how well they are accomplishing the tasks needed to cope effectively with chronic illness.

The Family Members:
A. Respond to the patient who is ill by acting:

0	1	2	1	0
insensitive		supportive		immobilized

B. Respond to the patient's emotional reaction to the illness with:

0	1	2	1	0
denial		empathy		being overwhelmed

C. Respond to the patient's specific disability by:

0	1	2	1	0
ignoring it		encouraging autonomy		being overprotective

D. Readjust expectations for the future by being:

0	1	2	1	0
overoptimistic		realistic & hopeful		pessimistic

E. Respond to help from outside the family by:

0	1	2	1	0
refusing it		accepting it		being overly dependent

F. Advocate for patient's and family's needs with health care providers by being:

0	1	2	1	0
passive		appropriately assertive		demanding & aggressive

G. Respond to the needs of all family members by:

0	1	2	1	0
denying patient's needs		balancing family members & patient needs		denying family's needs

Total Score

Greater than 10–The family is coping very well.

5–10–The family is having some difficulty adapting to the illness and are in need of primary care counseling.

Less than 5–The family is coping poorly and should be referred for family therapy.

CHAPTER 16

Integrating the Mind–Body Split
A Biopsychosocial Approach to Somatic Fixation

Somatic fixation is a process whereby a physician and/or a patient or family focuses exclusively and inappropriately on the somatic aspects of a complex problem (1). Somatic fixation can occur not only in hypochondriasis, somatization disorder, and psychosomatic disease, but in any illness, especially chronic illness, when there is a one-sided emphasis on the biomedical aspects of a multifaceted problem. In spite of very difficult life situations, somatically fixated patients tend not to present with anxiety, depression, or trouble coping, but with numerous physical symptoms. The number of patients in any family practice with some degree of somatic fixation is high. One study found that one-half of all medical patients had symptoms of undetermined cause (2). Another study found somatization disorder in a family practice to be not only a prevalent problem, but also an expensive and difficult one. deGruy et al. found that these patients had a 50% higher rate of office visits, 50% higher charges, charts that were close to twice as thick as the average chart, and significantly more diagnoses than matched controls (3).

The following example illustrates a common course for somatic fixation that can occur in association with a serious illness.

> Although Mr. Hammer's only biomedical problem was mild hypertension, he visited his family physician, Dr. E, frequently for numerous concerns about his health. Usually his anxiety could be reduced temporarily by a brief physical exam and reassurance by Dr. E. Unfortunately during one of these visits, a prostate nodule was detected, causing Mr. Hammer to become extremely fearful and upset.
>
> A biopsy of the nodule revealed cancer and Mr. Hammer underwent a radical prostatectomy. Immediately after surgery, he and his wife were reassured by the surgeon that he had "gotten it all." However, when the final pathology

report came back, the surgeon explained that all the malignant cells may not
have been removed, and that Mr. Hammer should receive radiation therapy.
Mr. Hammer agreed, but had great difficulty dealing with the news that there
might be some residual cancer. He became severely depressed and was
referred to a psychiatrist who hospitalized him for one week. Mr. Hammer
improved on antidepressants, and was discharged to Dr. E's care. The consulting psychiatrist felt Mr. Hammer should remain on antidepressants, but felt he
was "not a good candidate for psychotherapy."

During these events Mr. Hammer's level of somatic fixation escalated dramatically. Dr. E saw him frequently, monitored his physical state carefully, and
reassured him liberally. This seemed of only momentary benefit to Mr. Hammer. Mr. Hammer confessed his fears to his wife, who also reassured him,
speaking from her own experience of having two episodes of breast cancer
and a period of serious depression between the two episodes.

Mr. Hammer had worked all his life in construction and had retired several
years before this health event. He had prided himself in being active and
handy around the house. In the several years after his treatment for cancer, he
became inactive, withdrawn, and preoccupied with the prospect of a recurrence of his cancer. He reported pain and discomfort in the prostate area, difficulty concentrating, and dry eyes. Every time Mr. Hammer experienced a
new symptom, Dr. E evaluated him, always with negative findings. Often his
surgeon also evaluated him with similar results. Dr. E was concerned about
Mr. Hammer's persistent depression and tried several times to change him to
a more effective antidepressant. Each time Mr. Hammer had such difficulty
making the change and reported so many side effects that his physician maintained him on the original medication. Several years postsurgery, Mr. Hammer
was no longer severely depressed but he was quite markedly somatically fixated.

Because of the seriousness of Mr. Hammer's disease, he and his care providers had difficulty pursuing the psychosocial aspects of his adjustment. Mr.
Hammer had always been action-oriented rather than emotional or verbally
oriented, so he had little to draw on from his previous life to help him adjust
to his new status. His father, in fact, had a serious illness late in mid-life and
had not been able to make a healthy adjustment. He had become reclusive
and very difficult to deal with until his death some years later. In addition to
Mr. Hammer's somatic fixation, Dr. E struggled with her own tendency to
panic over her patient's symptoms. She was very fond of Mr. Hammer and felt
in some way responsible for not picking up the cancer earlier, so that when
he requested more tests to evaluate his symptoms she almost always con-
curred, with or without strong medical evidence to support the testing.

Why is somatic fixation, like that of Mr. Hammer, so widespread and so
difficult to manage? There are a number of **individual, family, and cultural factors that support the maintenance of somatic symptoms.**

• **Individual factors.** The first relevant individual factor is rooted in
the normal human experience of physical sensations. Kellner and
Sheffield found that 60–80% of healthy individuals experience some
somatic symptoms in any one week (4). If even a small proportion of
these people saw their physician, our offices would be flooded with

patients. Also, individuals' perceptions of a symptom are quite variable. It is well documented that the same amount of tissue pathology produces varying degrees of functional impairment and subjective distress in different individuals (5). Mr. Hammer, in the preceding case example, was very sensitive to any physical sensation in his body (and equally insensitive to emotional cues). After his surgery, he experienced a much greater degree of impairment and distress than most patients with similar disease and treatment.

• **Familial factors.** Many family factors can potentially support or reinforce somatic fixation. A subgroup of all people are raised in an environment where they receive some attention for physical pain but no attention for emotional pain. If families operate on a continuum from full encouragement and acceptance of emotional and physical experience to complete lack of acceptance of one or both, these repressed families condition children to experience any need or problem as physical. Physical symptoms become their language for a range of experiences, from physical to emotional. These patients may learn, as Barsky described, to amplify their bodily symptoms in an attempt to get their needs met (6). In keeping with this explanation, Katon found that chronic, severe somatizers also tend to have a developmental history of gross neglect and abuse as well as a family history of relatives using somatization or pain behavior as a way of coping or solving problems (7). Mr. Hammer came from a family in which his father was a somatizer. His family was emotionally unexpressive and communicated through physical symptoms. While he did not report a history of physical abuse, his parents did seem to be stressed and incapable of meeting many of his emotional needs.

• **Cultural factors.** In addition to the individual and family contributions to the development and maintenance of somatic fixation, our culture contributes to the problem by remaining rooted in the Cartesian notion of a mind–body dichotomy. Our language and much of our belief systems encourage patients like Mr. Hammer to conceptualize the physical as apart from and unrelated to the emotional. The notion that a physical symptom must have a primarily organic cause, or that an emotional feeling is determined primarily by some psychological experience, is well-accepted in our society. The idea that mind and body are an integrated, related, communicating whole has only recently, and tentatively, been considered by the wider society. Medicine itself has focused particularly on biomedicine in the twentieth century, in part because of the many scientific and technological advances that have occurred relatively recently. These advances make it that much more seductive to conclude that biomedicine *is* medicine, rather than it being one very important component of the diagnosis and treatment of a patient.

However, an alternative paradigm has emerged. The biopsychosocial approach is the medical model that operationalizes the systemic approach

| healthy & happy | sensitive to bodily sensations | the "worried well" | obsessed by symptoms | somatic delusion |

Range of Somatic Fixation by Patients

| biopsycho-social model | assess biomedical then psychosocial | uneasy with psychosocial | biomedical focus, refers psychosocial | purely biomedical |

Range of Somatic Fixation by Physicians

FIGURE 16.1.

to medicine; it is essential to the management and treatment of somatic fixation. **Every physical symptom has some biologic, some psychologic, and often some social component to it. A physician needs to be able to address each of these areas in a balanced and integrated way, without fixating inappropriately on any one component of the symptom.**

Figure 16.1 illustrates the range of somatic fixation possible for patients and for physicians. Patients may range from being comfortable with health and physical and emotional experience on one end of the continuum to amplifying symptoms and worrying over illness or expressing somatic delusions at the other extreme. Physicians may also express a range of behavior with regard to somatic fixation: from utilizing an integrated, biopsychosocial approach, to treating the biomedical and psychosocial separately and referring out most psychosocial problems, to the extreme position of perceiving and treating only biomedical problems.

This chapter will advocate for a biopsychosocial approach to somatic fixation, first describing the vicious cycle that physicians and patients can be drawn into and then elucidating principles of a successful biopsychosocial approach to the management and treatment of these problems.

The Battle of the Health Belief Systems

Somatic fixation can also be described as an interactional process that occurs when the health belief system of a patient and/or family does not match that of a physician. For example, in Mr. Hammer's case, postsurgery Dr. E believed that Mr. Hammer's symptoms were a result of his fear, depression, and ongoing sensitivity to bodily cues. Mr. Hammer, however, believed these symptoms indicated a recurrence of his cancer. These differing diagnoses made it difficult for the two individuals to understand each other or communicate without conflict.

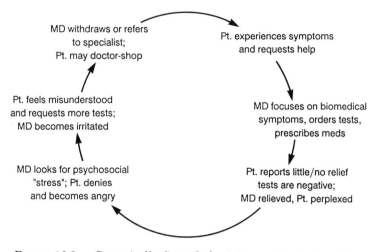

FIGURE 16.2.   Somatically fixated physician–patient interaction.

Figure 16.2 illustrates the vicious cycle that can occur in interactions between a somatically fixated patient and a physician who hold differing health belief systems. This cycle can begin when a patient experiences symptoms and seeks help from a medical provider. If we assume that the physician does not routinely use a biopsychosocial approach, that physician might review the patient's symptoms, listen sympathetically, and perhaps order some tests and prescribe some medication. In the next interaction, the tests may come back equivocal or negative. The physician then experiences relief, but notices that the patient is perplexed. With no biomedical answers, the physician turns to a psychosocial evaluation. The patient may then become angry and deny that the problem is "in my head." At this point the patient feels misunderstood and requests more tests, leading the physician to become irritated. Then, the physician may withdraw from the patient and/or refer out to a medical specialist, or the patient may drop out of the practice and begin a process of doctor-shopping. Either outcome sets the cycle into motion again as the patient presents his or her symptoms to a new physician. The lack of a shared belief system can result in a vicious cycle in which both physician and patient are locked into a battle over the patient's somatic fixation. The way out of the struggle involves adopting an integrated biopsychosocial approach from the beginning of the interaction with the patient. From a broad perspective, treatment consists of slowly educating and demonstrating to the patient the interconnections between biological and psychological systems. At the end of a course of treatment physician and patient are closer to sharing a common health belief system that recognizes this interdependency.

Twelve Principles for a Biopsychosocial Approach to Somatic Fixation

> Mr. and Mrs. Hunter were well known to Dr. B as patients who were extremely sensitive to physical symptoms and tended to worry about illness and disease. This couple had many strengths: they were devoted to parenting their three sons, they enjoyed their work, and they were committed to their church and their community. However, they were unusually conscious of their bodily cues. They and their sons each had occasional flu, colds, and headaches, which would send them to the office requesting medicine for benign diagnoses. On each visit Dr. B would treat the problem, reassure them, and check into other life events that might be stressing the family at the time. Until the last few years, this approach was effective. At that time, Mr. and Mrs. Hunter lost a second daughter to congenital heart defects soon after birth. Within a year, Mr. and Mrs. Hunter were making at least monthly visits to Dr. B with multiple somatic complaints. Reassurance and benign diagnoses no longer were effective in decreasing their anxiety.

Treating somatically fixated patients such as the Hunters requires careful and explicit attention to principles of biopsychosocial medicine:

1. **From the beginning, evaluate biomedical and psychosocial elements of the problem concurrently.** The physician can avoid operationalizing the mind–body split by mixing biomedical and psychosocial questions in the interview, a technique suggested by Doherty and Baird for all primary care interviewing (8). In particular, it is important to avoid working up the patient medically, finding nothing, then turning to a psychosocial evaluation. This dichotomy mimics the patient's belief that the two are separate, unrelated processes. It relegates the psychosocial to a position of lesser importance and leads to the common patient accusation: "You think this is all in my head." Interspersing questions about disease signs and symptoms with questions about recent stressful life events avoids this problem.

Try to do a balanced, reasonable work-up, neither overusing tests nor avoiding the biological aspects of the symptoms.

2. **Solicit the patient's symptoms, but do not let the symptoms run the interview.** It is important to respect the patient's somatic defenses; if these patients were able to tolerate direct expressions of emotion or distress, they would not have to somatize. By soliciting symptoms, the provider is able to speak these patients' language, enter their belief system, and metaphorically gain access to and validate their emotional experience. It is especially important to structure these interviews in such a way that the patient feels his or her concerns are heard and yet does not dominate the interview with long, rambling descriptions of pain and symptomatology. Several techniques can keep the physician active in the interview and prevent the patient from monologuing:

- Sit up and reflect or ask a question after each sentence or two by the patient
- Interrupt if necessary
- Assume a curious or perplexed posture rather than a frustrated, intimidated, or weary posture
- Unusual symptoms call for unusual diagnostic procedures – ask the patient to diagram symptoms, measure their length or intensity, and be active in the diagnostic process

The physician must be able to persist through what is typically a difficult early period of evaluation and heavy symptom focus by the patient. Requesting a symptom diary, especially one that includes both biomedical and psychosocial information about symptoms, can be useful in allowing the patient their concern about their symptoms, involving them in the diagnostic process, and providing information for the patient and the physician about the symptoms. The diary may be requested by explaining: "Your body is trying to signal us about something important. Unfortunately, we do not understand its signals just yet. We must work together to try and discover what it is telling us."

Early in treatment with the Hunters, Dr. B tried but had difficulty discussing the death of the couple's two daughters. Attempts to broach psychosocial issues were met with Mr. Hunter complaining, for example, that his right testicle was cold or that his semen was discolored. Mrs. Hunter usually accompanied her husband to see Dr. B and had her own litany of physical complaints. They included abdominal pain, ear pain, headaches, and unusual vaginal discharge. Mr. and Mrs. Hunter tended to be symptomatic simultaneously. Attention or attempted treatment of one inevitably led to symptoms and the need for treatment in the other. It seemed as if these patients may have had a chlamydia infection at some time, though no evidence existed of such an infection by the time of the consultations. Rather than increase the patient's resistance by focusing totally on the emotional, Dr. B carefully interspersed his psychosocial questions with more biomedical questions about Mr. Hunter's symptoms. Early in treatment, Mr. Hunter rarely answered the questions about stress directly, but continued to complain of various symptoms, including pains that shot up through his chest, being awakened by the sound of bubbles popping in his lungs, and being generally lethargic and unable to work. Dr. B asked both members of the couple to keep a symptom diary, and the patients brought in pages of symptoms and complaints, reporting little about their emotional states.

3. **Develop a relationship with the patient that is collaborative.** It is important with these patients to avoid an authoritarian position and any implication to the patient (or ourselves) that a "magic bullet" exists that would relieve them of their symptoms. It may be useful to describe these symptoms as mysterious and scientifically baffling; this approach underscores the physician's inability to treat these problems from a

purely biomedical perspective. These attitudes on the part of the physician also underline the importance of the patient's contribution to the diagnosis and treatment of these difficult problems.

4. **See the patient at regular intervals,** not dictated by symptom occurrence or intensification (9), **and discourage visits to other health care providers,** except upon specific referral. Regular and frequent appointments with the primary care physician are important to disconnect the patient's experience of crisis and symptoms resulting in attention and care. Instead the attention and care is given liberally without relation to acute symptoms. It is also important that these patients be routed through the primary care physician for all acute and chronic complaints, avoiding Emergency Department visits and referrals to medical specialists unless clearly indicated. Multiple work-ups and dispersal of these patients' care tend to reinforce biomedical fixation. When biomedical referral is necessary, it is important to talk with the consultant beforehand and be specific about the referral question.

> Dr. B was careful in the early stages to share his concern and confusion with the Hunters over their symptoms. He agreed with them that they deserved to have a "cure," but stated that an easy solution did not seem possible in their case. They would have to work together to manage these difficult and mysterious problems. Dr. B underlined his accessibility to the Hunters, telling them to see him every several weeks for the next few months until they began to function a little better. He encouraged them to bring any acute or chronic complaints to him rather than elsewhere. He told them other services, such as the Emergency Room or even other physicians unfamiliar with their cases, were likely to be ineffective with their problems and cost them more money because they would have to start from ground zero with each new evaluation. The Hunters agreed they did not wish more aggravation than they already had.

5. **Elicit the patient and family's diagnoses of the problem.** It is important to understand the meaning of the symptom to the patient, and the patients' explanations for the problem will often lead to what they expect from treatment. Following up on these concerns is important to develop a constructive relationship in which these patients feel heard. Over time, it is important to work toward mutually acceptable explanations for the symptoms.

6. **Elicit any recent stressful life events, life cycle challengers, or unresolved family problems.** Of particular importance to somatic fixation are problems such as early abuse or deprivation, unresolved grief, alcohol or drug abuse, and workaholism and other forms of overfunctioning. These questions may be best addressed during a family conference.

> Both Mr. and Mrs. Hunter initially worried that they had cancer. Mr. Hunter later reported that a friend had suggested perhaps he had AIDS, and Ms. Hunter continually worried that she had some serious "female problems"

or some other life-threatening illness. Testing and physical exams revealed no medical evidence for any of these concerns. Over 2–3 months of visits, these patients slowly began discussing the stressful events in their family life, which included long work hours and alcohol abuse by Mr. Hunter, and the difficulties that had occurred after their babies' deaths. Both provider and patients eventually agreed their symptoms were likely a result of some mixture of an early chlamydia infection, depression and unresolved grief after their daughters' deaths, alcohol abuse, and marital stress.

7. **Invite the family to participate early in treatment.** Including the family is important because symptoms can be maintained or intensified because they come to have meaning to significant others. Sometimes symptoms have interpersonal effects such as eliciting expressions of concern or sympathy and affording relief from responsibilities or work. At a family conference, it is useful to:

a. request each person's observations, diagnoses, and opinions about the illness and the treatment
b. listen for how the illness may have changed the typical roles or balance of power in the family
c. try to understand any marital and/or transgenerational meaning for the symptom by asking, "Has anyone else in the family had an illness that in any way resembles this one?"
d. ask what each person is doing to help the patient with the illness
e. ask how family life would be different if the patient's symptoms disappeared or improved
f. develop a treatment plan that the group can accept and request each person's help in its implementation.

> Interviewing Mr. and Mrs. Hunter together was both efficient and informative. Both Mr. and Mrs. Hunter reported that their illness had brought them closer together. Mr. Hunter had stopped working, the couple spent all their time together, and their fears of dying helped them readjust their priorities and realize how much they meant to each other. In fact, as Mr. and Mrs. Hunter improved, both worried that complete symptom relief would result in renewed marital stress or at least more distance between them, and in another episode of alcohol abuse by Mr. Hunter.
>
> A few months after their treatment began, Dr. B invited both spouses' parents in to share their concerns about their childrens' illnesses. An in-depth genogram taken in that session revealed that both Mr. and Mrs. Hunter's fathers were alcoholic and their mothers both had chronic medical problems that appeared to fit a pattern of somatic fixation. Both families agreed they had much in common. In this session, they arrived at a plan for the couple's parents to help with the grandchildren so the couple might return to work as their functioning improved.

8. **Solicit and constantly return to the patient and family's strengths and areas of competence.** Patients with severe somatic fix-

ation often have a history of deprivation or abuse; support is an important part of their treatment. Also, it is easier to build on strengths than to rectify deficiencies.

9. **Avoid psychosocial fixation; continue with an integrated approach.** In addition to the psychological aspects of somatic fixation, there are frequently biomedical components. Also, somatically fixated patients get sick at times, so remain fully alert for somatic signs of serious disease.

An ongoing integrated approach is both scientifically sound and an art form in itself. **The best interventions with somatically fixated patients are those that combine the biomedical and the psychosocial, i.e., biomedical interventions that make psychological sense and psychological interventions that make biomedical sense.** Similarly, explanations about scarring, stress, or a depressed immune system are attempts at integrating these two aspects of the illness.

> With the Hunters, continued focus on their devotion to each other and their commitment to good parenting of their children helped to support and balance the treatment. As an outgrowth of the focus on their good parenting, discussion of their daughters' deaths became somewhat easier. One very important intervention came when Dr. B reviewed the Hunters' daughters' autopsy report with them. While the couple had consistently had difficulty speaking directly about their sorrow, this medical approach facilitated their grieving and allowed them to ask questions that had heretofore not been asked.

10. **Find a way to enjoy somatically fixated cases.** These cases are traditionally frustrating and time-consuming for physicians, as demonstrated by the vicious cycle described in Fig. 16.2. These patients and their families often feel frustrated, angry at the medical establishment, and discouraged about the patients' illnesses. Finding a way to enjoy these cases allows one to stay connected to these difficult patients, and it prevents physician burnout. Cognitive and emotional strategies for enjoying these patients and their families include the following:

a. Listen to the patient's symptoms as metaphors for their larger problems.
b. Monitor both the patient's and your own discomfort with uncertainty. Somatic fixation offers many opportunities to rediscover that which we understand or have control over and that which we do not.
c. Discuss the case with a physician colleague, or invite that person to consult. Frustration with any patient or family is often dissipated when some respected colleague can offer support and another point of view.
d. Refer or collaborate closely with a family therapist or other mental health consultant. Many severe cases of somatic fixation require in-depth experience and expertise in both the biomedical and the psychosocial areas; collaboration offers an avenue of support and shared

responsibility for difficult cases; also, collaboration around this disorder can be the most cost-effective approach. Smith, Monson, and Ray, in a randomized controlled study, found that a psychiatric consultation coupled with recommendations for the primary care physician of patients with somatization disorder reduced these patients' medical costs by 53% (10). (See Chapter 22 for more on collaborating and referring to mental health professionals.)

> While Dr. B felt he had made considerable progress in helping Mr. and Mrs. Hunter, he remained concerned about lingering grief issues as well as continued signs of marital distress. As in some cases of severe somatic fixation, Dr. B decided that he needed to consult with a family therapist to provide effective biopsychosocial care to this couple.
>
> The therapist, Dr. T, and the physician, Dr. B, held a joint meeting with the couple for Dr. B to introduce Dr. T, make his referral, coordinate treatment with the couple, and lend his support to the new endeavor. Dr. B and Dr. T then discussed the session and developed a joint treatment plan. Dr. T met with the couple ten times over a nine month period. Several times over that period, the physician and the therapist met together with the patients. Dr. T was able to take the time to provide Mr. Hunter with the support he needed to discuss his daughters' deaths. In one of the early joint sessions, Mr. and Mrs. Hunter stated they had grown apart during the year after their daughters' deaths and Mr. Hunter revealed that he had increased his drinking behavior and had had an affair during this time. Mr. Hunter clearly felt very guilty about this experience. Between this issue and the death of their daughters, it became clear why many of their symptoms were either focused on their genitals or were related to pregnancy and reproduction in some way. As these issue were aired, Dr. B and Dr. T recognized the couple's commitment to each other, supported them each as individuals, and simultaneously dealt with their ongoing biomedical concerns. While Dr. T usually conducted the interviews around emotionally sensitive issues such as the affair or the couple's sex life, Dr. B provided support, checked into symptoms that seemed new or concerning, and provided some creative interventions such as reviewing the daughters' autopsy reports with the couple as a way of facilitating their grief work.

11. **Judge progress in these patients by monitoring changes in their level of functioning rather than in their symptoms.** Symptom-free living (i.e., a "cure") is unlikely in these patients. More realistic goals involve a decrease in symptoms and an increase in functioning in areas such as work and family relationships.

12. **Terminate the intense phase of treatment slowly.** It is always useful with these patients to restrain them from too-rapid improvement in their symptoms. If the physician keeps his or her expectations low, the patient is free to move at his or her own pace. When some improvement has occurred, it is helpful to wonder aloud what problems might emerge if the patient were to recover completely. In addition to a restrained, cautious approach to treatment, the physician may also realistically predict relapses as improvement occurs. These predictions prevent dis-

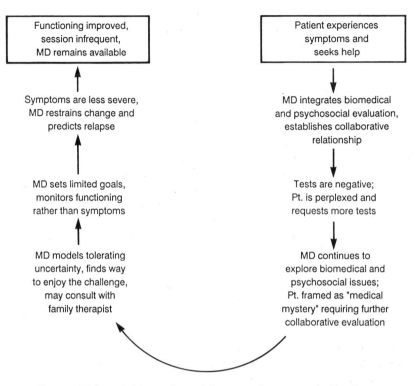

FIGURE 16.3.   A biopsychosocial approach to somatic fixation.

appointment and make the typical flare-ups in symptoms part of the
course of recovery.

With an increase in the patient's general level of functioning and a
decrease in the incapacitating nature of the symptoms, it is useful to
slowly lengthen the time between office visits. However, for the success
of this process, it is crucial that the patient feel the physician is available to him or her regardless of symptom states.

> By the end of nine months, Drs. B and T and the patients agreed that Dr. T no
> longer needed to meet with the couple. Mr. and Mrs. Hunter were not
> symptom-free, but the severity and frequency of their symptoms had
> diminished. Mr. Hunter was now working again, and Mrs. Hunter had a job
> for the first time since before her pregnancies. The couple reported their com-
> mitment to each other and their family was strong. Dr. B continued to see his
> patients, though less frequently, and Dr. T remained available for consultation
> if needed.

Figure 16.3 summarizes the biopsychosocial approach to somatic fixation. With this approach, the physician addresses a patient's complaints
with an integrated biomedical and psychosocial evaluation from the
beginning. The physician also solicits help from family members early

in the process. When the tests are equivocal or negative, patient, family, and the physician may be perplexed, and a collaborative relationship is established to manage the patient's mysterious symptoms. Of great importance is the message that the physician does not fully understand the symptoms, does not have a quick answer or pill that will solve the problem, and is able to tolerate the uncertainty while continuing to work up the various aspects of the patient's problem. At this point, the physician may or may not consult with a medical colleague or a family therapist to share in the evaluation. In either case, the physician should **set limited, concrete goals for treatment and measure outcome by monitoring the patient's functioning** in areas of work, family, and personal life rather than only the patient's symptom picture. As functioning improves and symptoms become less severe, the physician is cautious about a cure and predicts the inevitable relapse in the patient's symptomatology. When patient functioning has improved adequately, the patient and physician agree to make sessions less frequent. However, the physician gives a clear message that he or she will continue to remain available to the patient and the family.

This biopsychosocial approach to the management and treatment of somatic fixation offers physician, patient, and family a way out of the vicious cycle that can develop around this problem. Not only can it offer an effective alternative for treatment, but it can also provide the physician with a vehicle to enjoy working with this problem that is so often experienced as difficult and frustrating.

References

1. Van Eijk J, Grol R, Huygen F, et al.: The family doctor and the prevention of somatic fixation. *Fam Syst Med* 1983;**1**(2):5–15.
2. Stoeckle J, Zola I, Davidson G: The quantity and significance of psychological distress in medical patients. *J Chronic Dis* 1964;**17**:959–970.
3. deGruy F, Columbia L, Dickinson P: Somatization disorder in a family practice. *J Fam Pract* 1987;**25**(1):45–51.
4. Kellner R, Sheffield BR: The 1-week prevalence of symptoms in neurotic patients and normals. *Am J Psychiatry* 1973;**130**:102–105.
5. Eisenberg L: Interfaces between medicine and psychiatry. *Comprehensive Psychiatry* 1979;**20**:1–14.
6. Barksy AJ: Patients who amplify bodily sensations. *Ann Intern Med* 1970;**91**:63–70.
7. Katon W: Somatization in primary care. *J Fam Pract* 1985;**21**(4):257–258.
8. Doherty W, Baird M: Forming a therapeutic contract that involves the family, *Family Therapy and Family Medicine*. New York, Guilford Press, 1983.
9. Quill TE: Somatization disorder: One of medicine's blind spots. *JAMA* 1986;**254**(21):3075–3079.
10. Smith GR, Monson RA, Ray DC: Psychiatric consultation in somatization disorder. *New Engl J Med* 1986;**314**(22):1407–1413.

PROTOCOL

Twelve Principles for a Biopsychosocial Approach to Somatic Fixation

1. From the beginning, evaluate each element of the problem.
   a. Begin by interspersing biomedical and psychosocial questions in the interview.
   b. Do a balanced, reasonable work-up, neither overusing tests nor avoiding the biological aspects of the symptoms.
2. Solicit the patient's symptoms, but do not let the symptoms run the interview.
   a. Reflect or ask a question after each sentence or two by the patient.
   b. Interrupt if necessary.
   c. Assume a curious or perplexed posture rather than a frustrated, intimidated, or weary posture with unusual symptoms, use unusual diagnostic procedures that allow you to remain active, such as measuring the length or intensity of symptoms.
   d. Keep the patient active in the diagnostic process–for example, request a symptom diary including both biomedical and psychosocial information about symptoms.
3. Develop a relationship with the patient that is collaborative.
   a. Avoid taking a traditional, authoritarian position or promising any easy answers to the patient's problems.
   b. Consider framing the patient's symptoms as mysterious and scientifically baffling, requiring the patient and physician to work together to manage the problem.
4. See the patient at regular intervals and discourage visits to other health providers, except on specific referral.
   a. See patients at regular, frequent intervals, not dictated by symptom occurrence or intensification.
   b. Route all acute and chronic patient complaints through the primary care physician.
   c. Have patients avoid Emergency Department visits, medical specialists, and inpatient treatment, unless specifically recommended by the primary care physician.
   d. When referral is indicated, be sure to talk with the consultant beforehand and be specific about the referral question.
5. Elicit the patient and family's diagnoses of the problem.
   a. Explore the meaning of the symptom to the patient.
   b. Given their diagnoses, what treatment do they expect will be useful?
   c. Work toward mutually acceptable diagnoses or explanations for the symptoms.
6. Elicit any recent stressful life events, life cycle challenges, or unresolved family problems–look especially for:

    a. A history of early abuse or deprivation.

    b. Unresolved grief.

    c. Alcohol or drug abuse, workaholism or other forms of overfunctioning.

7. Invite the family to participate in the process early in treatment.

    a. Request each person's observations, diagnoses, and opinions about the illness and the treatment.

    b. Listen for how the illness may have changed the typical roles or balance of power in the family.

    c. Try to understand any marital and/or transgenerational meaning for the symptom by asking: "Has anyone else in the family had an illness that in any way resembles this one?"

    d. Ask what each person is doing to help the patient with the illness.

    e. Ask how family life would be different if the patient was asymptomatic.

    f. Develop a treatment plan that the group can accept and request each person's help in its implementation.

8. Solicit and constantly return to the patient's and family's strengths and areas of competence.

9. Avoid psychosocial fixation; continue with an integrated approach.

    a. Use interventions that combine the biomedical and the psychosocial.

    b. Use biomedical explanations that also have psychosocial meanings, such as stress, scarring, or depressed immune system.

10. Find a way to enjoy somatically fixated patients.

    a. Listen to the patient's symptoms as metaphors for their larger problems.

    b. Monitor both the patient's and your own discomfort with uncertainty.

    c. Discuss the case with a physician colleague or invite that person to consult.

    d. Refer or collaborate closely with a family therapist or other mental health consultant.

11. Judge progress in these patients by monitoring changes in their level of functioning rather than in their symptoms.

12. Terminate the intense phase of treatment slowly.

    a. Restrain patients from too-rapid improvement.

    b. Keep your own expectations low; set small, realistic goals.

    c. With some improvement ask, what problems might emerge if the patient were to recover completely?

    d. Predict relapses.

    e. Slowly lengthen the time between office visits when the patient experiences an increase in general level of functioning and a decrease in the incapacitating nature of the symptoms.

    f. Remain available to the patient.

CHAPTER 17

Mobilizing Resources
Treating Depression in Primary Care

Depression is among the most common problems of patients seen in primary care. A majority of all psychiatric conditions are treated in primary care and depression heads the list (1). One study indicated that 27% of patients coming to a primary care setting were depressed, but none of them indicated that depression was the reason for their visit (2). Because somatic complaints mask depression, the diagnosis can often be overlooked or missed.

While some primary care patients do receive a diagnosis of major depressive illness, the majority identified as depressed are experiencing an adjustment reaction due to situational stressors such as loss, marital discord, the birth of a child, job changes, and illness. Whether it is a major depressive disorder or an adjustment reaction, the physician's most important task is to identify the problem and mobilize the available resources to provide appropriate support for the patient and to initiate change.

In this chapter we will focus on how the physician can mobilize and integrate individual, interpersonal and pharmacological resources in the identification, assessment and treatment of depression.

An Interactional Approach to Depression

Strong evidence exists that interpersonal factors are both significant precipitants of depressive episodes, and significant determinants of how an episode will be resolved (3). In many cases stressful marital or family events precede the onset of depression (4). These findings corroborate the view that depressive symptoms serve as a "barometer for external tension" (5).

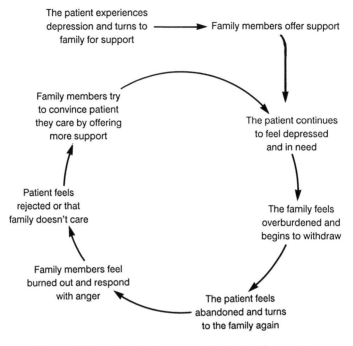

FIGURE 17.1.   The interpersonal spiral of depression

Coyne (6) suggests that depression results from social and interpersonal stressors that disrupt the patient's normal sources of support and nurturance. When these disruptions occur, the depressed person typically turns to his or her personal supports to gain the reassurance needed to restore a sense of security or worth. Partners and family members generally respond with support initially. Over time the depressed person may request increasing amounts of support and family members may begin to feel overburdened, irritated, or "burned out." These feelings often are not shared directly with the depressed person for fear of communicating rejection. The depressed person may become confused by family members' reassuring messages that are communicated in an angry tone or verbal support that is accompanied by withdrawing behavior. The patient then may respond by feeling more depressed and needy. This pattern may spiral over time as family members offer varying degrees of support which the patient may consistently experience as inadequate. In this way depressive symptoms can be maintained or intensified by patterns of behavior established between the depressed person and his or her significant others. (See Fig. 17.1.)

Studies indicate that depressed people whose relatives exhibit a high degree of critical comments have a greater incidence of relapse than those whose families demonstrate low levels of criticism (7,8). A good marital relationship can protect partners from depression when stressful life events occur, but when there is a poor marital relationship, women in particular are three times more likely to become depressed when facing life stressors (9).

Biochemical and intrapsychic factors have received much attention and validation in the treatment of depression. Coupled with the role of interpersonal factors, depressive symptoms can be understood as resulting from the interaction of factors on the biochemical, personal, interpersonal, and social levels of experience. Coyne (10) suggests that treatment should address three aspects of the system simultaneously: the depressed person, the partner, and any relationship problems between the two of them. In the following sections we will discuss guidelines for assessing and treating depressed persons from an interactional perspective.

Assessing Depression

> Mrs. Pulcino came to see Dr. X for the fourth time in two months. Mrs. Pulcino was married and had two children, one of whom was school aged. She worked outside the home as an aide in a nearby nursing home. Mr. Pulcino drove a delivery truck and also maintained a one-hundred-acre farm. Mrs. Pulcino reported symptoms of fatigue, headaches, and minor aches and pains. In the previous three months, she had seen Dr. X for a cold and an intestinal flu, as well.
>
> Mrs. Pulcino told Dr. X she was afraid there was something seriously wrong with her. None of Dr. X's tests revealed any organic causes for her symptoms. And yet Mrs. Pulcino was clearly feeling ill.

Some patients talk openly about their emotional or interpersonal problems with their physician, but others do not. Somatic complaints are often the primary way in which depressive symptoms are presented in a medical setting (11–13). The physician's first task is to recognize the signs that assessment for depression may be necessary. An increase in the number of office visits, functional complaints, infections and reports of pain and anxiety by the patient is often a harbinger of a depressive episode (14).

Assessment should focus on the patient in the context of his or her significant relationships. An interactional approach helps the physician gather a broad range of information and develop a treatment partnership that can include the patient and his or her main supports. Key elements in the assessment process include: evaluating the depressed individual, involving the partner, exploring difficulties, and measuring the effect of other life stressors.

Evaluating the Depressed Person

The following are important issues to assess:

1. How badly are you feeling? It is important to assess the severity of the patient's depression and how his or her symptoms are manifest in the patient's daily life:

• How long has the patient felt this way?
• Has the patient ever felt depressed before?
• Have any of his or her family members ever experienced similar difficulties?
• What does the patient feel is the cause of his or her depression?
• When the patient is depressed, does he or she ever drink or use other drugs to feel better?

In order to differentiate whether the patient is experiencing a major depression or an adjustment reaction, it is valuable to explore these areas (15):

• changes in appetite leading to weight gain or loss
• insomnia or hypersomnia
• psychomotor agitation or retardation
• loss of interest and pleasure in usual activities
• loss of energy
• poor concentration or indecisiveness
• feelings of guilt and worthlessness
• frequent fearfulness
• thoughts of death or suicide

A patient who reports continuous difficulty in at least **five of the areas** listed previously **during the same two week period** is experiencing a **major depressive episode.**

A patient who reports a strong **reaction to a life stressor** occurring in the **last few months** is experiencing an **adjustment reaction.** Patients who are having an adjustment reaction may experience social, occupational, or interpersonal impairment, but such impairment should remit once the period of stress if over. If an interview seems inconclusive, physicians may find it useful to administer a self-report instrument such as the Beck Depression Inventory (16).

2. Do you ever want to kill yourself? Depressed persons sometimes have suicidal thoughts. Do not assume that the patient will volunteer his or her suicidal thoughts or intentions. The physician should raise the question of suicidality with the patient and his or her spouse and family in a straightforward manner:

• Do you ever think of hurting yourself?
• Do you have a plan for killing yourself?
• How would you do it?

• When do you plan to act?
• Can you and your family maintain your safety?

Patients who have suicidal thoughts and a plan of action should be referred for a psychiatric evaluation immediately. The physician should involve the patient's spouse or family to support the patient and help maintain his or her safety until an evaluation can be done.

3. What do others think about your problems? In preparation for involving significant others in treatment, it is important to assess how the patient's symptoms may affect or be affected by his or her relationships with others:

• How do your spouse, family, and friends respond to how you are feeling?
• Who is most concerned about you?
• Who is most supportive of you?
• What do others suggest to remedy the situation?
• What do others think is the cause of your depression?

These questions explore the patient's view of interpersonal factors that may both contribute to the patient's depressive symptoms as well as help to alleviate them.

Dr. X begins the assessment of Mrs. Pulcino with these individual and interpersonal dimensions in mind.

> Dr. X learned that Mrs. Pulcino had been having difficulty sleeping for almost four months and that she had gained ten pounds over the same period. At times she felt confused and helpless to change her situation. Mrs. Pulcino often wished it would "all come to an end," but when Dr. X asked specifically if she wanted to hurt herself, Mrs. Pulcino said she had no intention of killing herself.
>
> Mrs. Pulcino said her husband worried about her and often suggested she rest more, but, at times, was impatient with her being tired so often. When asked if she considered herself depressed, Mrs. Pulcino said "yes." She also wondered if there was something physically wrong that made her feel depressed.
>
> Dr. X reiterated that none of the tests showed any significant physiological findings, but he agreed that Mrs. Pulcino definitely felt ill and was depressed. He suggested that it would be valuable to have Mr. Pulcino come with her to the next visit. Dr. X explained that Mr. Pulcino's input would help Dr. X get a broader picture of the problem and would be a chance for the three of them to work together on a treatment direction.

Involving the Partner

I would like your partner to come in with you. The inclusion of the patient's partner is an invaluable asset during assessment and treatment. A partner can provide information about depressive symptoms that the patient may not recognize. Also, in cases where antidepressant medication is indicated, patients in a supportive, satisfactory marital relationship respond more favorably (17).

By seeing the partners together the physician can gain a better understanding of how their interactions may play a part in the patient's depression. First, depressed patients behave differently with relative strangers, such as a physician, than they do with a spouse (18). Observation of the patient with a partner gives the physician a clearer picture of the patient's depressive behavior. Second, partners of depressed patients are often depressed themselves. Persons who have ongoing contact with depressed people often exhibit depressive symptoms themselves, such as anger (19). It is important to assess whether or not the partner may be depressed and, if so, to what degree the partner needs support. Third, relationship patterns often help maintain a patient's depressive symptoms (10). Even when partners do not report significant relational dissatisfaction they may still interact in ways that maintain the patient's depression. The patient who is needy and helpless may be made more so by a partner's willingness to meet his or her every need (20). On the other hand, a depressed person who is excessively demanding may find his or her partner's supportive behavior laced with subtle or open criticism, leaving the depressed person feeling rejected.

Questions of the partner which help the physician gather more information and understand the interpersonal dimension of the patient's depression include:

• How can you tell when your partner is depressed?
• What do you do when he or she is depressed? How does your partner respond?
• (to both partners) How do you think your relationship has been affected by this problem?
• Are there ever times when your partner does not feel depressed? Can you describe those times?
• Have you yourself ever felt depressed?

After getting to know Mr. Pulcino, Dr. X discusses Mrs. Pulcino's depression and her husband's perception of her illness:

> At the conjoint interview, Dr. X noticed immediately that Mrs. Pulcino was quieter and more withdrawn. Mr. Pulcino watched her continuously and spoke to her in soothing tones. When she appeared unresponsive, Mr. Pulcino sat back, looked at Dr. X and shrugged his shoulders.
>
> Mr. Pulcino said his wife had been depressed for several months. He knew she was having a bad day if she was not dressed when he returned from morning chores for breakfast. They both reported that Mr. Pulcino tried to talk to his wife or hug her, but sometimes she would not respond and he would fall silent or leave suddenly for the barn. Mr. and Mrs. Pulcino thought their marriage was a good one, but they were both exhausted and edgy with each other because Mrs. Pulcino's depression was not lifting. The only time her depressive behavior seemed to decrease was when they watched TV together

on Thursday nights. Then she might laugh and Mr. Pulcino would feel better. When Dr. X asked Mrs. Pulcino if she ever worried about her husband, she said she was concerned that he was becoming more moody. Mr. Pulcino agreed.

Mr. Pulcino's efforts to support his wife did not coincide with times when Mrs. Pulcino would accept his support. Consequently, Mr. Pulcino would feel frustrated and then withdraw while Ms. Pulcino would feel rejected and become more depressed. Mr. Pulcino would then try to support her again and the cycle would continue. Dr. X felt the Pulcinos had a strong marriage but that they were stuck in a pattern that supported rather than alleviated Mrs. Pulcino's depression.

Life Stressors

What other changes have occurred in your life? Depressed persons experience more stressful life events before the onset of depressive symptoms than nondepressed persons (21). These may include deaths, changes in work or financial status, the birth of a child, the departure of an offspring, geographical relocations, issues related to individual and family life cycles and recent illnesses.

Some questions to guide the discussion of life stressors include:

• What changes have occurred in your lives in the past year? Illnesses? Moves? Losses? Deaths?
• What impact have these changes had on you and your family?
• Do you feel these changes play a part in your depression?

Next, Dr. X helped the Pulcinos explore the significant events that have occurred in their lives in the recent past.

During the last year Mr. Pulcino had taken a part time job driving a delivery truck because of financial problems. To help out, Mrs. Pulcino had taken responsibility for keeping the books on the family business. It was not until then that she realized how serious their financial problems were. At the same time, Mrs. Pulcino's mother, who had lived down the road, moved to Florida after her retirement. This move had been particularly difficult for Mrs. Pulcino who depended on her mother for support and child care. As for the children, Emily, the oldest, had started kindergarten. Mr. and Mrs. Pulcino had not recognized how many stressful changes had occurred in the previous year. Mrs. Pulcino wondered if all the changes had been "too much" for her.

With a clearer understanding of Mrs. Pulcino's symptoms and their relationship to her interpersonal context and life situation, Dr. X began treatment with Mr. and Mrs. Pulcino.

Treating Depression in Primary Care

The severity of the patient's depression is a central factor in the physician's decision about treatment directions. **Patients who are experiencing an adjustment reaction are the best candidates for**

primary care counseling. Patients diagnosed with a major depression may receive a trial of antidepressant medication and primary care counseling. If either approach is not successful, the primary care provider should consider a referral to a specialist. Regardless, the primary care physician is in an excellent position to identify a patient's depression and mobilize the resources for treatment.

Our discussion of treatment will focus on how to change individual and interpersonal behavior that may perpetuate depression. We will conclude with guidelines for the use of antidepressant medication.

The Partner as a Collaborator in the Treatment of Depression

By involving the partner the physician can help the couple interact in ways that may alleviate some of the patient's depressive symptoms. To that end it is important to gauge any overinvolvement or underinvolvement the partner may have with the patient's problem (10). Overinvolved partners take too much responsibility for the depressed person, thus, inadvertently, supporting the depressed person's feeling of helplessness. Underinvolved partners appear distant or even hostile toward the depressed person who may then feel abandoned and hopeless. The physician can help the partner achieve a moderate level of involvement which is both supportive of the patient's needs and respectful of the patient's autonomy. For example, the partner who fixes all the meals for a depressed person may be encouraged by the physician to prepare one meal a day while assisting the depressed person in preparing the others. Or, to a partner who withdraws when the depressed person requests emotional support, the physician may suggest he or she offer encouragement once a day before it is even sought. In those ways the physician can help bring balance to the partner's involvement around the patient's symptoms. A more balanced approach may also reduce pressure on the partner and benefit the marital relationship as well. When relational discord makes it difficult for the couple to work together or is clearly a contributing factor in the patient's depression, the physician should engage the couple in primary care couples counseling or negotiate a referral to a marital therapist. (See Chapter 12 on counseling couples in primary care and Chapter 22 on collaboration and referral to a family-oriented mental health professional.)

When involving the partner in treatment, it is important to:

- **Maintain an alliance with the patient and the partner** – a relationship may already exist between the physician and patient so it is important to develop rapport with the partner in order to maintain a balanced relationship with the couple.
- **Avoid blaming the partner for the patient's depression or making the partner responsible for alleviating the patient's depres-**

sion—the partner often feels overburdened by the patient's depression and may need to be relieved of excessive guilt or responsibility.
- **Focus on ways in which the partner can be a resource in treatment**—emphasize the strengths in the relationship that may be utilized to help the patient.
- **Recognize and discuss the effect the patient's depression may have on the partner**—partners of depressed people often experience depressive symptoms themselves.
- **Support the partner in looking after his or her own needs**—by addressing his or her own needs the partner may find additional strength and energy to help the patient.

Working with the Depressed Individual

Depressed people tend to feel powerless and angry about changing their situation. Because they often depend on others to meet many of their personal needs, depressed people are extremely sensitive to criticism and rejection. At times, their perception of whether or not others are critical or rejecting is distorted. Depressed persons have often experienced many losses and their grief is frequently unresolved. The pain of these negative experiences may only confirm their feelings of worthlessness. To protect themselves depressed people may withdraw from what seems like a world that does not care, yet continue to hope that someone else will make things better. The further they withdraw, the more powerless they feel; the more powerless they feel, the more they count on others; the more they count on others, the more vulnerable they are to disappointment; the more disappointed they are, the more they withdraw, and so on.

Therapeutic approaches that are most effective with depressed patients are **brief, goal-oriented, and focused on behavioral change** (19). The central task of the physician is to help the patient interrupt the downward spiral of depressive symptoms that results from feelings of powerlessness and dependency on others. Primary care counseling should aid the patient in identifying small, manageable tasks that will increase his or her sense of personal mastery and competence. Below are some treatment strategies for working with the depressed individual:

- **Focus on changing behaviors**—an increase in meaningful activity has a positive effect on the patient's affect.
- **Go slowly**—do not facilitate too much change too quickly when the patient's resources may be depleted.
- **Take small measurable steps**—help the patient identify concrete, observable behavior which he or she can do (e.g., a patient who found it extremely difficult to leave the house started with a plan of going outside twice a week).

- **Emphasize self-monitoring** – encourage the patient to keep a journal of his or her periods of depression and what he or she is doing, thinking and feeling; the patient should also keep a record of the changes he or she is making and how he or she feels about them.
- **Utilize feedback from the patient's partner** – involve the partner in observing positive changes in the patient and in giving the patient feedback on these changes.

These strategies are designed to increase the patient's sense of autonomy and self-determination. The resulting positive feedback can help the patient internalize those changes and begin to feel more self-confident.

Utilizing Antidepressant Medication

Medication is a family issue. The effectiveness of antidepressant medication in treating most patients with major depression is well-established (22). This effectiveness can be greatly influenced by relationship factors in the patient's life. For that reason, pharmacological treatment should be approached as a family issue and integrated into an overall treatment plan that includes ongoing counseling with the patient and partner. The involvement of significant others can improve compliance and provide the support the patient will need in the early stages of pharmacological treatment. By the same token, antidepressant medication can increase the patient's concentration, energy, and motivation to work on relationship issues. Combining medication and family counseling has a beneficial effect on both modalities (23).

When utilizing antidepressant medication as part of a comprehensive treatment plan, it is important to:

- **Present the option of using medication to the patient and partner together whenever possible.** This provides the physician with the opportunity to educate the couple on the effects and side effects of antidepressant medication and to answer their questions.
- **Use only when indicated.** Antidepressants are most effective with vegetative signs of depression, such as weight loss and anorexia, insomnia, and psychomotor disturbance (23). Patients diagnosed with an adjustment reaction are not good candidates for antidepressants.
- **Clarify the patient's medical status.** Depression is common among the medically ill (24,25). It is important to assess whether or not the patient's depressive symptoms are the **result** of an underlying medical problem or a **response** to an acute or chronic medical condition. For example, depressive symptoms can result from cancer, endocrine problems, and neurological disorders. By the same token, stroke victims, post MI patients and those who suffer from chronic illnesses may experience depressive symptoms in response to their medical problems.

For these reasons, a complete physical is warranted for patients who have not been examined in the past six to twelve months.

• **Involve the patient and partner in a plan to monitor, decrease, and eventually discontinue the medication.** This may include planning a medication regimen together, monitoring signs of change, and continuing counseling during the transition from use to nonuse. The couples who work together around the use of medication can mirror and support other changes they are making in the relationship.

A valuable guide for the selection and use of antidepressant medications is provided in *Concise Guide to Somatic Therapies in Psychiatry* by Guttmacher (26). It may also be helpful for the physician to consult a psychiatrist regarding specific antidepressant medications.

The Pulcinos entered counseling with Dr. X to focus on alleviating Mrs. Pulcino's depressive symptoms. Mr. Pulcino agreed to attend these sessions as a resource to Dr. X and as a support to his wife.

During treatment Dr. X helped the patient choose small, observable tasks to accomplish what both partners felt would help Mrs. Pulcino feel less depressed. For example, Mrs. Pulcino's first goal was to get up each day by 7:00 a.m. Mr. Pulcino encouraged his wife and often reminded her of this goal. When she did not get up, he would become critical and they would argue. Dr. X helped Mr. Pulcino make changes in the way he offered support. Mr. Pulcino was encouraged by Dr. X to give positive verbal feedback to Mrs. Pulcino on days she met her goal but to say nothing when she did not. In discussing the issue, Mrs. Pulcino decided that getting up at 7:00 a.m. three times per week was a more reasonable goal.

Over the next few weeks Mrs. Pulcino was able to meet her new goal and the couple reported less conflict. Nevertheless, Mrs. Pulcino was still not sleeping well and had difficulty concentrating during the day. It was during this period that Mrs. Pulcino discussed feeling depressed at other times in her life, as had her mother. Mrs. Pulcino's father had died when she was two years old. She felt her mother was still sad about the loss. Mrs. Pulcino herself was tearful when discussing her father.

Dr. X discussed the use of antidepressant medication as a tool to help Mrs. Pulcino sleep better and regain some energy. He emphasized that the use of medication should be in conjunction with ongoing counseling to continue working on behavior changes and to monitor the effect of the medication.

Over the next two months Mrs. Pulcino began to sleep better and was able to accomplish her daily responsibilities, but the couple reported an increase in their arguing. Mrs. Pulcino felt her husband did not give her enough emotional support; and Mr. Pulcino said his wife demanded too much. Dr. X suggested the Pulcinos see a marriage counselor to address these issues. He clarified that he would continue to see them together periodically to monitor the medication and would be in regular contact with their counselor.

The Pulcinos accepted the referral and saw a marriage counselor for a year during which time they were able to improve their relationship. Dr. X proceeded cautiously with decreasing the medication and it was discontinued after nine months.

The primary care physician can do an excellent job treating the depressed patient, especially if he or she has developed a network of professional resources with which to collaborate. Mobilizing the resources of the patient and family is the key to a comprehensive, integrated treatment approach that is effective and efficient.

References

1. Rosenbaum JF, Polack MH: Anxiety, in Hacket TP, Cassem NJ (eds.): *Massachusetts General Hospital's Handbook of General Hospital Psychiatry*. Littleton, MA, PSG Publishing Co., 1987, pp 154–183.
2. Duer S, Schwenk TL, Coyne JC: Medical and psychosocial correlates of self-reported depressive symptoms in family practice. *J Fam Pract* 1988;**27**(6): 609–614.
3. Coyne JC: Depression, biology, marriage and marital therapy. *Fam Process* 1987;**13**(4):393–407.
4. Clarkin JF, Haas GL: Assesment of affective disorders and their interpersonal contexts, in Clarkin JF, Haas GL, Glick ID (eds.): *Affective Disorders and the Family*. New York, The Guilford Press, 1988, pp 29–50.
5. Bromet EJ, May S: Family environments of depressed outpatients. *Acta Psychiatr Scand* 1984;**69**:197–200.
6. Coyne JC: Toward an interactional description of depression. *Psychiatry* 1976; **39**:28–40.
7. Vaughn CE, Leff JP: The influence of family and social factors on the course of psychiatric illness. A comparison of schizophrenic and depressed neurotic patients. *Br J Psychiatry* 1976;**129**:125–137.
8. Hooley JM, Orley J, Teasdale JD: Levels of expressed emotion and relapse in depressed patients. *Br J Psychiatry* 1986;**148**:642–647.
9. Rousanville BJ, Weissman MW, Prusoff BA, Heraey-Baron RL: Marital disputes and treatment outcome in depressed women. *Compr Psych* 1979;**20**: 483–490.
10. Coyne JC: Strategic Therapy, in Clarkin JF, Haas GL, Glick ID (eds.): *Affective Disorders and the Family*. New York, The Guilford Press, 1988, pp 89–113.
11. Wittenborn JR, Buhlev MS: Somatic discomforts among depressed women. *Arch Gen Psychiatry* 1979;**36**:465–471.
12. Roy MJ, Weinman ML, Mirabi M: Physical symptoms of depression. *Br J Psychiatry* 1981;**139**:293–296.
13. Rodin G, Voshart K: Depression in the medically ill: An overview. *Am J Psychiatry* 1986;**143**(6):696–705.
14. Widmer RB, Cadoret RJ: Depression in family practice: Changes in pattern of visits and complaints during subsequent developing depression. *J Fam Prac* 1979;**9**(6):1017–1021.
15. American Psychiatric Association: *Diagnostic and Statistical Manual of Mental Disorders* (rev. 3rd ed.). Washington, DC, APA, 1987.
16. Beck AT, Ward CH, Mendelson M: An inventory for measuring depression. *Arch Gen Psychiatry* 1961;**4**:561–571.

17. Weissman MM, Prusoff BA, DiMascio A, Neu C, Gorklaney M, Klerman GL: The efficacy of drugs and psychotherapy in the treatment of acute depressive episodes. *Am J Psychiatry* 1979;**136**:555–558.
18. Hinchliffe M, Hooper D, Roberts FJ, Vaughan PM: A study of the interaction between depressed patients and their spouses. *Brit J Psychiatry* 1975;**126**:164–172.
19. Coyne JC, Kahn J, Gotlib IM: Depression, in Jacob T (ed.): *Family Interaction and Psychotherapy*. New York, Plenum, 1987, pp 509–534.
20. Watzlawick P, Weakland JH, Fisch R. *Change: Principles of Problem Formation and Problem Resolution*. New York: W.W. Norton and Co., 1974.
21. O'Neil MK, Lancee WJ, Freeman SJJ: Psychosocial factors and depressive symptoms. *J Nerv Mental Dis* 1986;**174**(1):15–23
22. Davis JM: Antidepressant drugs, in Kaplan HI, Freedman AM, Sadock BJ (eds.): *Comprehensive Textbook of Psychiatry* (3rd ed, vol 3). Baltimore, MD, Williams and Wilkins, 1980, pp 213–225.
23. Epstein NB, Keitner GI, Bishop DS, Miller IW: Combined use of pharmacological and family therapy, in Clarkin JF, Haas GL, Glick ID (eds.): *Affective Disorders and the Family*. New York, The Guilford Press, 1988, pp 153–172.
24. Nielsen AC, Williams TA: Depression in ambulatory medical patients: Prevalence by self-report questionnaire and recognition by nonpsychiatric physicians. *Arch Gen Psychiatry* 1980;**37**:999–1004.
25. Salkind MR: Beck depression inventory in general pratice. *J R Coll Gen Pract* 1969;**18**:267–271.
26. Guttmacher LB: *Concise Guide to Somatic Therapies in Psychiatry*. Washington, DC, American Psychiatric Press, 1988.

PROTOCOL

Treating Depression in Primary Care

The physician's most important task in treating a depressed patient is to mobilize the available resources to provide appropriate support for the patient and to initiate change.

Assessing Depression

A. Evaluating the depressed person.
1. How badly are you feeling?
   a. How long have you felt this way?
   b. Have you ever felt depressed before?
   c. Have any of your family members ever experienced similar difficulties?
   d. When you are depressed, do you ever drink or use other drugs to feel better?
   e. What do you feel is the cause of your depression?
   f. What, if any, changes have occurred in these areas:
      - weight loss or weight gain
      - insomnia or hypersomnia
      - psychomotor agitation or retardation
      - loss of interest and pleasure in usual activities
      - loss of energy
      - poor concentration or indecisiveness
      - feelings of guilt or worthlessness
      - frequent fearfulness
      - thoughts of death or suicide
2. Do you ever want to hurt yourself?
   a. Do you ever think of hurting yourself?
   b. Do you have a plan for killing yourself?
   c. How would you do it?
   d. When do you plan to act?
   e. Can you and your family maintain your safety at this time?
3. What do others think about your problem?
   a. How do your spouse, family, and friends respond to how you are feeling?
   b. Who is most concerned about you?
   c. Who is most supportive of you?
   d. What do others suggest to remedy the situation?
   e. What do others think is the cause of your depression?

B. Involving the Partner
1. How can you tell when the patient is depressed?
2. What do you do when he or she is depressed?

3. How does the patient respond?
4. (to both partners) How do you think your relationship has been affected by this problem?
5. Are there ever times when your partner does not feel depressed? Can you describe those times?
6. Have you yourself ever felt depressed?

C. Evaluating Life Stressors
   1. What change have occurred in your life in the past year? Illnesses? Moves? Losses? Deaths?
   2. What impact have these changes had on you and your family?
   3. Do you feel these changes play a part in your depression?

Treating Depression

A. The Partner as Collaborator in the Treatment of Depression
   1. Maintain an alliance with the patient and the partner
   2. Avoid blaming the partner for the patient's depression or making the partner responsible for alleviating the patient's depression.
   3. Focus on ways in which the partner can be resource in treatment.
   4. Recognize and discuss the effect the patient's depression may have on the partner.
   5. Support the partner in looking after his or her own needs.

B. Working with the Depressed Individual
   1. Focus on changing behaviors
   2. Go slowly
   3. Take small measurable steps
   4. Emphasize self-monitoring
   5. Utilize feedback from the patient's partner

C. Utilizing Antidepressant Medication
   1. Present the option of using medication to the patient and partner together whenever possible.
   2. Use only when clearly indicated.
   3. Clarify the patient's medical status.
   4. Involve the patient and partner in a plan to monitor, decrease, and eventually discontinue the medication.

CHAPTER 18

When Drinking Is Part of the Problem

A Family Approach to the Detection and Management of Alcohol Abuse

Alcohol abuse is one of the most serious and underrecognized health problems in primary care. One in ten Americans abuse alcohol (1) and one in three families report problems related to drinking (2). Alcohol abuse is the leading cause of death in 15 to 45 year olds and is associated with 10% of all deaths in the U.S. including suicide, homicide, and fatal accidents. Suicide is 30 times more common in alcoholics, and one half of all fatal automobile accidents are due to drunk driving. Patients who abuse alcohol use medical services much more often than other patients. The direct health costs related to alcohol misuse is estimated to be $15 billion, and indirect costs (lost productivity, MVAs, fires and crime) account for an additional $90 billion (3).

Despite its health consequences and economic costs, alcohol abuse is infrequently recognized or diagnosed in health care settings. Less than 20% of patients with alcohol problems are identified in any medical settings (4,5). Even in the hospital, where alcohol problems tend to be more severe and more common [approximately 20% of hospitalized patients abuse alcohol (6)], only a small fraction of alcohol abusers are diagnosed (7).

The reasons for the underrecognition of alcohol problems by health care providers are many:

1. Lack of education about alcohol abuse: Only 1% of medical school curriculum is devoted to substance abuse, and most are lectures on the medical complications of alcoholism (8). In one survey of practicing physicians, only 27% reported that they felt competent to manage alcoholism (9).

2. The early signs of alcohol abuse are mostly psychosocial, not biomedical. Medical students only learn about the medical problems associated with alcoholism, such as cirrhosis and alcoholic heart disease, which usually represent the end-stages of the disease. They are rarely encouraged to explore the psychosocial aspects of patient's lives and thereby recognize alcohol problems that are less severe or at an earlier stage.

3. Negative attitudes about alcoholism: Physicians in training often care for the skid-row, end-stage alcoholic who commonly evokes feelings of aversion, hostility, and depression. Physicians tend to see alcoholics as bad or morally weak individuals (10,11).

4. Pessimism about treatment. Many physicians feel that alcoholism is not treatable and feel helpless when confronted with a patient who has alcohol problems. Part of this pessimism comes from caring for hard-core alcoholics where treatment is less successful. It then becomes a self-fulfilling prophecy: the physician feels helpless and fails to offer appropriate treatment, the patient keeps drinking, and the physician's beliefs are confirmed. However, research demonstrates that treatment of alcoholism is often successful and cost-effective because it lowers medical care utilization and costs (12,13). As a result, more insurance plans are providing coverage of alcohol treatment; in some states this coverage is mandatory.

5. Denial. The distinction between social drinking and alcohol abuse is not always clear. To diagnose alcohol problems effectively, the primary care provider must address his or her own drinking or drug use, and this can be threatening. A recent study demonstrated that physicians are more likely to drink alcohol to excess than the general population, and heavy drinking by physicians is associated with job stress and burnout (14). A physician who drinks heavily is unlikely to recognize when a patient's drinking is problematic.

Alcoholism is a chronic and serious biopsychosocial disorder that involves problems at all levels of the system, from the physiologic effects of alcohol on organs and tissue, to the impact of drinking on society. In this chapter, we will focus on alcoholism as a family disorder and describe the role of the family-oriented physician in the detection, assessment, and management of alcohol problems. We will emphasize the importance of involving the family in all aspects of the problem. The abuse of substances other than alcohol, including illicit and prescription drugs, is beyond the scope of this chapter and covered by others (15,16). However, many of the concepts and interventions presented can be useful for other substance abusers.

Families and Alcohol Abuse

Over the past 20 years, there has been increasing recognition of the importance of the family in understanding and treating alcoholism. Theories of alcoholism that rely *solely* on individual psychopathology or genetics have been abandoned. Nearly all treatment programs involve families in some manner (17).

A family approach is important with alcohol problems for a number of reasons:

1. Alcoholics live in families. Most patients with minor or serious alcohol problems live in some kind of family. The stereotype of the "skid-row" alcoholic who lives in the street represents a very small percentage of people who abuse alcohol (18,19). In addition, the impact of alcoholism on the patient and the family is determined more by the family environment, its rules, attitudes, and beliefs, than by the amount or pattern of alcohol use (20).

2. Alcoholism runs in families. Patients who have two or more relatives with a history of alcohol abuse are at three times the normal risk of abusing alcohol themselves. Adoption and twin studies have demonstrated that both genetic and family environment increase this risk (20,21). One study demonstrated that families that are able to maintain healthy mealtime and holiday rituals in the face of alcoholism are less likely to transmit alcoholism to the next generation (22). These findings emphasize the importance of obtaining a family history of alcoholism with all patients to identify those who are at risk for alcohol problems.

3. A family approach allows earlier identification and treatment of alcohol problems. The earliest problems associated with alcohol abuse are usually interpersonal, and they occur long before any medical complications. Alcohol problems first present as marital disputes, parent–child conflicts, or work problems (20,23). Only by investigating these family problems will the physician identify underlying alcohol abuse (24). Family members are usually the first to recognize alcohol problems. They may alert the physician to the problem and ask for help, or they may present with problems related to the drinking in the family. One common example is the depressed woman with multiple somatic complaints and marital problems which are related to her husband's drinking. Caring for the entire family gives the family-oriented physician the chance to intervene early, when treatment is easier and more effective.

4. Families are a major asset in the assessment and treatment of alcohol problems. Patients who abuse alcohol often deny that they have a problem. They underreport both how much they drink and the adverse effects of their drinking. Family members can often provide a more accurate picture of alcohol use, although they may also share in the denial. Acting alone, the physician may have little impact on breaking down the alcoholic's denial, but allied with concerned family members, the physician can more effectively confront the alcoholic and begin treatment. The confrontation of Betty Ford by her family and friends is a classic example of the usefulness of this approach.

5. Families need treatment both to help cope with the effects of alcoholism on the family and to change family patterns that may have unwittingly contributed to the drinking. Alcoholism is a devastating illness that affects all members of the family. It often results in major family problems or disruptions, including marital conflict or divorce, child abuse or neglect, unemployment and poverty, and numerous mental and physical health problems. There is usually a tremendous amount of anger, blame and guilt in these families which persists even after abstinence if the family does not receive treatment.

In attempting to cope with the drinking, family members may inadvertently facilitate or "enable" the drinking. This most commonly occurs when a spouse thinks he or she is protecting the drinker by keeping the alcohol abuse a secret or covering up the adverse consequences, such as missing work. Drinking can be functional in some families in that it may be used as a solution to unresolved conflicts or unacceptable feelings. For example, anger or grief expressed while the person is drunk is often discounted by the drinker or the family because of the intoxication. These families often display stereotypic patterns of interaction which cycle between "dry" and "wet" phases (25,26). Alcoholic families need therapy to help them change these dysfunctional patterns of interaction.

Detection of Alcohol Problems in Primary Care

Alcohol abuse is best defined by the presence of adverse physical, family, social, or occupational consequences of drinking (DSM-IIIR, 27). The definition of alcohol abuse does not depend upon the amount, frequency, or pattern of drinking. In fact, Steinglass (28) found that the negative social and family consequences of drinking were not even correlated to the actual quantity or frequency of alcohol consumption. However, there is no clear-cut distinction between heavy alcohol use and alcohol abuse. The physician should have a high level of suspicion for alcohol problems in primary care and match interventions to the degree of the problem.

Because of the high prevalence of alcohol abuse and its serious impact on health, all patients should be screened for alcohol abuse. Studies have shown that patients with serious substance abuse rarely bring up these problems spontaneously to their physician (29). Unless the physicians specifically ask about drinking, alcoholics will remain anonymous (30). Alcohol use should be part of the basic medical history and data base. All patients should be asked:

"How much alcohol do you drink?" (not "do you drink alcohol?") and

"Have you ever had a problem with your health, your work, or your family because of drinking?"
Asking about alcohol problems has been shown to be particularly effective in identifying alcoholic patients (31). When obtaining a family history, ask

"Has anyone in your family ever had problems with alcohol use?"

The following guidelines should be used when inquiring about alcohol use:

1. Be as matter-of-fact as possible. Routinely include these questions about alcohol use with other health risks such as smoking. Show interest but not surprise or overconcern about the amount or pattern of use during screening or assessment. Avoid the terms "alcoholic" or "alcoholism," unless the patient brings them up. Many patients will admit that they or their family members have had problems with alcohol use, but they never considered it to be alcoholism. Be aware of the degree of defensiveness the patient exhibits in response to your questions. Patients with drinking problems may spontaneously deny that they abuse alcohol or question the relevance of discussing alcohol use.

2. Ask the patient to be very explicit about his or her alcohol use. Don't accept responses such as "just occasionally," "only on weekends and special occasions," or "maybe one drink when I get home from work." Ask "how often is occasionally?", "how much on weekends?" or "what is one drink?" If the patient responds that he or she "never drinks," find out why? Many abstainers have a personal or family history of alcohol abuse.

3. Inquire further about drinking in any patient who reports drinking daily or more than two drinks on an occasion. These patients need to be more closely screened for alcohol abuse. The CAGE questionnaire is a quick, reliable and easy to remember set of questions to use (32).

C Have you ever felt you ought to CUT DOWN on your drinking?
A Have people ANNOYED you by criticizing your drinking?
G Have you ever felt bad or GUILTY about your drinking?
E Have you ever had a drink first thing in the morning (EYE-OPENER) to steady your nerves or get rid of a hangover?

If the answers to the four questions are negative, it takes only a few minutes. Positive responses should be pursued further. Two or more affirmative answers to these questions indicates probable alcohol abuse with an 80 to 90 percent sensitivity and specificity (6,33,34). A "yes" answer to EYEOPENER suggests physical dependence on alcohol.

4. Record the patient's response in a prominent place in the medical chart. Alcohol and drug use should be on the front sheet of the chart with other basic medical history such as allergies, tobacco use, and previous surgeries.

Alcohol abusers visit their physicians more often than other patients with complaints and problems related to their drinking. These problems commonly include acute trauma, gastrointestinal symptoms, sleep disturbances, sexual dysfunction, and depression. Physicians should have a high degree of suspicion for alcohol or drug abuse when patients present with these types of problems.

Mrs. Seagram, a 44-year-old housewife and mother of three children, came to Dr. K for her yearly Pap Smear and check-up. She complained of feeling tired all the time, and having difficulty sleeping. She attributed it to caring for three young children and an aging parent, but wondered whether she was beginning menopause. Further questions by Dr. K revealed that Mrs. Seagram was mildly depressed and that her husband was rarely at home, spending more and more time at work. As part of his routine history, Dr. K asked how much alcohol she drank. She replied that she usually had a drink before dinner while waiting for her husband to come home, and occasionally had a brandy to help her sleep. With more specific questions, she admitted to regularly having 3–4 drinks each evening, but denied that it was causing any problems. At times she felt she ought to CUT DOWN on her drinking, and felt a little GUILTY about her drinking since she was very critical of her mother who drank to excess. (Two affirmative answers to CAGE questions.)

Negotiating with the Alcohol Abuser

All patients who report heavy drinking, answer yes to any of the CAGE questions, or present with a complaint related to alcohol use should have a more thorough assessment of alcohol use and problems associated with it.

The following guidelines are suggested for evaluating the problem and discussing it with the patient.

1. Focus on the patient's presenting problem during the assessment; link the drinking to the presenting problem. "I'm concerned that your drinking is contributing to your fatigue and sleeping problem." Focusing on the consequences of drinking reduces the patient's defensiveness and avoids blaming the patient for the drinking. However, treating a medical problem associated with alcohol abuse without addressing the underlying drinking reinforces the patient's denial. "Before doing further tests or giving you any medication, I'd like to see what happens after you've completely stopped drinking for two weeks."

2. When serious alcohol abuse is suspected, evaluation should proceed with care. Alcohol abuse develops over years, and unless there is some urgent problem, such as upper GI bleeding or suicide threats, the physician should spend the time over several sessions to gradually develop the patient's trust, by exhibiting a nonjudgmental approach.

3. Whenever possible, involve family members as part of the assessment and before suggesting that the patient abuses alcohol. Interviewing patients with family members present will usually provide more accurate information about the severity of the drinking and associated problems. Family members are the provider's most important allies in the treatment process. They have often been concerned about the problem for years, but have not known how to intervene. When you suspect significant alcohol abuse, ask the patient to return in two to three weeks with other family members to follow up on the presenting problem (see Chapter 5 on how to convene a family). With the patient and family members present, discuss the presenting problem and inquire about what seems to exacerbate the problem. If the family members do not bring up alcohol, present it as a contributing factor and ask their opinion. "One of the things that I think may be contributing to your wife's fatigue and sleep disturbance is her drinking. We know that alcohol disrupts sleep patterns and can cause chronic fatigue. What are your thoughts on this?"

4. Present your assessment as a problem with drinking or alcohol abuse, not alcoholism. Many patients and families will accept the former, but reject "alcoholism" because of its connotations with moral weakness and skid-row drunks. Ask family members whether they think the patient has a problem with drinking, and what should be done about it.

5. Educate the patient and family about alcohol and its abuse. Explain how drinking is related to the presenting problem and affects health in general. If there is a family history, it is often helpful to discuss the genetics of alcoholism. Emphasizing the disease concept of alcoholism can reduce the blame often felt by patients.

> Dr. K expressed concern about Mrs. Seagram's chronic fatigue and said that he thought it may be due to an underlying depression and made worse by her drinking. He asked her to return in two weeks to discuss the problem further and to review the results of the Pap Smear and lab tests. He further requested that her husband accompany her to the next visit, as "he may help us understand what's causing your fatigue."
>
> Mrs. Seagram returned for a follow-up visit with her husband. After thanking Mr. Seagram for coming in and socializing briefly with the couple, Dr. K asked for Mr. Seagram's perception of his wife's health. Mr. Seagram began by explaining that he wasn't home much because of work demands, but he was aware that his wife wasn't sleeping well and seemed more "run down" than usual. He thought she was worried about her mother who was having health problems. When he did not bring up his wife's drinking, Dr. K asked "What does your wife do to deal with all these pressures?" Mr. Seagram mentioned that sometimes she would have a nightcap to help sleep. Dr. K asked "How does her nighttime drinking affect her?" Mr. Seagram said he wondered whether some of her lack of sleep and grogginess in the morning was due to the brandy she drank at bedtime. He admitted being somewhat concerned about his wife's drinking. He thought that her mother was alcoholic and had read that there was a genetic component to alcoholism.

Management, Referral, and Follow-up of Alcohol Problems

Alcoholism is a complex biopsychosocial disorder that requires a specialized and multidisciplinary approach both for the patient and the family. Few primary care physicians have the specialized training or the time to treat patients and families with alcoholism. For that reason, the primary goal of the physician should be to facilitate a referral of the patient and family to a structured alcohol treatment program.

1. Recommend an evaluation by an alcohol counselor to determine whether there is a significant alcohol problem. Many patients and families are initially concerned enough to go for an evaluation, before they are ready to accept that alcohol is a problem. Attempts to refer directly for alcohol treatment or Alcoholics Anonymous are generally not successful. While a comprehensive treatment program and AA are essential to the successful treatment of alcohol abuse, premature referral can sometimes backfire, and make the patient more resistant to treatment.

> Dr. K spent a half hour with the couple, getting more history of Mrs. Seagram's symptoms and their effect upon the family. At the end of the session, Dr. K stated that he thought that Mrs. Seagram was suffering from mild depression and might be helped by some counseling. He also expressed concern that her drinking was making the problem worse, and thought that this should be evaluated further by an alcohol specialist. Mrs. Seagram didn't think it was necessary and said that she could stop on her own. Mr. Seagram also thought she should try to stop first on her own. At a followup appointment 2 weeks later, Mr. Seagram reported that his wife had consumed alcohol on several occasions, and he felt that she needed an evaluation. After some discussion, Mrs. Seagram agreed to go, and Mr. Seagram agreed to accompany her "for support." An appointment was made for one week with an alcohol counselor with whom Dr. K worked closely.

2. Know the community resources for alcohol treatment and establish a working relationship with an alcohol counselor. As with referring for family therapy (see Chapter 22) an alcohol referral is more likely to succeed if the physician can personally recommend a specific counselor and set up the appointment while the patient is still in the office. This counselor can also serve as a consultant to help the physician with patients who refuse an evaluation. Establishing a personal relationship with an alcohol counselor permits a collaborative approach to treating the alcoholic patient and family.

3. Refer to a alcohol treatment program that is family-oriented, whenever possible. Currently many programs claim to be family oriented, but may include only a family night with films about alcoholism. Ideally a family-oriented program should work with families throughout the treatment program, including them in the intake and the aftercare program. Also, all family members should be actively involved in Al Anon. Skilled family therapists should be available to work with the families. Multifamily groups are a particularly effective way for families to get support from others and learn ways to deal with the drinking family member.

> An alcohol evaluation revealed that Mrs. Seagram was abusing alcohol throughout the day and night, in part to treat her depression, to which it was contributing. She agreed to enter a 30 day family oriented alcohol treatment program as a "preventive measure" so that, in Mrs. Seagram's words, "I don't

become like my mother." During treatment, significant marital problems surfaced, and the couple began marital therapy as part of the aftercare program. During therapy, Mr. Seagram disclosed that he often stopped on his way home for a "couple of drinks" and was a heavy drinker. Several months later he entered the same treatment program. Dr. K saw the couple regularly throughout treatment and supported their progress. Although Mrs. Seagram's symptoms initially became worse with abstinence, over several months they gradually resolved without medication.

4. Closely follow alcoholic patients and their families, regardless of whether they go into treatment. When the patient enters a local inpatient treatment facility, the primary care physician should visit the patient to give support for the program and the patient's progress. Regular appointments should be scheduled for the patient and family during outpatient treatment and aftercare. Close communication with the patient's alcohol counselor is essential.

5. Detoxification with benzodiazepines should only be done in conjunction with an alcohol treatment program. Occasionally, the physician may be asked by the patient or an alcohol counselor to prescribe benzodiazepines or hospitalize a patient for detoxification. **The physician should not prescribe such medication to patients who claim that they can quit on their own.** If a patient is physically dependent upon alcohol the chance of self treatment is low, and likelihood of abuse of other drugs in quite high. Benzodiazepines can be prescribed as part of an outpatient treatment program, but patients should be seen at least every other day to be sure they are not drinking with the medication.

6. Anticipate relapses and intervene as quickly as possible to get the patient and family back into treatment. Alcoholism is a chronic, often lifelong disorder, and relapses are common. The patient, family and physician must recognize this, so that they do not feel demoralized and helpless if the patient resumes drinking. The physician should try to see the patient and family as soon as the renewed drinking is identified. Family members can be instructed to come in for an appointment if the patient starts drinking again. During the visit, the physician should support the patient, avoid criticism, and encourage the family to do the same. The physician can congratulate the drinker for abstaining as long as he or she did, and explain that relapse is common. The goal is to get the patient back into treatment as soon as possible. The alcoholism counselor should be contacted while the patient and family are in the office and a follow-up appointment made as soon as possible.

If a patient goes through an alcohol treatment program that does not include intensive family involvement and therapy, the drinking may stop without any change in dysfunctional family patterns. In these "dry drunk" families, alcohol has been removed, but the alcoholic behaviors remain. These families should be referred for family therapy.

Alcoholism in the Family: When Family Members Present

Family members of alcohol abusers use the health care services more often than other patients (35). On routine visits, the physician should screen for alcohol problems in the family as well as in the patient. Obtaining a genogram and asking about any family history of alcohol problems will often uncover alcohol in other family members. In addition, red flags may alert the physician that a patient is experiencing a problem related to drinking in the family. The most common problems include somatization, depression, physical and sexual abuse, and drug abuse. Alcohol abuse is particularly common in families where tranquilizers and other prescription drugs are being abused.

When further history reveals that there is probable alcohol abuse in another family member, the patient should be told the diagnosis and educated about alcoholism and its impact on the family. If the patient accepts that there is an alcohol problem in the family, he or she should be referred to Al-Anon (or Ala-Teen for adolescents) or to an alcohol counselor. Either resource can help such patients understand what role they play in the drinking pattern and how they must change to help the drinker. It is important that the focus be on what the family member should do for him- or herself, not on how to get the drinker into treatment.

If the patient does not accept that the drinking in the family is a problem, the physician should show how the presenting problem (e.g., depression, marital problems) is related to the drinking. This may be a slow and gradual process. As with the drinker, the physician can refer the patient to a family therapist for the presenting problem, letting the therapist know that there is drinking in the family. Over time the therapist can work to get the drinking family member into treatment and begin to confront the alcohol problem.

On occasion, a family member will try to get the physician to confront the alcohol abuser about their drinking. The family member may call the physician and explain that the family member is coming in for an appointment and that he or she has a "drinking problem." The implicit or explicit message is that the caller wants the physician to confront the drinker without revealing the source of the information. This effort to triangulate the physician into a family conflict can occur with any problem, but is particularly common in alcohol and drug abuse. In general, the physician should avoid taking the "bait" and encourage the caller to accompany the drinker for the appointment so that the concerns can be expressed directly by the family member.

> MRS. BUSCH: Dr. C, I just thought I should call you and let you know before you see my husband next week that he's been drinking a lot lately and I think it's affecting his health. You see he's . . .

DR. C: (interrupting) Mrs. Busch, I appreciate your concern about your husband's health, and I hope that you'll come in with your husband to express those concerns to him as well.

MRS. BUSCH: I can't do that. I just thought that as his doctor you could talk to him about his drinking.

DRS. C: I either need you to come and express your concerns directly to him or tell your husband you called me and why. You have good reasons for concern if your husband is drinking too much, but I need you to tell him so directly in front of me, so we can begin working on it. I realize that this is a difficult task for you, Mrs. Busch.

MRS. BUSCH: I don't know if I can do that. You won't tell him that I called, will you?

DR. C: Mrs. Busch, I never keep secrets. I am sure you would not want me to keep secrets from you. I must go now, but I suggest you use this opportunity to talk with your husband about your concerns. I hope to see you when he comes in next week. Goodbye now.

When the Patient Does Not Accept the Diagnosis of Alcohol Abuse Or Refuses Referral for Evaluation

Denial is a major defense in alcohol abuse, and many problem drinkers will not accept the diagnosis or will insist that they have their drinking under control. In such circumstances, the following can be helpful.

1. Remember that alcohol abuse is a *chronic problem* that may not respond to initial interventions. Do not give up if initial attempts to get a drinker into treatment fail. Sometimes it takes years for a successful referral and treatment.

2. Don't argue with the patient about the diagnosis or amount of alcohol consumed (36). If the patient refuses to accept any of the preceding interventions, acknowledge that you are concerned foremost about the patient's health, but that you disagree about the nature of the problem. The physician must find a balance between feeling overresponsible for the patient's drinking and its treatment and being underresponsible by ignoring the problem or prescribing tranquilizers.

3. Put the diagnosis, Alcohol Abuse *(currently refuses referral)*, on the patient's problem list and the front sheet of the chart. Once the diagnosis has been made, it should be dealt with in an open and nonjudgmental way. The patient should be told that the diagnosis appears on the problem list, so other physicians will be aware of the problem when they see the patient. Leaving the diagnosis off the problem list supports the patient's denial of the problem and thereby enables continued drinking (24,36).

4. Follow-up with the patient on each visit, and continue to link the presenting problem to alcohol. Screen for other alcohol related problems, especially common and bothersome ones such as gastrointestinal symptoms, sleep disturbance and sexual dysfunction.

5. Recommend a trial of abstinence for two weeks. This intervention is particularly useful when the patient insists that he is in control of his drinking and can stop at any time. It also can assess the effects of brief abstinence. If there is physical dependence, the patient will develop withdrawal symptoms. For some patients, there may be significant improvement in the presenting symptoms while abstaining. Insist that the patient's spouse or other family member come in with the patient for the two week followup to provide input about the presenting symptom and drinking. Discuss with the patient what he or she will do if he or she is unable to abstain during the two weeks. Try to get an agreement to go for an evaluation if he or she drinks during the trial. However, patients should be told that some drinkers who episodically abuse alcohol can go for two weeks without drinking, so that successful abstinence does not rule out alcohol abuse. In this circumstance, one can negotiate a program with the patient and family member to assess the drinking over a longer period with defined follow up appointments. Abstinence is not recommended as initial treatment, but as a way to get the patients and family to recognize when the drinking is no longer under control and alcohol treatment is necessary.

6. When possible, refer the patient or family to a family therapist for the presenting problem and let the therapist know about the alcohol abuse. If the patient or the family are unwilling to accept that there is an alcohol problem or to go for an evaluation, sometimes they will accept a referral for counseling around other problems, such as anxiety, depression, marital conflict or child behavior problem. If the therapist is alerted to the drinking problem, over time he or she may be able to work with the family to accept that drinking is a problem and can then refer them for an alcohol evaluation.

One effective method for confronting the alcoholic patient is called the Family Intervention (37). This intervention is designed to demonstrate the negative impact of the patient's drinking on family members and close friends. It involves getting the people closest to the drinker to confront him or her as a group and spell out specific consequences, including loss of family or job, if the drinker does not accept treatment. A treatment program needs to be available to begin treatment immediately. This forceful approach requires a committed family and should be organized by a therapist who has experience with the intervention. The primary care physician can play an important adjunct role in the intervention, but without specialized training, should not attempt to organize such an intervention. Most commonly the physician presents the health consequences of the patient's drinking at the time of confrontation and offers encouragement and assistance for treatment.

Primary care physicians should know which therapists or alcohol counselors in their community are experienced with interventions, so that family members can be referred to them. Before considering an intervention, family members should have attended Al-Anon and fully accept its principles. Attempting a family intervention before the family is really committed to following through with specific consequences can be demoralizing and counterproductive.

Physicians need to recognize that alcohol abuse is a common, serious, and treatable chronic illness. Primary care providers should be open and alert to the problem in all their patients. A family orientation gives the primary care provider an advantage in the early diagnosis and treatment of alcohol problems. Since alcohol abuse first causes problems within the family, access to the family allows for early recognition of the problem. Family members are the most important allies in the treatment process, and can provide the most leverage to get the alcohol abuser into treatment. Family-oriented alcohol treatment is essential to change the context within which the problem arose and to help families who are suffering from this problem.

References

1. *Fifth Special Report to the US Congress on Alcohol and Health*. Rockville, MD, DHHS publication No. (ADM)84-1291, 1983.
2. Fein R: *Alcohol in America: The Price We Pay*. Newport Beach: Care Institute, 1984, p 10.
3. Barnes HN, Aronson MD, Delbanco TL: *Alcoholism: A Guide for the Primary Care Physician*. New York, Springer-Verlag, 1987.
4. Kamerow DB, Pincus HA, Macdonald DI: Alcohol abuse, other drug abuse, and mental disorders in medical practice: Prevalence, costs, recognition, and treatment. *JAMA* 1986;**255**:2054–2057.
5. Soloman J, Vanga N, Morgan JP, Joseph P: Emergency room physicians' recognition of alcohol misuse. *J Stud Alcohol* 1980;**41**:583–586.
6. Bush B, Shaw S, Cleary P, et al.: Screening for alcohol abuse using the CAGE questionnaire. *Am J Med* 1987;**82**:231–235.
7. Lewis DC, Niven RG, Czecheowicz D, Trumble JG: A review of medical education in alcohol and other drug abuse. *JAMA* 1987;**257**:2945–2948.
8. Porkovay AD, Soloman J: A follow-up survey of drug abuse and alcoholism teaching in medical schools. *J Med Educ* 1983;**58**:316–321.
9. Sadler D: Poll finds MD attitudes on alcohol abuse changing. *Am Med News* 1984;**27**:60.
10. Clark WD: Alcoholism: Blocks to diagnosis and treatment. *Am J Med* 1981; **71**:275–286.
11. Groves JE: Taking care of the hateful patient. *N Engl J Med* 1978;**298**:883–887.
12. Holder HD, Blose JO: Alcohol treatment and total health care utilization and costs. *JAMA* 1986;**256**:1456–1460.
13. Jones KR, Vischi TR: The impact of alcohol, drug abuse and mental health treatment of medical care utilization. *Med Care* 1979;**17**:1–82.
14. Juntunen J, Asp S, Olkinuora N, et al.: Doctors' drinking habits and consumption of alcohol. *Br Med J* 1988;**297**:951–954.
15. Stanton MD, Todd TC, et al.: *The Family Therapy for Drug Abuse and Addiction*. New York, Guilford, 1982.

16. Stanton MD: The family and drug abuse: Concepts and rationale, in Bratter TE, Forrest GG (eds.): *Alcoholism and Substance Abuse: Strategies for Clinical Intervention*. New York, Free Press, 1985.
17. Coleman SB, Davis DI: Family therapy and drug abuse: A national survey. *Fam Proc* 1978;**17**:21–29.
18. Singer M: Family comes first: An examination of the social networks of skidrowment. *Human Organization* 1985;**44**:137–142.
19. Wolin SJ, Steinglass P: Interactional behavior in an alcoholic community. *Med Annals of D.C.* 1974;**43**:183–187.
20. Steinglass P, Bennett LA, Wolin SJ, Reiss D: *The Alcoholic Family*. New York, Basic Books, 1987.
21. Goodwin DW: Alcoholism and heredity: A review and hypothesis. *Arch Gen Psychiatry* 1979;**36**:57–61.
22. Wolin SJ, Bennett LA, Noonan DL: Family rituals and the recurrence of alcoholism over generations. *Am J Psychiatry* 1979;**136**:589–593.
23. Weinberg JR: Assessing drinking problems by history. *Postgrad Med* 1976;**59**:87–90.
24. Doherty WJ, Baird MA: Treating chemical dependency in a family context. *Family Therapy and Family Medicine*. New York, Guilford Press, 1983.
25. Steinglass P: The alcoholic family at home: Patterns of interaction in dry, wet and transitional stages of alcoholism. *Arch Gen Psychiatry* 1981;**38**:578–584.
26. Steinglass P, Davis DI, Berensen D: Observations of conjointly hospitalized "alcoholic couples" during sobriety and intoxication: Implications for theory and therapy. *Fam Proc* 1977;**16**:1–16.
27. American Psychiatric Association: *Diagnostic and Statistical Manual of Mental Disorders* (3rd ed. rev.). Washington, DC: American Psychiatric Association, 1987.
28. Steinglass P: The impact of alcoholism on the family: Relationship between degree of alcoholism and psychiatric symptomatology. *J Stud Alcohol* 1981;**42**:288–303.
29. Ford DE, Kamerow DB, Thompson JW: Who talks to physicians about mentl health and substance abuse problems? *J Gen Intern Med* 1988;**3**:363–369.
30. Woodall HE: Alcoholic remaining anonymous: Resident diagnosis of alcoholism in a family practice center. *J Fam Pract* 1988;**26**:293–296.
31. Cyr MG, Wartman SA: The effectiveness of routine screening questions in the detection of alcoholism. *JAMA* 1988;**259**:51–54.
32. Ewing JA: Detecting alcoholism: the CAGE questionnaire. *JAMA* 1984;**252**:1905–1907.
33. Bernadt MW, Mumford J, Taylor C, et al.: Comparison of questionnaire and laboratory tests in the detection of drinking and alcoholism. *Lancet* 1982;**1**:325–328.
34. Leckman AL, Umland BE, Blay M: Prevalence of alcoholism in a family practice center. *J Fam Pract* 1984;**18**:867–870.
35. Liepman M. Alcohol and drug abuse in the family, in Christie-Seeley J (ed.): *Working with the Family in Primary Care*. New York: Praeger Press, 1983.
36. Baird M: Chemical dependency: A protocol for involving the family. *Fam Syst Med* 1985;**3**:216–220.
37. Johnson V: *I'll Quit Tomorrow*. New York: Harper & Row, 1973.

PROTOCOL

A Family Approach to the Detection and Management of Alcohol Abuse

A. Screen all patients for alcohol problems with the following questions:
   1. "How much alcohol do you drink?"
   2. "Have you ever had a problem with your health, your work, or your family because of drinking?"
   3. "Has anyone in your family ever had problems with alcohol use?"

B. Guidelines for inquiring about alcohol use:
   1. Be as matter of fact as possible.
   2. Ask the patient to be very explicit about his or her alcohol use.
   3. Inquire further about drinking in any patient who reports drinking daily or more than two drinks on an occasion. Use the CAGE questions.

   C Have you ever felt you ought to CUT DOWN on your drinking?
   A Have people ANNOYED you by criticizing your drinking?
   G Have you ever felt bad or GUILTY about your drinking?
   E Have you ever had a drink first thing in the morning (EYEOPENER) to steady your nerves or get rid of a hangover?

   4. Record the patient's response in a prominent place in the medical record.

C. Negotiating with the alcohol abuser:
   1. Focus on the patient's presenting problem during the assessment; link the drinking to the presenting problem.
   2. When serious alcohol abuse is suspected, evaluation should proceed with care.
   3. Whenever possible, involve family members as part of the assessment and before suggesting that the patient abuses alcohol.
   4. Present your diagnosis as a problem with drinking or alcohol abuse, not alcoholism.
   5. Educate the patient and family about alcohol and its abuse.

D. Management, referral and follow-up of alcohol problems:
   1. Recommend an evaluation by an alcohol counselor to determine whether there is a significant alcohol problem.
   2. Know the community resources for alcohol treatment and establish a working relationship with an alcohol counselor.
   3. Refer to an alcohol treatment program that is family-oriented, whenever possible.

4. Closely follow alcoholic patients and their families, regardless of whether they go into treatment.
5. Detoxification with benzodiazepines should only be done in conjunction with an alcohol treatment program.
6. Anticipate relapse and intervene as quickly as possible to get the patient and family back into treatment.

E. When the patient does not accept the diagnosis of alcohol abuse or refuses a referral for evaluation.
1. Remember that alcohol abuse is a chronic problem that may not respond to initial interventions.
2. Don't argue with the patient about the diagnosis or the amount of alcohol consumed.
3. Put the diagnosis, *Alcohol Abuse (currently refuses referral)*, on the patient's problem list and the front sheet of the chart.
4. Follow-up with the patient on each visit and continue to link the presenting problem to alcohol use.
5. Recommend a trial of abstinence for two weeks.
6. When possible, refer the patient or family to a family therapist for the presenting problem, and let the therapist know about the alcohol abuse.

CHAPTER 19

Protecting the Family
Child Abuse and Primary Care

In Collaboration with Barbara Gawinski*

Violence occurs more frequently within the family than any other place in society. Since Kempe et al. (1) first introduced the "battered child syndrome" into the social consciousness, increasing attention has been given to domestic violence in all its forms: spouse abuse, child abuse, and abuse of elders. Our focus in this chapter will be on child abuse, especially cases in which the abuse is committed by a family member.

Child abuse is the infliction of injury on a person under 18 years of age by a parent, legally responsible guardian, or other adult. Such abuse must be reported when acts of physical or sexual injury occur, or are suspected, or when children are exposed to substantial risk for any of the above. Over one and a half million children and adolescents are reported abused each year (2). These figures may reflect only a small percentage of the total amount of abuse which occurs but is never reported.

The physician's main job is to recognize the signs of abuse and then utilize those resources which exist within the family and community to protect the child and family. Individuals in abusive families lack the internal controls needed to create a safe environment for their family. Consequently, external controls by community agencies are often required. The primary care physician's role in treatment is to mobilize a safety network for the family that can protect the child or children and can initiate the work of change and healing that must occur in the family. With the help of the legal system, community agencies, and mental health providers, the physician can set a process in motion that can result in successful treatment for these families.

*Barbara Gawinski, Ph.D., is a Family Therapist and Instructor in the Departments of Family Medicine and Psychiatry, University of Rochester School of Medicine and Dentistry, Rochester, New York.

In this chapter we will focus our attention on the specifics of identification, assessment, reporting, and follow-up with the family. Recognizing that physical abuse and sexual abuse have some very different features, we will address both in this chapter, drawing on their commonalities and specifying their distinctions. We will begin by discussing the nature of families in which any type of abuse occurs.

Abuse in the Family—Common Elements

Child abuse is a complex family problem that is the result of multiple factors. An understanding of these factors can help a physician recognize families that may be vulnerable to abuse. The most common factors include: a history of abuse across generations, marital discord, blurred or confused generational boundaries, and family isolation.

1. A History of Abuse. A parent's primary model for parenting is his or her own mother and father. Most parents who abuse their children come from families in which they experienced some degree of abuse or neglect (2–5). As children, they may not have had many of their own needs met. Parents who themselves feel emotionally depleted may utilize parenting approaches that they have learned from their own childhood. Such responses can be impulsive and based on unrealistic expectations for their child's behavior. Substance abuse is often a significant contributing factor to the parent's impulsive behavior with the child (6).

2. Marital Discord. Many of these parents have entered their marriage with the hope that long unmet needs will finally be met by their partner. Unfortunately, because both partners' needs are so great in these families, neither person has the resources to fulfill their mate's needs. Physical violence and sexual distance can result from the frustration of these needs. Children are often drawn into these marital problems, being recipients of their parents' violence or being targeted as substitute sexual partners.

3. Blurred Generational Boundaries. In families where abuse occurs the boundary between the parent generation and the child generation is often unclear and at times nonexistent. Children may be seen as sources of reassurance about the parents' personal adequacy or self-esteem (4). When the child is unable to nurture the parent, the parent may feel rejected and may respond in a punitive manner.

The oldest daughter in families where incest occurs is often subtly encouraged to replace her mother as a parent and a spouse. These daughters function as parentified children, handling many of the maternal and domestic responsibilities in the household and meeting the sexual and emotional needs of their fathers as well. While the sexual relationship between the father and daughter remains a secret, it sometimes reduces tension that exists between the mother and father (5).

4. Family Isolation. These families as units, and their members individually, tend to be socially isolated. Fathers in families with incest are often overly protective of their daughters. They may block their daughters from developing relationships outside the family, especially with males. Incest is frequently reported for the first time when the daughter enters adolescence and is prohibited by her father from developing peer relationship or boyfriends. A study comparing abusive and nonabusive mothers found that abusive mothers were more socially isolated, had partners who were less available, and had parents who were more critical and rejecting (7). Social isolation fosters the belief that all the needs of family members must be met within the family. This belief increases the burden on already overburdened families and also blocks members from reporting problems to those outside the family who may be able to help.

Families in which abuse occurs frequently want help but do not know how to seek it. Physical symptoms of abused children can be the first opening that the community has to engage the family. Since these symptoms are often first presented to a medical provider, the medical provider's capacity to identify the problem is critical. It is to that task that we turn next.

Identifying the Signs of Abuse

Physicians may be the first to bring the problem of abuse to light. Identification depends on recognizing key signs of possible sexual and physical abuse.

Sexual Abuse

The signs of sexual abuse will vary according to the age of the child (8,9). Most of these symptoms are nonspecific to abuse; however, presentation of any combination of these symptoms should signal to the provider the need to rule out abuse. In children who are **five years old or under** the physician should watch for:

- symptoms of failure to thrive
- extreme clinging behavior
- sleep disturbances
- enuresis and encopresis
- appetite changes, stomach aches, and vomiting
- fear and night terrors
- poorly explained sores or bruises in genital area
- severe anxiety around physical examination

Preteen school-age children often present:

- anxiety, fear, depression
- insomnia
- conversion disorder
- sudden weight loss or gain
- school failure or truancy
- knowledge of sexual behavior inappropriate to the child's age
- preoccupation with or fear of sexual activity
- excessive masturbation
- running away
- inconsistent stories about bruises and sores in genital areas

Adolescent girls who are or have been abused often exhibit significant rebellious behavior, especially toward their mothers. They may be more forgiving of their fathers than of their mothers who they feel have not protected them. Other possible signs of sexual abuse of adolescents are:

- psychosomatic complaints
- changes in appetite
- assumption of responsibilities in the house previously held by the mother
- chronic depression and suicidality
- social isolation and running away
- sexual promiscuity

Physiological symptoms common to all age groups include (10–14):

- genital and rectal injuries, irritations or discharges
- sexually transmitted diseases
- recurrent urinary tract infections
- foreign body in vagina, urethra, or rectum
- bruises on the breasts, buttocks, abdomen, or thighs
- abnormal dilation of urethral, vaginal, or rectal openings
- pelvic pain
- pregnancy

Some researchers believe that physicians often overlook sexual abuse of boys (15). While father–daughter incest is the most frequently reported form of abuse, one in ten victims of sexual abuse will be male. It is important for physicians to apply many of the same identification criteria to both their female and male patients.

In the following case the physician's suspicion of sexual abuse is first aroused by the nature of the child's behavioral symptoms.

> Mrs. Wooden brought Madeline, age 9, to see Dr. H because she had been complaining of stomach aches at night and vaginal itchiness. Mrs. Wooden

also took Dr. H aside to say she was concerned about a report from the school that Madeline had written a note to a boy in her class asking if he wanted to "put his finger in her hole."

Dr. H asked Mrs. Wooden if she had noticed any other changes in Madeline's behavior. Mrs. Wooden reported that Madeline was often afraid to go to bed at night and wanted her mother to sleep with her. Madeline's teachers also reported that her grades were going down and that she seemed preoccupied and anxious. With this information in mind, Dr. H proceeded with a complete physical of Madeline.

The principles of such a physical will be discussed in detail later in the chapter. We turn now to some of the characteristic signs of physical abuse.

Physical Abuse

Signs of physical abuse depend not only on the evidence of injury on the child but also on the nature of the parent's presentation to the physician. Parents of children who have been physically abused are often less distraught by their child's injuries than one would expect. As for the child, the location and type of injury often help the physician differentiate between accidental and non-accidental cause.

Parental behaviors that may be evidence of child abuse include (3):

- unexplained delay in bringing the child for treatment
- implausible or contradictory explanation of the injury
- a history of the child having unusual injuries
- the parent blaming the child for injury
- the parent having history of previous abusive behavior

Common **physical findings** that are indicative of abuse are:

- bruises on the buttocks or lower back
- bruises in the genital area or lower thigh
- multiple bruises at different stages of healing (a sign of repeated abuse)
- hand marks, strap marks, pinch marks, bite marks
- burns (cigarette, scalding on hands and feet)
- abdominal trauma
- subdural hematoma with or without skull fracture

In the following case the physician's concern about possible abuse is raised by both the mother's behavior and the visible signs of injury on the child.

Mrs. Campanis came to see Dr. M with her son Joey, age 2, because of bruises he sustained in a fall at home. Mrs. Campanis could not give an accurate account of the fall because she was not in the room when it happened. Joey had a bruise and swelling over his right eye.

Mrs. Campanis appeared agitated but not overly concerned about Joey's injury. She said Joey was often clumsy and fell a lot. She didn't know what to do with him. Dr. M also noticed finger marks on both of Joey's arms.

If there are signs of abuse that strengthen the physician's suspicion, then he or she should proceed with further assessment and examination of the child. Based on the information gathered during the assessment and examination, the physician can make his or her decision about a treatment intervention.

Interviewing the Parent and Child

Begin with the parent and the child together and clarify that the goal is to understand thoroughly the concerns of the parent and the symptoms or injuries of the child. Gather a detailed history of the most recent symptomatology as well as previous incidents of a similar kind in the family. Explain that it is also necessary to talk with and examine the child alone.

In child abuse cases it is helpful to have **aids for interviewing and assessing the child** that can make communication easier and documentation more accurate. These include (14,17):

- **Anatomically correct dolls** for gathering information concerning a sexual assault. Dolls can also help desensitize children to a physical examination.
- **Paper, crayons, and pencils** to help younger children draw pictures of their families or incidents that may be difficult to verbalize. Older children may also find it easier to communicate through the written word.
- **A color camera** to take pictures of any injuries incurred by the child.

When talking with the child it is important for the physician to (17):

- **Develop a relationship with the child.** Conversation should focus initially on less threatening topics such as friends, school, and the child's interests.
- **Proceed at a relaxed pace.** If the physician is too hurried or anxious, the child will become anxious as well.
- **Listen to what the child is willing to share.** It is important not to pressure the child for information about anything; for example, the identity of the perpetrator.
- **Clarify the child's understanding of anatomy.** Regarding sexual abuse in particular, use the child's language when referring to parts of the body ("pee pee", "wee wee", "butt", etc.).
- **Not assume the child is angry at the person who committed the abuse.** Abused children are often very attached to the abusive parent.

- **Encourage the child to share his or her feelings.** This may be the youngster's first opportunity to discuss a family problem.
- **Reassure the youngster** that his or her safety is very important and that you are hopeful things will work out for the child and family.

> Dr. H talked alone with nine-year-old Madeline whom he suspected had been sexually abused. Dr. H found Madeline to be very talkative about her friends and her collection of dolls. Dr. H explained that he was concerned about the difficulties she was having and wanted to understand Madeline's situation so he could help. During their conversation Dr. H learned that Mrs. Wooden often worked at night and Madeline's father would put her to bed. Madeline reluctantly shared that during the past several months he often stayed with her and touched her "wee wee." Sometimes he would ask her to hold his "thing" until "stuff" came out. Twice recently he told her to put it in her mouth which she did. Dr. H learned that Madeline's father had tried to penetrate her vagina once but it hurt too much so he stopped. Madeline said she loved her father but was afraid sometimes. Madeline reported trying to tell her mother once but her mother "didn't seem to understand."

The interview provides the physician with invaluable information and also helps the child feel comfortable with the physician before he or she proceeds with a physical examination.

The Physical Examination

The **physical examination** should be complete, from head to toe, in order to reduce the child's anxiety about examining any particular area of the body. A general exam can also be used to reassure the child that he or she is physically all right.

Examinations in potential **physical abuse** cases should include (18):

- **A record of all bruises and burns** according to size, shape, position, color, and age. Color photographs are required by law in many states.
- **Special attention to retinal hemorrhaging** that may be evidence of subdural hematomas due to shaking injuries.
- **An X-ray survey of children under the age of five** because clinical findings of fractures often disappear after a week.

In cases of suspected **sexual abuse** the examination should include:

- **A careful description of genital anatomy.**
- **A test for the presence of sperm** in the vagina of females.
- **A rectal exam** to assess reflex relaxation in males.
- **Documentation of any foreign objects** in the geniturinary and rectal areas.
- **A pregnancy test** for adolescent girls.

- **Tests for sexually transmitted disease** in children of both sexes. These should include blood tests for syphilis and cultures for gonorrhea from the throat, urethra, urine, vagina, and rectum (17).

Whenever possible the physical exam should be conducted with both a nurse and the parent present. The parent can provide valuable support for the child. Having the parent present also gives the physician the opportunity to clarify what he or she will be doing and why.

> Dr. H invited Mrs. Wooden and the nurse into the room for Madeline's physical. He explained to Mrs. Wooden and Madeline that a thorough physical was needed to help find out why Madeline was having stomach pain and vaginal itchiness. Noticing Madeline had brought a doll with her, Dr. H examined her doll first to help Madeline understand what he would be doing. He then did a general screening physical of Madeline before examining her genital area and taking a culture from her vagina. His examination revealed some bruising around the vagina and evidence of an old hymenal tear.

It is very important that the physician document his or her findings clearly and in detail (16). If the physician's findings support his or her suspicion of abuse, the next step is to report the problem to a family member and, in many cases, to the appropriate child protective agency.

Reporting Suspected Child Abuse

All states require physicians and other professionals to report suspected child abuse to the appropriate authorities, usually a local child protective agency or police. This is often a difficult step for a physician to take because he or she may not feel completely convinced that abuse has occurred. One study indicates that only 42% of physicians who suspect abuse report it (15). Reporting one's suspicion is a legal responsibility and a critical step in providing for a child's safety as well as involving other professionals who can help strengthen the family's childrearing abilities.

The physician should report suspicion of abuse when he or she suspects that:

• **A family member has committed an act of sexual or physical abuse.** The physician needs to decide whether or not to inform the parents beforehand of his or her intention to report suspected abuse. In most cases the physician should tell the parents first and then call Child Protective Services while the parents are in the office. Unless there is a family member available who supports the child's story and can protect him or her the child should not be allowed to return home until Child Protective has made a determination about the case. This reduces the risk of further abuse, punishment, kidnapping or efforts to persuade the child to change his or her story. In extreme cases of physical abuse in which the injuries are severe, it may be necessary to hospitalize the child to further assess his or her health as well as to maintain the child in a safe environment.

> It was apparent to Dr. H from Madeline's story and the physical examination that she had been sexually abused for at least six months by her father. Dr. H told Mrs. Wooden that he was concerned that Madeline may have been sexually abused and that she was required by law to notify Child Protective Services. Dr. H called Child Protective Services while Mrs. Wooden was still present. The protective worker said someone would come as soon as possible. Mrs. Wooden and Madeline waited two hours at Dr. H's office until the Child Protective worker arrived.

In these circumstances, it helps for the physician to emphasize his or her legal responsibility to report any suspicion of abuse. Reporting is not intended as a personal judgment of the parents but as a necessary step to clarify whether or not abuse has occurred. Abuse that is substantiated often leads to removal of the child from the home by Child Protective Services. There is some evidence indicating that removal of the abusing parent from the home decreases the child's trauma and increases the focus on the parent's accountability (19). Whenever possible, the reporting physician should encourage Child Protective Services to take such action.

• **The parents have not provided for the child's safety and welfare in cases of extrafamilial abuse.** When the perpetrator is not a family member, the physician should immediately report his or her suspicion to both parents. It is important to have the parents take action and report the incident to the police. If the parents are unwilling, the physician should let the parents know he or she will have to report them to the local Child Protective Agency for child neglect. The physician should encourage the parents to support and reassure the child that they will protect him or her. In cases of sexual abuse the parents should emphasize that the child is not at fault.

> Mr. and Mrs. Lemanski brought Jim, age 11, to Dr. X because he was complaining of headaches and refusing to go to school. During the interview alone with Jim, Dr. X learned that his gym teacher had been fondling Jim in the shower at school. Dr. X had Jim's parents return to the exam room where he helped Jim share what had happened to him at school. Mr. and Mrs. Lemanski were shocked and hesitant to believe their son at first. With Dr. X's help Jim talked to his parents and they assured him they would protect him and that something would be done. Mr. and Mrs. Lemanski did not know what steps to take. Dr. X encouraged them to contact the police and to talk to school officials. Dr. X also recommended that the Lemanski's return in a few days to discuss the situation further.

In cases such as this the physician should also encourage the family to see a family therapist to help all the family members work through the crisis. It is important to include non-abused siblings in the therapy because of the confusion and symptomatic behavior they may be experiencing (20).

• **Involvement of Child Protective Services can provide parenting support and education.** In some cases the involvement of child protective services can help parents develop more effective parenting skills and prevent more serious harm to their children. For example, a physician may suggest referral for preventive services to parents who use corporal punishment and may be at risk of seriously abusing their children.

> Dr. M was concerned that two-year-old Joey's bruises were inflicted by his mother. He asked Mrs. Campanis how it was to be raising a two-year-old. Mrs. Campanis began to cry. She reported being tired all of the time and having little or no support. She and her husband had separated while she was pregnant with Joey. Mrs. Campanis worried that she could hurt Joey. Dr. M said Mrs. Campanis deserved to have additional support and that Child Protective Services could be a resource to her. Mrs. Campanis was fearful that Child Protective would remove Joey from the home. Dr. M said he would call Child Protective while Mrs. Campanis was in the office. Dr. M learned that Child Protective often referred cases to a parent education program run by social services. The program provided home visits by a social worker as well as a child care program. Child Protective would meet with Mrs. Campanis to investigate the situation first and make a referral if it was warranted. Mrs. Campanis was still anxious after the call but was willing to go ahead with the plan. Dr. M maintained contact with Mrs. Campanis and Child Protective during the assessment. Mrs. Campanis was referred to the parent education program.

It is **important for the physician to maintain contact with the family** especially when reporting is necessary. This can be difficult when the physician has reported abuse without notifying the parents beforehand. Families may react initially with intense anger but almost always remain in the physician's practice and can benefit from his or her ongoing involvement. The physician can provide important continuity of support for families who may be involved with a variety of legal, social service, and therapeutic agencies and professionals. Lawyers, therapists, social service workers, and judges may change frequently during the investigation and treatment of child abuse. The primary care physician may be the one stable, ongoing contact with the family who can provide support and help the family work with these multiple systems.

> Dr. H contacted Mr. and Mrs. Wooden after Child Protective had seen them regarding possible sexual abuse of Madeline. Mr. Wooden was furious with Dr. H and refused her offer to meet with them. Dr. H called the Woodens again in a week. Madeline had been removed from the home and Mr. Wooden was scheduled to appear in both Criminal and Family Courts. The Woodens were very distraught and were now more open to meeting with Dr. H. Dr. H met with the Woodens periodically over the next three years to

provide support and help them understand and work with the judicial, social service and therapeutic systems. Dr. H talked with the Protective officer frequently and also attended a meeting with the Wooden family and their family therapist. Eventually Madeline was returned to her family and they continued in therapy for a year. Dr. H maintained contact throughout the process and continued to provide medical care and support to the Wooden family.

Physicians can play a pivotal role in stopping the cycle of child abuse in families. Recognizing the signs of abuse is the first step. By reporting one's suspicions to the appropriate authorities, the physician can help provide safety for the child and support to the family in a time of crisis. This step can also lead to involving resources that can strengthen the family's capacity to raise their children in a secure environment. In that sense the physician's actions are protective of both the child and the entire family.

References

1. Kempe CH, Silverman F, Steele B, Droegemueller W, Silver H: The battered child syndrome. *JAMA* 1962;**131**:17–24.
2. Segal J: Child abuse: A review of research, in *NIMH Science Monographs: Families Today: Volume II*. Washington, DC, U.S. Department of Health, Education and Welfare, 1982, pp 577–606.
3. Green AH: Current perspectives on child maltreatment. *Resident and Staff Physician* May 1979:150–163.
4. Kent JT, Blehar MG: Helping abused children and their families, in *NIMH Science Monographs: Families Today: Volume II*. Washington, DC, U.S. Department of Health, Education, and Welfare, 1982, pp 607–630.
5. Shapshay R, Vines DW: Father-daughter incest: Detection of cases. *J Psychoc Nurs Ment Health Serv* 1982;**20**(1):23–26.
6. Batten DA: Incest–A review of the literature. *Med Sci Law* 1983;**23**(4):245–253.
7. Green AH: A psychodynamic approach to the study and treatment of abusing parents. *J Am Acad Child Psychiat* 1976;**15**:414–429.
8. Kempe CH: Sexual abuse, another hidden pediatric problem: The 1977 C. Anderson Aldrich Lecture. *Pediatrics* 1978;**62**(3):382–389.
9. Pascoe DJ: Management of sexually abused children. *Ped Annals* 1979;**8**(5):44–58.
10. Emans SJH, Goldstein DP: *Pediatric and Adolescent Gynecology*. Boston, Little, Brown and Co., 1982.
11. Kempe CH: Incest and other forms of sexual abuse, in Kempe CH, Helfer RE (eds.): *The Battered Child*. Chicago, University of Chicago Press, 1980, pp 198–214.
12. Rosenfeld AA: Sexual abuse of children: Personal and professional responses, in Newberger EH (ed.): *Child Abuse*. Boston, Little, Brown and Co., 1982,pp 57–87.
13. Sgroi SM: *Handbook of Clinical Intervention in Child Sexual Abuse*. Lexington, MA, Lexington Books, 1982.

14. Duringer JJ, Kriepe RE, Kempe A: Protocol for the evaluation and management of sexual misuse of children and adolescents. Rochester, NY, University of Rochester, 1984.
15. James J, Womack WM, Strauss F: Physician reporting of sexual abuse of children. *JAMA* 1978;**240**(11):1145–1146.
16. Mrazek PB, Kempe CH: *Sexually Abused Children and Their Families.* London, Pergammon Press, 1981.
17. Sgroi SM: Comprehensive examination for child sexual assault: Diagnostic, therapeutic, and child protection issues, in Burgess AW, Groth AN, Holmstrom LL, Sgroi SM: *Sexual Assault of Children and Adolescents.* Lexington, MA, Lexington Books, 1978, pp 143–157.
18. Schmitt BD: The child with nonaccidental trauma, in Kempe CH, Helfer RE: *The Battered Child.* Chicago, University of Chicago Press, 1980, pp 128–146.
19. Galinas GJ: Unexpected resources in treating incest families, in Karpel MA (ed.): *Family Resources: The Hidden Partner in Family Therapy.* New York, The Guilford Press, 1986, pp 327–358.
20. Gawinski BA: Five families descriptions of experiences with a social service agency: A mini-ethnography of father-daughter incest. Unpublished dissertation. Texas Tech University, 1987.

PROTOCOL

Assessing and Reporting Child Sexual and Physical Abuse

The physician's main job is to recognize the signs of abuse and then utilize those resources which exist within the family and community to protect the child and family.

Sexual Abuse

A. Identifying the Signs

 1. Children five years old or under
    - symptoms of failure to thrive
    - extreme clinging behavior
    - sleep disturbances
    - enuresis and encopresis
    - appetite changes, stomach aches, and vomiting
    - fears and night terrors

 2. Preteen

    - anxiety, fear, depression
    - insomnia
    - conversion disorder
    - sudden weight loss or gain
    - school failure or truancy
    - knowledge of sexual behavior inappropriate to the child's age
    - preoccupation with or fear of sexual activity
    - excessive masturbation
    - running away

 3. Adolescent

    - psychosomatic complaints
    - changes in appetite
    - assumption of responsibilities in the house previously held by the mother or father
    - chronic depression and suicidality
    - social isolation and running away
    - sexual promiscuity

 4. Physiological symptoms – all ages
    - genital and rectal injuries, irritations, or discharges
    - sexually transmitted diseases
    - recurrent urinary tract infections
    - foreign body in vagina, urethra or rectum

- bruises on the breasts, buttocks, abdomen or thighs
- abnormal dilitation of urethral, vaginal or rectal openings

B. Guidelines for the Physical Exam

1. Carefully describe genital anatomy
2. Test for sperm in the vagina
3. Perform rectal exam to assess reflex relaxation in boys
4. Test for venereal disease in males and females
5. Document foreign objects in the geniturinary and rectal areas
6. Perform a pregnancy test for adolescent girls

Physical Abuse

A. Identifying the Signs

1. Parental behaviors

- unexplained delay in bringing the child for treatment
- implausible or contradictory explanation of the injury
- a history of the child having unusual injuries
- the parent blaming the child for injury
- the parent having history of previous abusive behavior

2. Common physical findings

- bruises on buttocks or lower back
- bruises in genital area or lower thigh
- multiple bruises at different stages of healing (a sign of repeated abuse)
- hand marks, strap marks, pinch marks, bite marks
- burns (cigarette, scalding on hands and feet)
- abdominal trauma
- subdural hematoma with or without skull fracture

B. Guidelines for the Physical Examination

1. Record all bruises according to size, shape, position and color
2. Pay special attention to retinal hemorrhaging
3. Have an X-ray survey of children under the age of five

Interviewing the Parent and Child

A. Begin with parent and child together in order to:

1. Clarify the goal: to understand the parents' concerns and the symptoms and injuries of the child

    2. Gather a detailed history of recent symptomatology as well as history of previous incidents in family
    3. Explain the necessity of speaking alone with the child

B. When talking with the child:

    1. Develop a relationship with the child
    2. Proceed at a relaxed pace
    3. Listen to what the child is willing to share
    4. Clarify the child's understanding of anatomy
    5. Do not assume the child is angry at the person who committed the abuse
    6. Encourage the child to share his or her feelings
    7. Reassure the child about his or her safety and your hopefulness that things will work out for the child and family

Reporting Suspected Child Abuse

A. The physician should report suspicion of abuse to local Child Protective Services when there is evidence that:

    1. A family member has committed an act of sexual or physical abuse
    2. The parents have not provided for the child's safety and welfare in cases of extrafamilial abuse
    3. Involvement of Child Protective Services can provide parenting support and education

B. In all cases the physician should make every effort to maintain contact with the family to provide continuity of support as the family works with various legal, social service, and therapeutic agencies and professionals.

Implementing
Family-Oriented
Primary Care

CHAPTER 20

Family-Oriented Primary Care in the Real World

Ethical and Practical Issues

This book presents a family-oriented approach to primary care, including the biopsychosocial assessment of the family, the health care of families through the life cycle, and a family-oriented approach to specific medical problems. Implementing this family-oriented approach in daily clinical practice raises broad ethical concerns ("Are family-oriented interventions ethical?") and specific practical issues ("How will I find the time? Who will pay for this approach?"). These are important issues that we will address in this chapter, starting with common ethical dilemmas, then discussing how to maintain a family-oriented approach when seeing individual patients, and finally presenting specific practical recommendations for establishing a family orientation in primary care.

Ethical Issues in Family-Oriented Primary Care

Three commonly raised ethical concerns in family-oriented medical care deal with the perception of conflicting interests between the individual patient and other family members, the issue of confidentiality and the involvement of the family in an individual patient's care. The following case example illustrates the first two of these dilemmas.

> Martha McNabb, a 65-year-old woman, first presented to Dr. D with a malignant breast lump which was widely metastatic. She and her husband, Chuck, had longstanding marital conflicts, and shortly after the diagnosis of cancer was made, Chuck began making daily visits to care for a disabled woman in a nearby apartment. Mrs. McNabb became upset by his lack of attention. Mrs. McNabb's daughter, Cheryl, defended her mother and accused her stepfather of spending more time with his "girlfriend" than with his wife.

> As Martha's condition gradually deteriorated over the next year, the marital conflict increased, until Martha left her husband and moved in with her daughter. Her daughter felt overwhelmed by the responsibilities of caring for her mother, as well as her own two small children.
>
> After several months, Martha was admitted to the hospital with back pain from her metastases. Although the pain was easily controlled with medication and Martha's condition appeared stable, Cheryl felt that she could no longer care for her mother. Chuck wanted her to return home with him which Cheryl adamantly opposed. Martha said she wanted to return to her daughter's home and did not want to live with her husband or in a nursing home. After a few days, Dr. D was informed by the hospital that Martha no longer needed acute care and should be discharged. Dr. D felt that it would be best for her to return to her daughter's, but wondered if the best outcome for the daughter and her family was for Martha to be placed in a nursing home. He was uncertain what to do.

One of the most common ethical concerns of the family-oriented physician is **what to do when the interests of the family appear to conflict with the interests of the individual patient.** This concern arises in cases in which the family is overwhelmed by the care of an elderly person, and the patient does not want to go into a nursing home. The physician is often asked by the family or by other caregivers to decide what should be done. In these circumstances, the physician should avoid being drawn into the role of decision-maker, unless the decision is clearly a medical one (e.g., whether it is medically safe to return home). Instead, the provider should bring all relevant parties together and facilitate a process in which the group can discuss the problem (1). The best solution occurs when all parties can agree to support the outcome. If not, the patient retains the right to make his or her own decision, but does so fully informed as to what others are willing to do (2–4).

> Dr. D convened the McNabb family to discuss discharge planning with the social worker and visiting nurse at the hospital. He laid out the options to the patient and the family. Starting with the patient, he asked each family member to say what he or she wanted to happen. He encouraged Martha and her daughter to discuss the problems of returning to the daughter's home. Cheryl told her mother that she wished she could continue to care for her, but the strain was too much for her and her family. She felt that her mother could not return to her home. Martha was at first quite angry and upset, but finally agreed that she could not return to her daughter's. She said that she did not want to live with her husband and that her only alternative was to go into a nursing home.

In these situations the role of the physician is not to determine what is right or best for the patient or family, but to help the patient and family discuss the problem together and, when possible, to reach an agreement. Advocating for the needs of the patient by pitting them against those of the family is rarely helpful for the patient. This situation is analogous to winning the battle and losing the war, in that it is in the long-term best interest of the patient to reach a solution that the family can support, or at least accept.

Confidentiality is another concern that often arises in family-oriented medical care.

> Several weeks later, Chuck McNabb appeared for an appointment with Dr. D. He was upset that his stepdaughter Cheryl had told him that his wife did not want him to visit her in the nursing home, and Cheryl would not tell him which nursing home she was in. Dr. D was reluctant to reveal this information to Chuck without his wife's permission. He also feared that telling Chuck might put him in a coalition with Chuck against his stepdaughter and possibly Martha. Yet he thought Chuck should know where his wife was, so he was uncertain what to do.

In family-oriented primary care, it is sometimes difficult to **determine the difference between preserving legitimate confidentiality and colluding with family members about a secret that may fuel individual and family dysfunction.** Confidentiality is an essential ethical standard in medical practice, but secrets are destructive to healthy family functioning (5). To deal with this ethical dilemma, the physician should never provide information about an adult patient to another family member except when the patient has given explicit permission (or is in immediate danger to him or herself, i.e., suicide, or others) (6). Even with permission, this process is best accomplished with all relevant parties present. When the physician suspects a secret that may be damaging to family relationships (e.g., an affair, or a serious or terminal diagnosis), the physician can use his or her influence to advise the patient or family to disclose any important information. However, the physician should not be the party to actually reveal the confidential information. If the information is likely to be provocative, one should consider referral to a psychotherapist to manage any serious fallout.

> Dr. D suggested to Chuck that he and his stepdaughter meet at the nursing home to discuss with Martha whether Chuck could visit his wife. Chuck agreed to abide by whatever decision Martha made about his visiting. Dr. D called the daughter who reluctantly agreed to tell Chuck which nursing home her mother was in and to attend a family conference, as long as Chuck promised to respect Martha's wishes.
>   Dr. D met with the three of them at the nursing home. Martha said that she did not want her husband visiting often or for long periods of time, but told Chuck that he could visit every two weeks as long as Cheryl was not visiting. Chuck agreed to come every other Sunday afternoon for one-half hour. After several months of this schedule, Martha invited him to visit every Sunday for up to one hour.

By maintaining simultaneous strong alliances with each family member, the family-oriented physician can be the most helpful to the patient and the family. In this case, Dr. D avoided getting drawn into taking sides in the family feud and helped the McNabb family successfully deal with some of their conflicts.

Finally there are situations where it may be **unethical not to encourage the family to be involved** in the management of a health problem (7). In certain circumstances, failure to inform or involve the family can result in serious harm to the patient or family members. When a patient is suicidal, family members should be informed and involved in treatment planning to help protect the patient's life, even if the patient does not want them told. The sexual partners of patients with AIDS or other serious sexual transmitted disease should be informed of the risk, even when the patient refuses. Most state laws now permit or even mandate such disclosure. More commonly, there may be situations where the physician should strongly urge the patient to involve or inform the family, such as when the diagnosis of a serious, fatal, or genetic disease is made, or when the patient decides to refuse treatment. In general, when the patient refuses or is reluctant to inform or involve the family in his or her health care, **the physician should inform the patient of the potential harm that may occur to the patient or the family if the family is not involved** and balance these risks with the patient's reluctance to involve the family.

A Family-Oriented Approach to the Individual Patient

One of the basic premises of a family-oriented approach is that the primary focus of medical care is the patient in the context of the family. (See Chapter 1.) Most family oriented physicians primarily see individual patients in their medical practices. Although many patients, especially the young and the old, often come to the physician's office with another family member, patients usually come by themselves. However, a family orientation involves thinking about patients and their problems within the context of the family: how do the health issues affect the family and how does the family influence the health problems? The family-oriented physician often encourages other family members to come to medical appointments and periodically convenes the family for important issues that need family involvement. Most of the time, however, the family-oriented physician will see individual patients within the context of the family.

Whether or not a family member accompanies the patient to the visit is important information. For example, when a 9-year-old boy comes for an appointment by himself or a parent insists on accompanying an 18-year-old into the exam room, the physician should suspect that these families are having difficulty establishing appropriate levels of independence for their children. These red flags suggest, but do not indicate family problems, and require further evaluation. For example, there may be multiple reasons why a mother or a father consistently is the parent to bring their child in for a well child visit: one parent may want to be more involved in their medical care than the other; one may be working outside the home while the other is not; the parents may be divorced with one parent having sole custody, or one of the parents may have died. Whatever the reason or combination of reasons, they are usually relevant to the medical care of the children.

Earlier chapters in this book provide suggestions for helping to maintain a family orientation when seeing individual patients. These include: obtaining basic family information, especially the genogram, on all patients (see Chapter 3); being aware of red flags that suggest family problems or dysfunction that need further evaluation; assessing problems within the context of the family (see Chapter 3); involving family members in the care of the patient when appropriate (see Chapter 4); and convening a family conference whenever it may be helpful for the patient's medical care (see Chapters 5 and 6).

Practical Aspects of Family-Oriented Medical Care

This section presents a list of suggestions that we have found useful to implementing a family-oriented medical practice. Few physicians or medical practices can adopt all these suggestions but many can implement most of them. Some of these suggested apply only to starting a new practice while others can be incorporated into existing practices. Individual providers need to decide which ones can be used for their particular practices.

A Family-Oriented Image

First impressions are important. Medical providers should advertise their family-orientation by including the word "family" in the name of the practice or group. Examples include Family Medicine Group, Family Health Associates, Family Practice Center, Family Health Clinic. A logo for the practice which represents the family is a useful way to communicate the family orientation. Many family medicine practices adapt the American Academy of Family Physicians' or Society of Teachers of Family Medicine's logo for their use. Promotional material about the practice should emphasize its family-orientation and services for families, and sensitivity to nontraditional families.

The staff of the practice should support and encourage a family-oriented approach. Staff members should attempt to get to know family members of patients, even if they are not members of the practice. Phone calls and visits by family members should be encouraged and not viewed as intrusive. Family members in the waiting room should be invited into the examination room with the patient if the patient so desires.

Range of Available Services

A family-oriented medical practice should offer the services that a family most often needs. Pregnancy care is an important part of family oriented health care. Pregnancy and childbirth (described in Chapter 8) is a crucial stage in the development of the family during which a family orientation and continuity of care is important. In addition, family physicians who practice obstetrics have a more balanced mix of ages of patients, with more children in their practices than family physicians who do not (8). Unfortunately high malpractice premiums are forcing many family physicians to stop practicing obstetrics (9). In cases where the family-oriented physician does not do obstetrics, it is helpful if he or she works closely with a family-oriented family physician who does deliver babies or an obstetrician to ensure as much continuity of care as possible. In some situations, the family-oriented physician may participate in some of the prenatal care to maintain the continuity, even though he or she will not do the delivery.

Family-oriented practices should either directly provide or have access to other health related services, such as social work or nutrition counseling. These other health professionals, like nurse practitioners, social workers, or dieticians, should be family-oriented. For example, the dietician should be aware that the families usually share the same diet (10), that dietary interventions must consider the entire family, and counseling the family about diet is more efficient and effective than counseling one individual. Whenever possible, a family therapist should be part of the health care team (11), with an office in the same practice or building as the medical practice. (See below for discussion of incorporating a family therapist into a medical practice.)

The family-oriented physician should have a list of resources with telephone numbers for services not provided by the practice. These resources would commonly include other family-oriented mental health professionals, alcohol and drug services (including detoxification, inpatient and outpatient treatment facilities, AA, Alanon meetings, Adult Children of Alcoholic's groups), self-help and support groups for chronic illness, bereavement, divorce, and advocacy organizations. Many communities maintain directories of these services. One should consider renting out space in the office after hours to organizations that offer services that are beneficial to patients and families, such as Weight

Watchers, Childhood Education Association, Alcoholics Anonymous, and other support groups. Patients and families may be more likely to go if the group meets in their physician's office. Larger multiprovider practices may want to organize their own family-oriented groups focused on specific areas, such as dealing with normative family development (e.g., prenatal and parenting classes), nonnormative family crises (e.g., divorce and separation) or chronic illness. Gonzales, Steinglass, and Reiss (12) have described the development of multi-family discussion groups for families dealing with chronic illness.

Enrollment of Patients and Families

A family orientation begins with the first visit (13). Whenever possible the entire family should be encouraged to register together with the same physician and at the same time. Even when all members of the family do not have the same physician, sufficient information about the entire family should be obtained at registration to construct a basic genogram. There are now available self-administered genograms (14) and computerized genograms (15,16) that can be completed at the time of registration. At the time of registration, families should be encouraged to come in together for an initial family session. This may involve meeting with the entire family for the first session to introduce them to the practice, to get some background health information about the family, to construct a routine genogram, and to plan follow-up visits and examinations. This type of meeting gives the strong impression to the patients and families that the provider is family oriented and will want to include the family in health care.

Commonly, the initial visit to the physician will be by the individual patient. Obtaining a basic three generation genogram is essential for adequate background and history to implement a family oriented approach.

Family Charts

An essential tool in family-oriented care is the family chart or folder (17), in which the charts of all members of the family are filed together in the family folder or chart. Family is defined here for convenience as "a group of persons sharing a common household". A relationship (not necessarily by blood or marriage) is implied (18). The University of Rochester Family Medicine Program has successfully used family charts for over 20 years and details of this charting system have been described (17). In addition to each family member's chart, the family folder includes a separate family card that goes in the front of the chart and is made of sturdy yellow cardboard to be easily identified and accessible for each visit. On one side, there is space for the genogram with a brief list of standard symbols and a section for family history. Family problems or family assessments are written on the back.

The advantages of a family chart are many. Information about the family, especially the genogram, can be obtained from different family members and is available for each family member's visit. This important data does not need to be duplicated for each family member's chart. Information gathered during visits by different family members can be entered onto the genogram. Without a family chart, the physician may not otherwise know that two patients with different last names are closely related. Having a genogram readily available in the family chart is particularly valuable when caring for remarried or blended families where relationships may be quite complex.

Having all the family members' charts in one family folder facilitates the detection of patterns of health care utilization which may reflect family stress or dysfunction. Widmer (19) has shown that when one family member is depressed, other family members visit the doctor more frequently. These visits by different family members can be graphically illustrated by a family care journal (20) in which dates and diagnoses (using a code such as ICD-9) for all family members is recorded graphically. Huygens (21) kept very meticulous and elegant journals or charts of familial patterns of illness for over three decades in his practice in the Netherlands. In their classic study of family stress and illness, Meyer and Haggerty (22) used similar charts to demonstrate that streptococcal pharyngitis is often preceded by stressful family events.

Knowing about another family member's health problem at the time of a visit can be quite helpful to the physician. Another family member may have been seen recently with illness due to a common exposure, such as an infectious or toxic agent. A family chart makes it easier to identify whether more than one family member has a cardiac risk factor, such as smoking or hypercholesterolemia. In such cases, an intervention aimed at the entire family may be more effective and efficient. Family charts also makes family research easier to conduct. One can easily retrieve and compare information about the family.

Often a family member requests information about another family member's health care. For example, a mother at her yearly gynecological visit, may inquire when her children should come in for their next visit or immunization. This information is readily available in the family chart. However, with family charts, the physician must be particularly careful about the confidentiality of information. The physician should not provide information about an adult family member without that person's consent; a patient should not have access to the entire family chart without permission of the other members of the family.

The major disadvantage of family charts is their bulk. For a large family with multiple medical problems, these charts can get quite thick and heavy. This problem can be reduced by using flow sheets for pertinent clinical information and laboratory results, and periodically pruning non-essential material from the chart.

Physical Layout

Whenever possible, the physical layout of the medical office should be designed or adapted to accommodate families. Waiting rooms should be large enough to accommodate several families and have reading material that is oriented to families. They should be accessible to the elderly and disabled and have separate play areas with toys for children. Pictures of families in the practice or babies delivered by the provider can add a family touch to the waiting area or nurses' station. Exam rooms should be large enough to comfortably seat at least two family members, preferably three. Many standard exam rooms are not equipped with a third chair. Often careful planning and rearrangement of furniture will permit more chairs for family members. It is very helpful to have at least one family conference or consultation room that can accommodate eight to ten people comfortably.

Videotaping

The physician who is involved in teaching medical students or residents, or who wishes to study his or her own work, should consider having one or more rooms set up for videotaping. Simple and versatile video equipment can be purchased inexpensively. A basic system can be set up in the family conference room with a videocassette recorder, a camera with attached microphone (for small rooms a wide angle lens is preferable) and a small TV monitor. This system may be built upon by adding a separate microphone for better audio or an additional camera for an examination room. If patients and families are approached in an open and matter of fact manner, they are usually very willing to have sessions videotaped. Consent forms should be available and signed by all adult patients who are videotaped.

Scheduling

Scheduling appointments in a family-oriented practice should be flexible to accommodate the different needs of families and of the physician. Because of school and work conflicts, many families have difficulty coming in during the usual nine to five hours. The office should be open for appointments on some evenings and/or Saturdays for these families. However, the physician must also balance this with the need to be home with his or her own family. Sometime early morning or noon time appointments can be good times for family conferences. Scheduling should also be flexible enough to allow for several 15 to 30 minute appointments with couples or families throughout the day. These are often best scheduled at the beginning of the morning or afternoon session when the physician's pace is usually less rushed. Many practices reserve a half day per week especially for family conferences or counseling sessions. These appointments can be scheduled every 30 to 45 minutes throughout the half day allowing for a more predictable and relaxed pace. These afternoons can also be used for making home visits.

Home Visits

Home visits or house calls are an important part of any family-oriented medical practice. They offer an opportunity to see the patient or family in their own natural setting and can provide valuable information about how the patient is functioning and how the family is adapting to the health problem. Siwek (23) has argued that house calls may be the best form of intervention during a family crisis. Home visits are particularly important for the frail elderly where a visit to the physician's office during the winter may actually be dangerous. For home-bound elderly, it can be helpful to arrange to meet other family members or the Public Health nurse at the home to get their assessments of how the patient is doing.

We recommend regular home visits for all two week well-child/post partum visits. This can be a difficult time for the family to get to the office, and a home visit avoids exposing the newborn to infectious illnesses in the waiting room. A home visit is also the best way to assess how the family is adapting to the new baby (see Chapter 8 for family-oriented pregnancy care), how the feeding is going and what kind of help and support the mother is receiving. Finally, making home visits is a very quick way to become known in a community. Word spreads through the neighborhood that the doctor is making a home visit, and one commonly has neighbors come by to meet this unusual doctor.

Sometimes for multiproblem or chaotic families, making a home visit may be the only way to assemble the entire family for a meeting. Such a home visit may provide insights into the problems that the family is facing.

Billing and Finances

A common concern about a family-oriented approach to medical care is that it takes too much time to implement and is not financially feasible. Involving the family in medical care takes some additional time which pays itself back in the long run with reduced visits. Any additional time can and should be billed for. Inviting the father to prenatal and well-child visits should not take additional time; having both parents present when discussing problems is usually the most efficient way to proceed.

Similarly, involving the spouse of a patient with a chronic illness in his or her care, does not take additional time and can be very helpful.

Family conferences do take additional time, and that time should be billed for at the same rate as other visits. Unfortunately, the present reimbursement system overvalues technical skills and therapies and undervalues educating and counseling patients. Some of this bias will change with implementation of the Resource-based Relative Value Scale for reimbursement (24). Physicians should not themselves undervalue the worth of these family conferences or counseling by undercharging for them. The billing procedure should be flexible enough to take account of the family's income and insurance. The physician should be familiar with the different insurance plans and what services are covered. In some cases the patient may be billed for an extended visit or consultation, or if appropriate, for a counseling session. In other situations, different family members can be billed for portions of the session. Whatever method is used, it should be acceptable to the insurance company and discussed and negotiated in advance with the family so that the method of billing and payment is clear to everyone involved.

Incorporating a Family Therapist into a Medical Practice

Collaboration and referrals to family-oriented mental health professionals is discussed in detail in Chapter 22. The most successful collaboration occurs when the family therapist practices under the same roof as the physician. With such an arrangement, referrals are easier and more successful. The physician can personally introduce the patient or family to the therapist and can attend part or all of the first session. The therapist can more easily meet with the physician during a family conference or a regular office visit. Patients and families often feel more comfortable coming for counseling sessions at the physician's office, than going to a therapist's office or to a mental health center. Communication between therapist and physician is improved, each learns more about the other's work when they are practicing under the same roof.

There are several different models of collaborative family health care (11). In the most traditional model, the therapist has a private practice in the same building as the physician. In a more collaborative model, the therapist may rent space within the physician's office, but conduct a private practice, financially independent of the physician's practice. The therapist may do his or her own scheduling and billing or may contract with the physician for secretarial and billing services. A therapist may be fully integrated into the medical practice as a partner or employee and treated as other health care providers in the practice. Services are billed by the practice and the therapist is paid either on a straight salary or based upon a formula involving productivity or the overall profits of the practice. One unique model of collaborative practice is when a family physician and family therapist see patients together as a team. Dym and Berman (25,26) have described the theoretical and practical aspects of this innovative approach. Regardless of the model used, the different theoretical orientation and style of practice between family-oriented medical practitioners and family therapists must be addressed directly (27).

When the therapist is seeing patients in a medical practice, a decision must be made whether the therapist's notes are included in the medical chart or are kept in a separate mental health chart. We prefer and use the former approach in which all the therapist's notes are written or typed in the regular medical chart in chronological order with the medical notes. The initial consultation and the termination notes are typed on a different colored paper, so that it can be easily found. Subsequent notes are marked with a stamp identifying them as a Mental Health Visit. This method encourages both the physician and the therapist to be aware of what the other is doing. The therapist can see what medical visits and problems have occurred since the last therapy session, and the physician is kept up to date with the course of therapy. At the time of referral, the therapist receives a referral note and the medical record containing the family card with genogram and the medical records of other family members. This method of charting encourages the integration of physical and mental health care. However with this method, the physician must be careful not to release the mental health notes to other physicians or insurance companies unless the patient specifically permits their release in addition to the medical records.

This chapter has reviewed some of the most common ethical and practical issues in family-oriented primary care. Many physicians are concerned that family-oriented approach is not practical. And, it is true that a family-oriented medical practice does require some reorganization of space and time. However, with some creativity and attention to the details of scheduling, billings, space needs and other practical issues, a family-oriented practice can be created that is both efficient for the practitioner and effective for the patient and their families.

References

1. Sherlock R, Dingus CM: *Families and the Gravely Ill: Roles, Rules, and Rights.* New York, Greenwood Press, 1988.
2. Brody H: Ethics in family medicine: Patient autonomy and the family unit. *J Fam Pract* 1983;**17**:973–975.
3. Sider R, Clements C: Family or individual therapy: The ethics of modality choice. *Am J Psychiatry* 1983;**139**:1455.
4. Williamson P, McCormick T, Taylor T: Who is the patient? A family case study of recurrent dilemma in family practice. *J Fam Pract* 1983;**17**:1039–1043.

5. Karpel M, Strauss E: Family secrets, in *Family Evaluation*. New York, Gardner Press, 1983.

6. Christianson CE: Ethical issues in family-centered primary care. *Counseling and Values* 1985;**30**:62–73.

7. Boszormenyi-Nagy I: Ethics of human relationships and the treatment contract, in Lennard HL, Lennard SC (eds.): *Ethics of Health Care*. New York, Gondolier, 1979.

8. Mehl LE, Bruce C, Renner JH: Importance of obstetrics in a comprehensive family practice. *J Fam Pract* 1976;**3**:385–389.

9. Weiss BD: The effect of malpractice insurance costs on family physicians' hospital practices. *J Fam Pract* 1986;**23**:55–58.

10. Eastwood MA, Brydon WG, Smith DM, Smith JH: A study of diet, serum lipids, and fecal constituents in spouses. *Am J Clin Nutr* 1982;**36**:290–293.

11. Glenn M: *Collaborative Health Care: A Family-Oriented Model*. New York, Praeger, 1987.

12. Gonzales S, Steinglass P, Reiss D: Putting the illness in its place: Discussion groups for families with chronic medical illnesses. *Fam Proc* 1989;**28**:69–88.

13. Christie-Seeley J: Establishing a family orientation, in Christie-Steeley J (ed.): *Working with Families in Primary Care*. New York, Praeger Press, 1983.

14. Rogers JC, Cohn P: Impact of a screening family genogram on first encounters in primary care. *Fam Pract* 1987;**4**:291–301.

15. Ebell MH, Heaton CJ: Development and evaluation of a computer genogram. *J Fam Pract* 1988;**27**:536–537.

16. Gerson R, McGoldrick M: The computerized genogram. *Primary Care* 1985;**12**:535–545.

17. Froom J, Culpepper L, Kirkwood RC, Boisseau V, Mangone D: An integrated medical record and data system for primary care, Part 4: Family information. *J Fam Pract* 1977;**5**:265–270.

18. A Glossary for Primary Care. Report of the North American Primary Care Research Group (NAPCGR). Presented at the Annual Meeting of NAPCRG, Williamsburg, VA, March 1977.

19. Widmer RB, Cadoret RJ: Depression in family practice: Changes in patterns of patient visits and complaints during subsequent developing depression. *J Fam Pract* 1979;**9**:1017–1021.

20. Froom J: An integrated system for the recording and retrieval of medical data in a primary care setting: Part 4: Family folders. *J Fam Pract* 1974;**1**: 49–51.

21. Huygens FJA: *Family Medicine: The Medical Life History of Families*. New York, Brunner-Mazel, 1978.

22. Meyer RJ, Haggerty RJ: Streptococcal infections in families: Factors altering individual susceptibility. *Pediatrics* 1962;**29**:539–549.

23. Siwek J: House calls: Current status and rationale. *Am Fam Physician* 1985;**31**(4):169–174.

24. Wsiao W, Braun P, Dunn P, Becker E: Resource based relative value scale: An overview. *JAMA* 1988;**260**:2347–2353.

25. Dym B, Berman S: Family systems medicine: Family therapy's next frontier? *Fam Ther Networker* 1985;**9**:20.

26. Dym B, Berman S: The primary health care team: Family physician and family therapist in joint practice. *Fam Syst Med* 1986;4:9–21
27. McDaniel S, Campbell T: Physician and family therapists: The risks of collaboration. *Fam Syst Med* 1986;4:1–4

PROTOCOL
How to Set Up a Family-Oriented Practice

1. Use a family-oriented image
   a. The practice name should contain the word "family".
   b. Staff should support and encourage a family-oriented approach.
2. Provide a range of available services
   a. The practice should offer pregnancy care when possible.
   b. Social work and nutritional services should be offered.
   c. A family therapist should be part of the practice or available for close collaboration.
   d. A comprehensive list of other family-oriented resources in the community should be available to the provider, patients and families.
3. Enroll patients with their families
   a. The entire family should be enrolled together with an initial joint visit whenever possible.
   b. A genogram should be obtained on all families at the time of their first visit.
4. Use family charts
   a. The charts of all members of the household should be filed together in one family folder.
   b. The family folder should have an easily accessible location for the genogram and other essential family information.
5. Plan the physical layout to support a family orientation.
   a. The waiting room should be able to accommodate families with all age members, including small children and disabled elderly.
   b. Examination rooms should be large enough to accommodate three chairs comfortably.
6. Implement flexible scheduling
   a. Patient scheduling should be flexible enough to meet the needs of the families and allow longer appointments for family counseling.
7. Use home visits
   a. Home visits should be an integral part of the practice.
   b. Home bound elderly and post-partum families should be seen in the home when possible.
8. Bill for family-oriented services
   a. Family conferences and counseling should be billed at the same rate as other visits.
   b. Billing procedures should be flexible enough to take account of families' incomes and insurances.
9. Incorporate a family therapist into a medical practice
   a. Establish a close collaboration with a family therapist.

    b. Options for collaborative practice include having a family therapist.
- with a private office in the same building
- rent space from the medical practice
- become an employee or partner in the practice
- see patients with the medical provider

    c. When possible, include the therapist's notes in the medical record.

CHAPTER 21

Acute Hospital Care
Letting the Family In

George Mayer did not look well when he arrived at the emergency room. Clutching his chest, he was pale, anxious, and sweating. "The pain in my chest started several hours ago and just won't go away," he told the nurse as she attached him to a cardiac monitor. "I thought it was just indigestion, but maybe it's my heart." The nurse hooked up the oxygen, adeptly inserted an intravenous catheter, and called for the physician.

George's wife, Sarah, accompanied her husband to the emergency room and remained by his stretcher trying to reassure him that everything would be okay. The nurse asked her to leave and wait in the ER waiting room while her husband was being evaluated. As she left the room, her husband slumped over, the cardiac monitor showed ventricular fibrillation, and the nurse shouted "Code Blue."

Cardiopulmonary resuscitation was begun, as Sarah was escorted to the waiting room. George responded to intravenous lidocaine and electric cardioversion and regained consciousness as his rhythm became regular again. His EKG showed he had suffered a large anterior wall myocardial infarction. He was sedated and transferred to the Intensive Care Unit.

Sarah remained in the waiting room throughout this time. Each time she went to the emergency desk to get information, she was told her husband was being evaluated, and the doctor would be out shortly to talk with her. After an hour, the emergency room physician appeared and spoke with her. He explained that her husband had suffered a serious heart attack, that his heart had briefly stopped, but they had been able to restart it, and now he was stable and on his way to the intensive care unit. He directed her to the ICU waiting area and said that she could see her husband as soon as he was stable.

Admission to an acute care hospital is usually a crisis for patients and their families. It may occur because of a new acute illness, such as pneumonia, myocardial infarction or a newly diagnosed cancer or because of an exacerbation of a chronic illness, such as asthma, congestive heart failure, or renal failure. It is a time when families usually pull together: family members come from out of town, old conflicts are put aside and the family tries to do whatever they can to help (1).

Family support is particularly important during such a crisis, but unfortunately, hospital procedures often result in families being cut off from their hospitalized member and from his or her medical care. When a patient is admitted to the hospital, the family literally hands the care of the patient to the hospital. The hospital staff takes over, and provides everything from meals and personal care to intensive medical procedures and surgery. Families are only allowed to visit during restricted visiting hours. They may even be viewed as interference or a nuisance by the hospital staff.

Families often encounter difficulty getting information about the health condition and medical care of the patient. Physicians are usually hard to contact, and nurses may be unfamiliar with the details of care or reluctant to share them with the family. This communication problem is compounded when there are multiple medical specialists involved, some of whom have different recommendations for the patient. Unless the patient is unable to make decisions about care, families are rarely consulted about treatment plans and typically participate little in the care of the patient. By contrast, after leaving the hospital, most of a patient's health care is provided by family members. The family reassumes their roles as the primary health care givers. There is often little coordination of care during this transition from the home to the hospital and back again, and the care of the patient and the well-being of the family may suffer as a result.

A family-oriented health care system cares for the patient in a way that encourages families to actively assist in hospital care and prepares families to care for the patient in the home. To implement this, a team approach involving the physician, other ambulatory health care providers, the hospital and all its services, staff, and the family is necessary. As part of the team, the physician needs to have knowledge and understanding of the family and the hospital system, and be able to work as a negotiator between the two systems. Most community physicians communicate regularly with the families of their hospitalized patients and acknowledge the importance of their support to the patient. This chapter provides a framework for thinking about this family orientation and extending it in new ways.

The Changing Hospital Scene

Gone are the days when a physician could electively admit a patient to the hospital for the evaluation of a worrisome symptom and discharge the patient when the physician, patient or family thought the patient was ready. Economic pressures at national, state and local levels are restricting the use of hospitalization for briefer periods of time and for only the most serious medical problems. Hospitalization rates and lengths of stay in the hospital have dropped dramatically in the last decade (2). Patients in the hospital now are sicker, and require more intensive and high technology care. Hospital staffs are providing more services with fewer personnel and are busier than ever before. Nurses and physicians complain that they have less time for the "caring" part of their work such as talking to and consoling ill patients and their families.

While DRGs and other cost containment measures have had some benefits, serious problems have emerged. Many patients, especially the elderly, are being discharged from the hospital before they are able to function independently (3). With less time for adequate discharge planning, patients are sent home when they no longer need acute hospital care, regardless of whether they are ready to return home or adequate services have been set up. These patients are sicker and have more health care needs than before. Unfortunately community and home services have not been developed to adequately care for these patients, and families are left to provide care the best they can. Medicare and most other third party payers generally reimburse for acute medical and nursing care and rarely for adequate preventive, rehabilitative or custodial care.

The lack of support for community-based services and other changes in the pattern of hospital utilization make the role of the family even more important in the care of patients in the hospital. To ease the transitions in and out of the hospital, outpatient services need to be coordinated with in-hospital care. Families should be viewed as an integral part of the health care system and supported and attended to by family oriented practitioners; they should be involved at the time of hospital admission, throughout hospitalization and after discharge. Adequate services in the community need to be available and affordable to patients and their families, so that families can adequately care for their sick members.

Involving Parents in the Care of the Hospitalized Child

Pediatrics has been in the forefront in involving the family in hospital care. Until the 1950s, hospitalized children were isolated from their parents, and parents were discouraged from visiting. Because the children cried after their parents visited, it was believed that seeing their parents was emotionally upsetting and therefore unhealthy for the children! As a result of studies by Robertson (4) and others (5), the adverse effect of the child's separation from his or her parents was recognized, and dramatic changes have occurred in hospital policies concerning the involvement of parents in the care of their children. In most hospitals today, parents may stay with their child continuously throughout the hospitalization. Cots or beds are provided for parents to sleep with the child. Parents may accompany their child for tests. Some hospitals even allow a parent to accompany a child into the operating room while anesthesia is being induced and into the recovery room to be present when the child awakens. All these policies have helped to make the hospital visit a less traumatic experience for the child and parents. The child is less anxious when accompanied by the parent, and parents feel they can help and care for their child. (6)

Adult health care has not yet caught up with pediatrics in this domain. Children are not the only ones who need their families at their bedside in the hospital. We need to open up hospitals to families, not just the pediatrics or obstetric wards, but the entire hospital; so that families can be used as a resource in the care of patients, rather than a nuisance that interferes with appropriate care. To accomplish this will involve changes in hospital policies and the attitudes and behavior of all medical professionals. As advocates for patients and their families, primary care providers should lead the way in this movement by modeling appropriate behavior for hospital staff and using their influence to change hospital policies.

Family-Oriented Hospital Care

The primary goal of family oriented hospital care is to address the needs of the patient and the family and utilize the family's resources in the care of the patient throughout the hospitalization. Working with the family can directly benefit the patient in several ways:

1. Families can assist in the medical evaluation of the patient. As in most medical situations, family members are usually excellent observers and can provide additional valuable information about the patient at the time of admission and throughout the hospitalization. The acutely ill patient is often less able to give a reliable report of the illness. Interviewing family members may be especially useful in the hospital setting for several reasons.

a. A family member may give critical historical information about the illness which the patient may have forgotten or neglected. For example, a middle-aged man was admitted with severe abdominal pain and diarrhea. During an interview with the family, his son recalled a camping trip with his father to the Adirondack's a month earlier. Giardia cysts were found on microscopic examination of the patient's stool.

b. The family may recognize a pattern that the patient does not. A young woman was admitted to the hospital with another exacerbation of her asthma. Her husband commented to her physician, that her wheezing became much worse whenever the heat was on in their house. Upon checking the furnace, a mold was found growing on the filter.

c. The patient may minimize symptoms. The wife of a cardiac patient contradicted her husband's claim that he was having very little chest pain. She explained to his physician that he went through three bottles of nitroglycerin tablets each week. On cardiac catherization, he had severe triple vessel coronary artery disease.

d. The patient may completely deny symptoms or behaviors. A 60-year-old woman was admitted with unexplained ataxia. On the second hospital day, when the patient developed a tremor and hallucinations, her son admitted that the patient had been a heavy drinker for many years, something unknown to her primary care physician. She was diagnosed as having alcoholic cerebellar degeneration.

e. The patient may be unaware of some symptoms. An 80-year-old man was seen in the emergency room after an apparent black out spell at home. After interviewing the patient's wife, the physician learned that the patient had fallen and struck his head three days previously, and that morning he had had a grand mal seizure, not syncope. A CT scan revealed a subdural hematoma.

In each of these cases, the family provided essential information which led to the diagnosis. Even during hospitalization, family members can provide important information about the patient, information the hospital staff may be unaware of. For example, a 78-year-old man was having episodes of unexplained confusion for several days after a hip replacement. His wife, who had been at his bedside each day, said that she thought he became confused shortly after receiving one of his medications. She reported a similar reaction had occurred several years previously after surgery on his prostate. The offending medication was stopped and the confusion resolved.

2. Reducing the family's anxiety will reduce the patient's anxiety and speed recovery. Children are strongly influenced by their parents' perception of health problems and medical procedures. Pediatricians have long recognized that a child's fear of doctors or immunizations often reflects parental fears transmitted (usually unconsciously) to the child. Dealing with the parent's anxiety can be more effective than trying to directly allay the fears of the child. Studies have shown that adults are similarly influenced by perceptions of those closest to them, especially family members (7–9). Some surgeons realize the importance of speaking with the spouse or adult child of a patient about a planned operation. Family members who have doubts or concerns about the surgeon or the operation will often communicate these to the patient either directly ("I don't think you should have this operation, Mom") or indirectly ("This is a pretty small hospital to be doing this kind of surgery. I wonder how many of these procedures they've done?").

Keeping the family informed and addressing their emotional needs will help them to be more supportive and confident to the patient.

3. **Involving family members in the hospital will help them to assume the appropriate health care responsibilities after discharge.** With shorter hospital stays, patients are returning home with greater nursing and health care needs. While some of these are met by home health services, most are provided by family members. If family members are not involved in the care of the patient while in the hospital, they are unlikely to be prepared physically or emotionally to care for the patient when he or she returns home. Family members who develop the skills and confidence to provide for the patient while still in the hospital will provide better care at home and hasten recovery.

> Although she was 86 years old, Mrs. Phemore had never been hospitalized before, until she fell and broke her hip. On admission she was very agitated and mildly confused. She initially refused to consider surgery, saying that she would rather die at home than in the hospital. The orthopedic surgeon met with the patient and the daughter and son-in-law with whom she lived, and explained the procedure, its risks and benefits, and how it would speed her recovery and return home. The patient's daughter and son-in-law told Mrs. Phemore that they wanted her to return home as soon as she was able, and the operation would help her do this. She consented to the surgery which was uneventful. Mrs. Phemore's daughter participated in her mother's physical therapy and learned the exercises and how to help her to walk. With the help of the hospital social worker, the daughter set up home services that included Meals on Wheels, physical therapy and public health nurse visits to supervise her rehabilitation, and two weeks after admission, Mrs. Phemore was discharged back to her home.

Several surveys of the families of acutely ill or dying patients have identified what families want most during hospitalization (10–12). In order of priority, these include:

1. to be with the ill person
2. to be helpful to the ill person
3. to be assured of the comfort of the ill person
4. to be kept informed of the medical status of the ill person
5. to be able to share their emotions
6. to receive acceptance and support from the hospital staff

The family-oriented physician can assist family members in getting these needs met. The physician is directly responsible for some, such as keeping the family informed of the patient's medical status and maintaining the maximal comfort of the patient. For others, the physician must work with the hospital staff to provide emotional support to families, encourage them to share their feelings, and find ways that they can be helpful to the patient. Finally, physicians can influence hospitals to become more family oriented with unlimited visiting hours for close family members and family participation in patient care. The rest of the chapter will present specific suggestions for implementing a family-oriented approach to hospital care that meet the needs of patients and their families.

Initial Hospital Family Conference

Family conferences are an efficient and effective way to deal with family and patient anxiety that occurs around a hospitalization. It is important to meet with the family as soon after hospital admission as possible. The family has often brought the patient to the hospital and desires more information about the patient. (The basic skills of convening and conducting a family conference are covered in Chapters 5 and 6.) This section will cover aspects of the family conference that are particular to the hospital setting.

Family meetings at the time of hospitalization are often quite impromptu and informal. They may be as simple as talking to a spouse in the emergency room to obtain more history or as complex as meeting with an extended family of a dying patient about limiting treatment or whether to resuscitate (DNR). Several principles are useful:

1. Involve the patient in family meetings whenever possible. Health care providers and family members often exclude the patient from these family meetings feeling that the patient either is too sick to participate or will become emotionally upset. Some families have a rule not to discuss health problems directly with an ill family member. Although sometimes a patient may be too ill to participate or may be undergoing a procedure, in most cases the patient can listen and often actively participate. Involving the patient in the family conference can be helpful because it:

a. is more time efficient. The physician can give medical information to the patient and family at the same time and does not have to repeat it.
b. allows the patient to comment on and correct important medical information.
c. encourages the family to discuss the illness and hospitalization together, and to share information and emotional reactions.
d. helps to keep the family focused on the immediate and specific issues faced by the patient and the family.
e. prevents secrets from developing (e.g., the physician gives the family a prognosis and the patient is not told or vice versa).
f. allows the physician to see how the family interacts with the patient (e.g., blaming, overprotective, etc.).

Occasionally it is necessary to meet briefly with the patient or family alone after a family meeting with the patient. The family may not be willing to share information or feelings with the patient present, despite the physician's urging. For example, Mrs. Bramer was admitted with "falling spells." After a meeting with the patient and the family, Mr. Bramer pulled her doctor aside and explained that she "drank a lot." In such cases, the physician should be clear about not keeping secrets, and should address these issues directly with the patient and the family together. Dr. C met again with the family and the patient and asked the family to share this information with the patient. He thanked her family for being so concerned about her health that they would tell him about the drinking and he emphasized that this information was very important in understanding her health problems and treating her successfully in the hospital.

   2. Take time to find the best place to meet with the family. It is often difficult to find a quiet, private place to meet with patients and their families. Patients may be bedbound and unable to travel to a family conference room. The best place to meet with the family is often at the patient's bedside, whether the patient is in the emergency room, the intensive care unit or a private room. This may require assembling enough chairs for everyone or remaining standing in the emergency room or intensive care unit. If the patient is in a semi-private room and the roommate is ambulatory, the roommate can be asked to leave the room during the conference. Otherwise, using the curtain to separate the room provides some privacy. Failure to attend to this basic, but often overlooked need for a quiet and private place to meet with families can interfere with best work done with patients and families.

   3. Always invite the patient's nurse to the family conference. If the hospital has a primary nurse system, in which one nurse is responsible for developing and coordinating a nursing care plan, the primary nurse is a key person to get involved with the family. Nurses, not physicians, provide most of the care for patients in the hospital, and have the most contact with families (13).

   4. Obtain a skeletal genogram to identify important family members and their relationship to the patient. This common outpatient tool can be especially valuable to inpatient care. Constructing such a genogram usually takes several minutes and becomes invaluable during later contacts with the family. It should be placed prominently in the chart to help other care providers (e.g., nurses, residents, dietician, physical therapist) orient themselves to the family, and can be developed further during the hospitalization. For many families, the primary care physician will already have a genogram that can be shared with the rest of the health care team. (See the Appendix of Chapter 6, for further information on constructing genograms.)

   5. Briefly review the events leading up to the hospitalization acknowledging the helpful information provided by the family, and then state the current assessment and treatment plan for the patient. Reviewing the history gives the patient and family the opportunity to correct any misinformation or confusion about the events prior to admission, and reassures the family that you have a clear understanding of what's going on. Pertinent test results should be explained and a simple, clear assessment of the illness presented. The treatment plan, the prognosis and anticipated length of stay in the hospital should be discussed. The patient and family members are encouraged to ask questions and express their concerns. Depending upon the complexities of the problem, family conferences can last from a few minutes to an hour. When decisions regarding options such as surgery or whether to resuscitate must be made by the patient and family, extra time is necessary to be sure that all family members understand the issues involved. (See Chapter 14 for a discussion of DNR conferences.) If the illness is of sudden onset or the diagnosis is grave, the patient and family are often in a state of shock or disbelief and may not remember or seem to understand what is told to them. Explanations must be kept quite simple and non technical, and repeated several times over the ensuing days.

6. Clarify the channels of communication among you, the family and the primary nurse. Families are reassured when they have a name and telephone number of someone who will be with the patient during the day or night. With unstable patients, the nurse may want to call the family at certain times during the day or when there is any change in the patient's status. Giving the family a way to reach the primary physician for urgent questions is very reassuring to the family and is rarely abused.

> Shortly after George Mayer was transferred to the intensive care unit, his family physician, Dr. T arrived at the hospital. After examining George, reviewing his test results and discussing the case with the senior resident in the ICU, Dr. T and his primary nurse spoke with his wife Sarah in George's room. Although George was mildly sedated, he was well oriented and could participate in the meeting. While reviewing the events leading up to the hospitalization, Sarah added that her husband had been having chest pain for several weeks prior to this episode, something George had not mentioned.
>
> Dr. T explained the heart attack, the cardiac arrest and the resuscitation to George and Sarah. He said that George's cardiac rhythm was now stable and he was through the riskiest part of a heart attack. "You will be in the intensive care unit for about three days while your heart begins to heal," he explained. "After you are transferred to a regular floor, we will develop a plan to get you on your feet and home." George's nurse demonstrated how the cardiac monitor and other equipment worked, and gave Sarah the ICU telephone number to call at any time. Sarah was allowed to sit with her husband in the ICU for an hour while he slept. She was comforted to see how much care he was receiving and how well he slept. She felt that simply holding his hand was helping him during this critical period.

While it is best for the physician or nurse to give information directly to as many family members as possible, this is not always possible. It is helpful to have the family choose one member who will be responsible for communicating with the health care providers and passing on information to the family. This person can be so designated on the genogram. This approach helps to prevent getting phone calls and messages from numerous family members requesting the same information. If the family has difficulty choosing one spokesperson or the physician still gets calls from several family members, it may be a sign of a distressed or dysfunctional family and may warrant reassembling the family to explore what is going on. Occasionally there will be a family member who lives out of town but plays a particularly important role in the family, such as someone in a health profession. It may be necessary to talk with these family members directly to be sure they understand what is happening and that they support the treatment plan.

> While George Mayer was still in the ICU, Sarah asked Dr. T whether George should be considered for coronary artery bypass surgery. She explained that her daughter was a surgical resident in a distant hospital and had raised this question to her. Dr. T explained why George was not being considered for CABG surgery at that time, but agreed to call her daughter and discuss this question directly with her. After calling the daughter and discussing her father's care with her, the daughter was reassured by Dr. T's competence and supported his plans to the rest of the family.

Involving the Family During the Course of the Hospitalization

The family-oriented physician can help the family to be actively involved in the hospital care in a number of ways.

1. Maintain regular contact with the family during hospital rounds. One efficient way to do this is to inform the family when you plan to visit the patient each day and encourage them to be present at that time. An update on test results and further plans can be given to the patient and family at the same time.

2. Encourage family members to be present and supportive of the patient when they can. All departments in the hospital should have the most liberal possible visiting policies for family members as possible. Close family members should be allowed unrestricted visiting hours as long as they do not disrupt essential hospital care or disturb the patient, decisions that can be best made by the patient's physician and primary nurse. Even in the intensive care unit where routine policies allow visiting for 10 minutes out of each hour, policies should be developed that allow for a spouse, child or parent to stay with the patient for longer periods of time. Small children free of communicable disease should be allowed and encouraged to visit a parent in the hospital.

When visiting policies are more restrictive, the physician can assist the family in requesting extended visiting hours.

> An elderly woman with Alzheimer's Disease became quite agitated during the first few nights in the hospital. Despite attempts to restrain and medicate her, she screamed throughout the night and crawled out of bed on several occasions. Finally, the patient's daughter spent the night with her mother sleeping on a cot provided by the staff. When her mother awoke during the night, her daughter would reassure her, coax her back to bed, and sing her a song to help her sleep. Sleep medication and restraints were stopped and the woman's day–night reversal improved. After two nights, the hospital staff tape recorded the daughter's voice and singing and played it to the woman at night to help her sleep.

Participating in the hospital care of a family member can be stressful. If children or others are at home, the family member may feel pulled between responsibility to the hospitalized patient and those at home. Routine family care is disrupted. Family members may have to take time off from work to be in the hospital with resulting loss of income and financial stress. At times, it is important to encourage a family member to attend to their own needs: to go home, get adequate sleep, take care of their own health problems or care for others in the family.

3. Find ways in which the family can participate in the routine care of the patient. Hospital policies should promote and encourage this participation. Some elderly patients require help to feed themselves, a time-consuming task for the nursing staff, but one that family members may enjoy. If visiting hours start in the afternoon, family members cannot help at breakfast or lunch. In addition to helping with hospital meals, family members can bring in appropriate foods for the patient. Not only are home cooked foods generally more appetizing and likely to be eaten, but family members who learn from the dietician what foods are allowed in the diet and how to prepare them will be more likely to incorporate them into the diet at home. Family members can also help with other aspects of care of the patient. During physical or occupational therapy, family members can learn what activities the patient participates in and which exercises the patient should do after discharge. When dressing changes or other simple procedures will continue after discharge, a member of the family can work along side the nurse and learn the procedure in the hospital. What kinds of procedures and care the family can participate in will depend upon the desires of the patient and the interests and capabilities of the family.

In one randomized clinical trial, women participated in their husbands' post MI exercise stress test. The women who actually walked on the treadmill were more confident of their husbands' physical and cardiac capacity and less fearful of another MI than women who did not participate or simply observed the test (14). However, participating in some aspects of care may be too stressful for families and have an adverse effect. Another study of high risk cardiac patients and their families found that family members who learned cardiopulmonary resuscitation were more anxious about the patient's health than those who did not, and the patients in these families were also more anxious and had poorer adjustment to their illness (15). The investigators suggested that the CPR sessions had a "rehearsal component" that made the normal and healthy repression of thoughts of sudden death more difficult to maintain. In addition, family members reported feeling responsible for keeping the patient alive, and in some cases feared leaving the patient least he have a cardiac arrest while alone. In general, it appears that family involvement is most beneficial for procedures and treatments that emphasize the patient's recovery and wellness, rather than potential adverse outcomes.

Several hospitals have developed innovative programs which involve family members in every aspect of hospital care (16). Patients are admitted with their spouse or other relative and stay in apartment-style rooms. The family members are taught to perform many of the tasks traditionally performed by the nursing staff. These units are very popular with patients and their families. Patients report reduced anxiety, and family members feel more competent to handle medical problems when the patient returns home. In addition, these units require fewer nurses (an important advantage during the current nursing shortage) and cost approximately half as much to run as traditional hospital units.

Even in the intensive care unit, family members can help with personal care, such as bathing, as well as the emotional support that is important to a patient's recovery. Such simple measures like holding the patient's hand can have powerfully reassuring effect on both the patient and the family and help humanize this frightening and highly technical environment. Cardiologist James Lynch (17), has documented the importance of human touch in the ICU: how it can reduce the resting heart rate and improve or abolish some arrhythmias.

Involving the family in a patient's care helps to meet the needs of both the patient and the family. It provides the patient with additional care and family support to reduce anxiety and speed recovery. It permits the family to be with the patient and feel that they are being helpful to him or her. And it provides the physician with the necessary information and resources to successfully treat the patient.

Three days after his heart attack, George Mayer was transferred to a regular medical floor and began cardiac rehabilitation. He and his wife attended several cardiac teaching classes together in the hospital. They learned about the role of diet and exercise in cardiac rehabilitation and met with the dietician to review their diet. Together they negotiated which high cholesterol foods would be eliminated from both of their diets and which only George would avoid. (Sarah did not want to give up ice cream.) Sarah purchased the American Heart Association cookbook and brought a couple of home cooked meals to George in the hospital. On his seventh hospital day, George underwent a limited stress test which revealed no ischemia or arrhythmia. Sarah accompanied him to the exercise lab and after watching him on the treadmill, was invited by the cardiologist to try the treadmill out to experience what her husband had endured. She was amazed at how strenuous the exercise was and felt reassured that George could safely tolerate it.

Discharge Planning

With shorter hospital stays and patients being discharged with greater medical needs, planning for home care by the family has become an increasingly important aspect of hospital care.

1. Discuss discharge plans with the family early and on a regular basis. This may be as simple as telling the patient and family how many additional days the patient is likely to be in the hospital or as complex as discussing nursing home placement. Discuss this as early as possible. Unfortunately patients or families are given less than 24 hours notice that the patient will be discharged.

2. Ask the family to meet with the social worker or public health nurse early to determine their post-discharge needs. This can be useful even when there are no obvious home care needs. A social worker or public health nurse is usually better able to assess home care needs and more aware of the resources in the community. For instance, the patient may benefit from a hospital bed or commode, or be able to take advantage of a community service (such as Friendly Visitors, Meals-on-Wheels) or group (such as Multiple Sclerosis Association). In addition, these professionals can help the family determine what they can afford and what services their insurance will cover.

3. Discharge the patient home when both the patient and the family are ready. Patients should not be discharged simply when they no longer need acute medical care in the hospital. Sending a patient home when there are insufficient services or the family is unprepared to care for the patient is bad medical care. If discharge planning is started early, an adequate plan can usually be set up prior to the time the patient no longer needs acute hospital care.

4. Convene a family discharge conference one or two days prior to discharge. Try to get all the members of patient's household to be present, but encourage as many other family members as possible to attend. Invite the hospital staff that have been involved with the patient's care or helped with discharge planning. This usually includes the primary nurse and the social worker or public health nurse, but may also involve other consulting physicians, physical, occupational or speech therapists, or the dietician.

a. Update the current medical status of the patient (diagnosis, treatment received and prognosis). Have the other staff report on their areas of involvement.
b. Outline the treatment plan (including medications), the needs of the patient at home and services to be provided.
c. Elicit the patient's and family's understanding, questions and reactions to the patient's discharge and the discharge plan. Anticipate difficulties by asking how they think the plan will work, and what problems are likely to arise.
d. Encourage the patient and family to negotiate what roles and responsibilities they will assume in the patient's care. (See Chapter 15 on chronic illness for details of this negotiation.)

5. Set up a postdischarge appointment with the patient and family. Depending upon the nature and severity of the problems, this may occur in the office or the home one to six weeks after discharge. Patients and their families should be encouraged to call sooner if problems arise.

> The day before George's discharge from the hospital, Dr. T met with the couple, their daughter who had flown in from out of town, George's primary nurse, the cardiac nurse educator, and the dietician. George's medical condition, diet, medication, and exercise program were all reviewed with the family. George and his wife were referred to a cardiac rehabilitation program at the local YMCA. The family was encouraged to share their feelings and concerns about George and his health. Sarah was most concerned that George would push himself too hard and not tell anyone if he was having any chest pain. Dr. T helped the couple negotiate how they would handle these issues. George agreed to tell his wife if he was having chest pain. Sarah agreed that he would be responsible for his level of activity, but that she would give him one reminder if she felt he was overdoing it.
>
> Dr. T briefly met with the couple alone to discuss guidelines for sexual activity. He took a brief sexual history and explained that based upon George's stress test and his level of activity, they could safely return to their normal sex life. He said that they may experience some anxiety or even some sexual difficulties in the beginning, and that this was normal. He scheduled them for a follow-up visit in the office for one month. If all was going well at that time, he told George that he would be able to gradually return to work after that.

Family-oriented care in the hospital offers special opportunities and challenges for the primary care provider. Because families are often in a state of crisis, they can greatly benefit from regular communication and support from the physician. During the hospitalization, they have the opportunity to learn more about their family member's illness and how to assist in the patient's care.

References

1. Steinglass P, Temple S, Lisman S, Reiss D: Coping with spinal cord injury: The family perspective. *Gen Hosp Psychiatry* 1982;**4**:259–264.
2. Blumental D, Shlesinger M, Drumheller PB et al.: The future of medicare. *New Engl J Med* 1986;**314**:722–728.
3. Newcomer R, Wood J, Samkar A: Medicare prospective payment: Anticipated effect on hospitals other community agencies and families. *J Health Polit Policy Law* 1985;**10**:275–282.
4. Robertson J, Robertson J: Young children on brief separation. *Psychoanalytic Study of the Child* 1971;**26**:264–315.
5. MacCarthy D, Lindsay M, Morris I: Children in hospital with mothers. *Lancet* 1962;**i**:603–608.
6. Hardgrove C, Healy D: The care-through-parent program at Moffit Hospital, University of California, San Francisco. *Nursing Clin North America* 1984;**19**:145–160.
7. Chatham M: The effect of family involvement on patients' manifestations of postcardiotomy psychosis. *Heart Lung* 1978;**7**:995–999.
8. Schwartz L, Brenner Z: Critical care unit transfer: Reducing patient stress through nursing interventions. *Heart Lung* 1979;**8**:540–546.
9. Wishnie H, Hackett T, Cassem N: Psychological hazards of convalescence following myocardial infarction. *JAMA* 1971;**215**:1292–1296.
10. Hampe SC: Needs of the grieving spouse in a hospital setting. *Nursing Research* 1975;**24**:113–120.
11. Breu C, Dracup K: Helping the spouse of critically ill patients. *Am J Nursing* 1978;**78**:50–53.
12. Daley L: The perceived immediate needs of families with relatives in the intensive care unit setting. *Heart Lung* 1984;**7**:231–237.
13. Leahy M, Wright LM: *Families and Life-Threatening Illness.* Springhouse, PA: Springhouse Corp., 1987.
14. Taylor CB, Bandura A, Ewart CK, Miller NH, DeBusk RF: Exercise testing to enhance wives' confidence in their husbands' cardiac capability soon after clinically uncomplicated acute myocardial infarction. *Am J Cardiol* 1985;**55**:635–638.
15. Dracup K, Guzy PM, Taylor SE, Barry J: Cardiopulmonary resuscitation (CPR) training: Consequences for family members of high-risk cardiac patients. *Arch Intern Med* 1986;**146**:1757–1761.
16. Berg B: A touch of home in hospital care. *NY Times Magazine* No. 27, 1983;90–98.
17. Lynch JJ: *The Broken Heart: The Medical Consequences of Loneliness.* New York, Basic Books, 1977.

PROTOCOL

Checklist for Family Involvement during Hospitalization

☐ Meet with the family as soon as possible, at least within the first 24 hours of hospitalization.

☐ Establish a method for the family to communicate with the treatment team.

☐ Make contact with family members during hospital rounds.

☐ Encourage the family to support and assist the patient in the following ways:

  ☐ visit as much as possible.

  ☐ help with meals and bathing or other grooming needs.

  ☐ assist with dressing changes and other medical treatments.

  ☐ participate in physical, occupational and speech therapy.

  ☐ learn about any special dietary needs and bring in home-cooked meals.

  ☐ accompany the patient to medical tests and procedures.

  ☐ stay overnight when appropriate.

  ☐ attend educational courses and instruction on the patient's illness.

  ☐ obtain books and other written material about the illness.

☐ Discuss discharge planning with the patient and family, as early as possible and on a regular basis.

☐ In anticipation of discharge, encourage the family to:

  ☐ meet early with social worker to determine needs at home.

  ☐ learn from the patient's nurse about medication to be taken after discharge.

  ☐ obtain dietary instructions from the nutritionist.

  ☐ learn about post discharge treatments and therapies.

☐ Meet with the family prior to discharge to be certain they have the necessary information and are prepared for home care.

☐ Schedule a follow-up appointment for the patient and family.

CHAPTER 22

Working Together
Collaboration and Referral to Family-Oriented Mental Health Professionals

Collaboration between family-oriented primary care physicians and mental health professionals has generated much interest and enthusiasm in recent years, providing new opportunities for improved care for our patients. The development of the biopsychosocial model (1) has provided a theoretical foundation that can be shared by both primary care and mental health. The field of family systems medicine has begun to articulate the implementation of this theory, including issues around collaborative health care (2–4). Several kinds of collaborative relationships are possible between the primary care physician and the mental health specialist, ranging from consultation (for mysterious or stuck cases) to cotherapy sessions (for especially difficult cases like somatic fixation or dysfunctions around chronic illness) to referral (for serious or time-consuming cases) (5,6). (See Fig. 22.1.) This chapter will make practical suggestions for building a collaborative model that increases the ability of primary care providers to work with mental health professionals to maximize outcome for the patient and the provider.

Several studies have demonstrated the ability of mental health services to reduce the cost and frequency of other medical services (7,8). These studies suggest that good outpatient psychotherapy can save the primary care provider time and save the patient money. Family-oriented mental health care has begun to demonstrate its effectiveness through a body of research studies (9). In particular, family therapy has been shown to be effective in several specific mental and physical disorders. (See Chapter 2.) However, like family-oriented primary care, it is a relatively new discipline that needs to further develop its research base. Research on the even more specialized area of collaboration between family-oriented primary care and mental health specialists has only

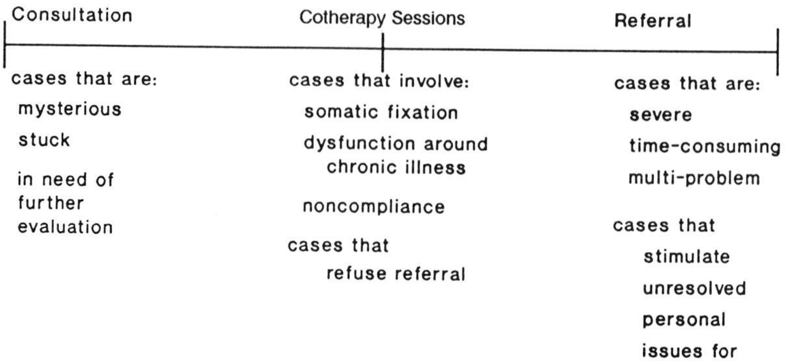

Consultation	Cotherapy Sessions	Referral
cases that are:	cases that involve:	cases that are:
mysterious	somatic fixation	severe
stuck	dysfunction around chronic illness	time-consuming
in need of further evaluation	noncompliance	multi-problem
	cases that refuse referral	cases that stimulate unresolved personal issues for

FIGURE 22.1. Types of collaborative relationships between primary care providers and mental health specialists.

recently begun. One clinical study by the Dutch family practitioner Huygen looked at the role of family therapy in providing better care to family medicine patients. Huygen found that patients referred from his practice who were frequent utilizers of medical services improved their health status and used fewer medications after family therapy than did a matched group of controls (10). Research on the effects of family-oriented mental health services on family-oriented primary care is an important area for future study.

How to Find a Good Psychotherapist

Many practitioners are convinced of the importance of having good mental health specialists to work with; the problem is finding them. Finding good psychotherapists to work with patients can be more challenging than finding other specialists because the technical skills that define a good psychotherapist are subjective and interpersonal, unlike those of a good general surgeon or opthalmologist. Successful use of mental health professionals depends on a good knowledge of community resources (11). Providers new to a community have several avenues to track down reliable, competent family-oriented therapists.

1. The most frequently used method of finding a good therapist is to **ask respected colleagues whom they use and why.** Professionals who have been in the community for a long time will know who they believe to be competent and how reliable these people are over time. Of course, physicians differ in what they want from a therapist, so asking the colleague to describe the therapist may help you to decide if that is the kind of service you wish.

2. **Arrange a face-to-face meeting with the therapist** to discuss his or her orientation to evaluation and treatment. This can be the most useful method of finding a good therapist. A lunch or a meeting at either professional's office provides first-hand information about how the therapist interacts, his or her theoretical orientation, beliefs about treatment, ability and experience interfacing with the medical system, and how well he or she can cooperate with you.

3. **Use the American Association for Marriage and Family Therapy Directory to find a family-oriented mental health professional in your community.** Psychotherapists come in what can be a bewildering array of professional degrees and theoretical orientations. Family-oriented physicians will find that family-oriented mental health professionals often share their perspective and philosophy on patient care, regardless of whether their training resulted in an M.D., a Ph.D., an M.S.W., or some other counseling degree. The American Association for Marriage and Family Therapy certifies that its members have had intensive and in-depth training in a systems or family approach to mental health problems. Only those mental health professionals who can demonstrate substantial supervised experience with families may join this organization. These therapists are also well qualified to deal with individual patients, though they are likely to do so with the family in mind, no different from the practice of a family-oriented medical provider who sees many individual patients but carries a family perspective into any interview. Write to the American Association for Marriage and Family Therapy, 1717 K Street NW, Suite 407, Washington, D.C. 20006, to secure the most recent copy of their Membership Directory.

Avoiding Potential Problems in Collaboration

While much recent progress has been made in building a successful collaborative model with mental health professionals, problems have traditionally plagued this relationship and sometimes still result in misunderstandings that block effective patient care (12). These problems are rooted in differences in training and differences in the goals and purpose of the work each professional does. These differences need to be understood in order to be complementary and for effective collaboration to take place. Table 22.1 describes the differences in the working styles and goals of primary care and mental health professionals.

The following is an extreme example that illustrates the ways these differences can plague collaboration and referral. It is, in a sense, a lesson in how to prevent collaboration and bring out the worst in your colleagues. In it, a stereotyped primary care physician is calling a stereotyped mental health professional to make a referral.

TABLE 22.1.   Differences in the Working Styles of Primary Care and Mental Health Professionals

	Primary care	Mental health
Language	Medical	Humanistic, psychoanalytic, or systems
Traditional paradigm	Biomedical	Psychoanalytic
New paradigm	Biopsychosocial	Family systems
Professional style	Action-oriented	Process-oriented
	Advice-giving	Avoids advice
	M.D. takes initiative	Patient takes initiative
Standard session time	10–15 minutes	45–50 minutes
Demand for services	Around the clock	Scheduled sessions (excepting emergencies)
Use of medications	Frequent	Infrequent
Use of individual and family history	Basic	Extensive
At risk for	Somatic fixation	Psychosocial fixation

Dr. P: Hello, this is Dr. Psycho.

Dr. M: Hi, Sue? This is Dr. Medic at the Family Medicine Center. I have this patient I'd like you to see, but I just have a minute to tell you about her as I'm already 45 minutes behind in my appointments. She's a 16-year-old primigravida at 34 weeks gestation complicated by some intrauterine growth retardation and mild preeclampsia. The problem is that this lady just won't come in for her prenatal visits or any of the tests she needs. I've tried everything to get her in. She's really impossible! I keep telling her that the baby is going to die if she doesn't do what I tell her. Can you see her? Maybe you can convince her that she's got to come in for these appointments.

Dr. P: Well, Dr. Medic, I can hear you're really upset. What do you think is going on? Could she be depressed?

Dr. M: I don't know, that's your department. She doesn't look very happy, but who would in her situation? Say, if you want to put her on an antidepressant, let me know so I can be sure it's a safe one for pregnancy.

Dr. P: Seems like you're jumping to medications rather quickly, Dr. Medic. I feel I need to know something about the patient, you know, her history and her family, before we rush into pharmacotherapy. What do you know about her family?

Dr. M: I don't have time for that stuff. It's hard enough dealing with all her medical problems. All I know is that I've seen her boyfriend and I'm sure he's on drugs. I've checked the lady for AIDS and she's okay so far, but she's not cooperating with me.

Dr. P: Boy, sounds like this case is really getting to you. You're pretty angry at her, you know.

Dr. M: I am not the patient here. Will you see this patient or not? Just convince her to come back for her tests.

DR. P: Calm down, Dr. Medic. I'm going to need some time to do a complete evaluation on this patient. I've got an opening in two weeks.

DR. M: Two weeks—she'll have a dead baby by then! Besides she probably won't show up. I'm calling now to get an appointment for her, which I'll give to her social worker so I can be sure she'll get there.

DR. P: That's being too directive. We need to use her ability to secure an appointment and get to my office as a measure of her motivation for change. I can't badger her to come. That's her decision.

DR. M: Look, I don't have time for this. Forget about seeing the patient. I'll just call Child Protective. They'll do something about this.

DR. P: I'm sorry, Dr. Medic. I'm trying to be helpful to you. I have to tell you I'm concerned you're falling back on strongarm tactics instead of demonstrating the caring and sensitivity that's supposed to be part of being a health professional.

DR. M: Big help. Thanks a lot.

DR. P: Good-bye.

This extreme example illustrates the many ways primary care and mental health professionals can misunderstand and miscommunicate with each other because of their differing job demands and their differing expectations of each other. Recognizing and appreciating our differences can facilitate collaboration and reduce miscommunications around referrals.

What Triggers a Referral to a Therapist

Once an effective professional network has been established, referral to a psychotherapist can be expedient. When is referral necessary? Individual and family assessment are fundamental tools for managing the psychosocial needs of primary care patients and deciding when to refer. (Chapter 3 provides a guide to assessing families in primary care.)

Many psychosocial problems lend themselves to **primary care counseling** (11,13), for those providers who feel interested and trained to do counseling with their patients These problems include **adjustment to the diagnosis of a new illness, the range of situational or adjustment problems** (e.g., problems after the birth of the first child), **individual, marital, or family crises of limited severity and duration** (e.g., an accident or unexpected surgery), **many behavior problems, mild depressive or anxiety reactions, and uncomplicated grief.** In addition to the problems that may be treated in primary care, other problems exist such as somatization and substance abuse that often require a lengthy period of primary care counseling to mobilize the patient and family for a specialist referral. A multiplicity of factors involving the patient, the problem, and the provider combine to dictate the decision about whether and when to refer to a mental health specialist (11).

Patient Factors that Trigger a Referral

1. Severity of the problem. The problems in this category, by definition, require time, specialized training, and an intensity of treatment not typically practical in a primary care setting. They include:

• suicidal or homicidal ideation, intent, or behavior
• psychotic behavior
• recent sexual abuse (incest or rape), or a history of abuse that continues to influence the patient's feelings or behavior
• recent physical abuse (child, spouse, or elder), or a history of abuse that continues to influence the patient's feelings or behavior
• substance abuse (alcohol or drugs)
• somatic fixation
• most marital or sexual problems (especially those involving affairs, separation, or divorce, or active consideration of any of the above)
• multi-problem, complex family situations (two pathognomonic signs of these situations are when the family is so complicated you cannot figure out how to draw the genogram, or when the chart is extremely thick)

Some of these problems can be referred easily in the heat of a crisis. For example, the family with a patient experiencing an acute psychotic break or suicidal episode, a patient who has been recently raped, or a couple considering divorce are all situations in which people are sufficiently anxious and motivated that they will typically agree (or even request) to see a mental health specialist. (See Chapters 12 and 17 for suggestions about referral for marital, sexual, or depressive problems.)

Other situations may involve more long-standing problems such that the patient and family are less anxious and more familiar with their dysfunction. Problems in this category may include substance abuse, a history of sexual or physical abuse, somatization, and some multi-problem family situations. While these patients may be very unhappy about their problem, they may be reluctant or frightened by the idea of a referral. They may require more lengthy support and counseling, or the situation may have to escalate into a crisis, before the patient or family will successfully connect with a mental health specialist. (See Chapters 16, 18, and 19 for suggestions about referral of somatization, substance abuse, and physical and sexual abuse.)

2. Chronicity of the problem. One trigger for a referral is a severe and acute problem. Another is a serious and chronic problem. If the provider or the patient has been concerned about a psychosocial problem for greater than six months to one year, this by itself may indicate the need for an evaluation or referral to a specialist. For example, a patient may report behavior problems with her son in school, problems she and her husband tried to manage unsuccessfully over the last school year.

Now, at the beginning of a new year with a new teacher, the same problems emerge. Or, a physician may contract for six primary care counseling sessions over six months with a couple experiencing marital problems in their first year of marriage. At the end of that time, both the provider and the couple agree some moderate improvement has occurred but on the whole the problems still exist. Another example might be a patient with a drinking problem who denies he is alcoholic and requests a period of time to prove it to his provider and his family by abstaining from any alcohol. At the end of a six month contract with the provider, both patient and family report he reduced his drinking but was unable to abstain altogether. All of these situations call for referral based on the chronicity of the problem.

   3. **Patient request.** At times a patient or family will request a referral to a mental health specialist out of concern for themselves or one of their members. Sometimes the problems that concern them are serious and would trigger a referral from most providers. Other times the provider may feel comfortable suggesting primary care counseling, but the patient wishes the privacy of counseling with a specialist because of his or her discomfort discussing the problems with the physician he or she routinely sees. (Rape or divorce fall in this category for some patients.) Patient readiness, family support, and type of problem are all factors in whether or when a problem is referred. Equally important are the provider's considerations about the evaluation and treatment of any given patient or problem.

Physician Factors that Trigger a Referral

   1. **Constraints on the physician's time or energy.** Most physicians that do primary care counseling feel they must limit this practice to, say, an afternoon a week or to one or two appointments per day. Other physicians prefer to do much less counseling in their practices. Whatever the preference, physicians with little time for or interest in primary care counseling may have a lower threshold for referring their patients with psychosocial difficulties and want to collaborate more frequently with mental health specialists.

   2. **The limits of a provider's training.** Physicians differ in the amount and kind of training they receive in assessing and treating psychosocial problems. Some obtain specialized training in marital and family problems, or alcohol counseling, or hypnosis. Others have basic training in the management of psychiatric disorders but no interest in or access to other more specialized training. The trigger for referral may occur with the sense that "I'm in over my head" or "This is out of my league." As in other areas of primary care, the training of the provider will often determine his or her threshold for referral.

3. Recognition of a need for further assessment of the problem. Even with specialized training, a provider may recognize that something is missing from the current assessment. The treatment that logically follows from the initial assessment is not working, or the information just does not "add up." In these cases, a referral for further evaluation can be helpful.

4. Stagnation or failure of primary care counseling (11). It is always useful to contract for a specific number of sessions for primary care counseling (somewhere between 3 and 6). This contract serves to increase the patient's or family's motivation if they wish to avoid referral, and it also provides a set time to evaluate whether the patient's goals are being reached. If either the provider or the patient is dissatisfied with the treatment at the time of this evaluation, referral should be considered. (If not, a new contract with similar limits may be negotiated.)

5. Personal issues that make it difficult to work effectively with a particular patient, family, or problem. The provider who is feeling very stressed in his or her own life may have little energy for assessing or treating patients' psychosocial problems. It is important to protect ourselves (and our patients) at those times and use our referral network more liberally than perhaps at other times. Problems that "hit close to home," such as alcoholism for a physician from an alcoholic family, or marital problems for the physician separating from her husband, may require early referral. Other signs may signal potential countertransference problems, such as the feeling that "this patient is driving me crazy" or a sense of dread when a particular name appears on the day's roster of patients. At a minimum, a consultation in these situations might be useful to ensure that the primary care provider is able to separate out his or her personal issues from those of the patient. The consultation might then result in either a referral to the consultant or in new ideas for how to handle the case. The positive side of identification between the provider and the patient is that the provider tends to have a high investment in helping the patient and the patient may feel understood. The negative side is that the provider may lose a clear view of the patient's problem because of his or her own difficulties. (See Chapter 23 for further discussion of physician's own family issues and how they influence practice.) Consultation with colleagues or specialists is a very important mechanism to provide support for the physician and to increase the likelihood of a positive outcome for the patient.

How to Make a Successful Referral

A successful referral begins with a successful contact between the primary care physician and the mental health specialist.

MENTAL HEALTH SPECIALIST: Hello, this is Dr. Frank.

PRIMARY CARE PHYSICIAN: Hello, Dr. Frank, this is Dr. Kim at the Primary Care Unit. I have a patient over here that I'm scheduled to see again tomorrow and I'd like some help with her. She is a 35-year-old married woman with three children who has become pregnant again. She is unsure about carrying the pregnancy, and I think it is unwise. Her husband favors an abortion for this reason and because he does not wish to have more children. I have tried to talk to this patient, but she says unless the pregnancy is life-threatening she doesn't think she wants an abortion. I can't tell her she'll die for sure, but another pregnancy does jeopardize this woman's health. I wonder if it would be possible for you to see her and provide another perspective.

THERAPIST: That sounds like a very interesting and difficult situation, Dr. Kim. Could you clarify for me the medical implications of this woman carrying another child?

PHYSICIAN: I wish I knew for sure. In her last pregnancy, she had severe toxemia and bad gestational diabetes. I warned her against getting pregnant again. She states the timing is bad, in the best of circumstances, and is not morally opposed to abortion, but says she herself would rather not go that route. I suppose we could manage it if she does decide to carry the pregnancy, but it is risky.

THERAPIST: I would be happy to meet with this woman and her husband to discuss their decision. At least if the two of them could agree one way or the other, we could be assured this woman would have some family support whatever they decided. I would see my role as protecting this woman's right to make a final decision on this, but I would try to help her remain open to her husband's input and to clearly understand the medical implications of both decisions. Please have the patient call me after your appointment tomorrow. Then, if I or either member of the couple have any further medical questions, we will call you, as that's your area. Otherwise I'll try to see the couple before your next scheduled appointment with them, and get back to you immediately. Would you rather I drop you a note, or give you a call?

PHYSICIAN: The best would be to call me right after the session just to let me know where things stand, then drop me a short note for the chart.

THERAPIST: Fine, and if they wish to pursue this beyond one session, I'll let you know. I do understand there is time pressure here if the possibility of abortion is to be a real option, so I'll get right on it. Thank you for your call.

PHYSICIAN: I'll look forward to hearing from you. Good-bye.

Having clarified the request to the specialist, secured his or her agreement to see the patient, and gotten the specialist's input on making the referral, the next step is to present the referral in a way that makes sense and is palatable to the patient.

DR. KIM: Hello, Mrs. Fortune. I'm sorry to see your husband was unable to join us today.

MRS. FORTUNE: He had to work. He said to tell you maybe he could come next time.

DR. KIM: I know from our last conversation that you have a lot of mixed feelings about your current pregnancy. How are you feeling about it now?

MRS. FORTUNE: About the same. My husband and I have been round and round about it. We've even had a few arguments. I just don't know what to do. Now his mother is getting involved, telling me I have to get an abortion. I'm really angry that he even told her.

DR. KIM: Sounds like it's hard to figure out exactly how you feel with so many people around you having strong opinions.

MRS. FORTUNE: Yeah, that's right.

DR. KIM: I wonder if you and your husband have ever considered seeing a counselor?

MRS. FORTUNE: No, we've never had a big problem.

DR. KIM: You certainly don't have to have a big problem to be helped by seeing a good counselor. You and your husband have a lot of strengths; I think the two of you could make good use of seeing a counselor colleague of mine for a consultation. She has seen other patients in similar circumstances and has sometimes been able to help them sort out what they really want to do. She will not make the decision for you, but she may help you and your husband see the situation a little more clearly so you can support each other whichever way you decide. As you know, from a medical perspective, the pregnancy is risky so I would really like to be sure that you and your family have the information and the support you need to make the best decision you can. I have worked before with Dr. Frank and I think you like her.

MRS. FORTUNE: Isn't this something we could just talk out on our own?

DR. KIM: That's certainly a possibility. However, I know you're having a rough time and I think it's a difficult enough situation that it might be useful to accept some special support and expertise.

MRS. FORTUNE: Well, maybe you're right. I haven't been sleeping well I've been so worried.

DR. KIM: Please give Dr. Frank a call today for an appointment. She'll be expecting to hear from you. And be sure to make it for a time when your husband can go as well. Do you think that will be a problem?

MRS. FORTUNE: He may not like the idea initially, but he has been very upset about this whole thing.

DR. KIM: How about if I give him a call and tell him why I think it might be a good idea? That way if he has questions I could answer them.

MRS. FORTUNE: Okay, you could reach him at home late this afternoon.

This example illustrates the importance of the primary care physician, the specialist, and the patient having clear communications around the time of the referral. This clarity helps to avoid problems such as the primary care physician feeling the specialist did not focus on the referral request, the specialist not communicating with the primary physician after the consultation, or the patient feeling abandoned by the primary care physician. The following summarize the **guidelines for making a successful referral:**

1. Clarify the consultation or referral question in your own mind. If it is not clear, say so in the initial call to the specialist so that person might help with clarification.

2. Refer to someone you know and trust whenever possible. Suggest a meeting if the person is unknown.

3. Consult with the intended therapist as early as possible to share ideas and strategy, even prior to the time of presenting the referral to the patient.

4. If the referral is your idea rather than the patient's, **work to maximize the patient's motivation to use the referral** in a productive way.

- **Use the patient's language** and the patient's understanding of the problem to pitch the referral (e.g., "You are very worried about whether to carry this pregnancy. I am also concerned about you. I think you and your husband deserve to discuss this with someone who has special expertise in this area.")
- **Refer for "evaluation", "consultation", or "counseling". AVOID** referring for "family therapy", unless the patient or family specifically requests it (14). (It is often premature to refer for any kind of "therapy" before the patient(s) has had an opportunity to find out if they feel working with a particular therapist will be helpful to them.) Some patients hear a referral for "family therapy" as meaning that their family is bad or in some way responsible for the current problem, rather than that the family can be a resource in helping to find a solution. Interaction around these issues can be tricky and is best avoided altogether by just referring for "consultation" around the presenting problem as it is understood by the patient.
- **Refer to the specialist as a "counselor" or an "expert** on helping patients with problems such as yours". It is most helpful to use a generic description of the mental health specialist, rather than terms such as "family therapist", or even "psychiatrist" or psychologist". For people knowledgeable and interested in these distinctions, such information can be helpful. For others, it can be confusing and scary.

5. Elicit family support for the referral. Have a family meeting or conference to assess and discuss the problem. Get the family to support the referral and be a part of the treatment process, if possible. If the family is resistant or refuses to attend the family conference, inform the psychotherapist and let that person manage who will or will not be a part of the treatment (10).

6. Have the patient call the therapist for an appointment before he or she leaves your office (11).

7. Join the therapist for the first session, in your office or in the therapist's office, for those patients who are difficult and need your support to accept the referral (e.g., somatic fixation cases).

8. **When a patient strongly resists a referral,** in spite of using the principles listed in numbers 4–7:
   - Make your recommendation to the patient and family, but **do not battle about it.**
   - **Take a longer view of the problem.** Some difficult referrals take 1–2 years to accomplish. State that you are sure this will be something the patient will decide can be useful in the future. Get the patient to agree that if they do not improve over a specific time period, they will agree to see a specialist.
   - **Wait for a crisis to occur,** when referral is typically easier.
9. **Support treatment with the mental health specialist.**
   - **Communicate regularly with the therapist.**
   - **Let the patient know you and the therapist are a team** and that you communicate regularly. Reassure the patient that if specific information exists that he or she wishes to remain confidential in therapy, that will be respected.
   - **When a patient complains about the specialist early on:**
     a. Encourage the patient to talk directly to the therapist about whatever is concerning him or her.
     b. Reassure the patient that the beginning of treatment is often difficult.
     c. Encourage them to attend at least three sessions to "give it a fair try."
     d. Report the difficulty to the therapist.
   - **When a patient complains about the specialist later in treatment:**
     a. Encourage the patient to talk directly to the therapist about whatever is concerning him or her.
     b. If the patient is very distressed and refusing to return, suggest that you will talk to the therapist and get back to the patient.
     c. Tell the therapist the patient is reporting difficulty. Try to assess whether the problem is that
        •• the process is painful but necessary (in which case the patient should be strongly encouraged to continue)
        •• the treatment has been helpful but now is stalemated or stuck (in which case a meeting with the therapist, the family, and an outside consultant might help), or
        •• the treatment is not useful (in which case the patient may want to quit treatment altogether or be referred to different specialist)
10. **Follow-up with the patient after making the referral.**
   - **Set up an appointment with the patient soon after the counseling begins** to support treatment and reassure the patient of your interest.

- **Set up an appointment with the patient soon after counseling ends** to debrief and help perpetuate the changes that have occurred.

Your Rights and Responsibilities as a Referring Physician

A collaborative relationship works well because both people manage their part in the relationship in a responsible and responsive way. Because mental health care consists primarily of an interpersonal "procedures," referrals to mental health specialists are somewhat different from referrals to other medical specialists and need to be given some distinctive consideration. The following are what we see to be the **responsibilities of the referring physician in collaborating with a mental health specialist around a referral:**

1. **Contact the therapist before the patient's first visit.**
2. **Clarify the reasons for the referral.**
3. **Send any records or reports the therapist may need** to understand or treat the patient and family.
4. **Make explicit what kind of communication you want from the therapist:**
    - **letter and/or phone contact**–Some providers wish to be called after the first session or two, then receive a report for the chart at the beginning and end of treatment.
    - **frequency of contact**–Providers vary in how frequently they wish to be contacted. Be specific about your wishes. Minimally, request reports at the beginning and end of therapy, and calls about any crisis or issue that might affect the primary care of this patient.
    - **how much information you want**–Providers vary in the amount of information they want from a mental health specialist. Again, be specific if you wish a brief, one-paragraph report, or if you want a lengthier description of the case that might illuminate the patient and family's dynamics and difficulties in a way that could be helpful in formulating new strategies for your own relationship and care for the patient.
5. **Clarify your own availability with regard to the case.** "I am very busy right now in my practice. This is the second time this adolescent has run away. I would like you to see this family and take charge of these issues. I would see myself as providing support and back-up for your treatment, as you work to help this family establish a different way of relating."
6. **Negotiate and clarify what you will work on with the patient, what the therapist will work on, and how you will work together.**

Patients often bring the same issue to their primary physician that they bring to their therapist, in part to see if they both say the same thing. While it can be useful to solicit different opinions about the same problem, this process can undermine the therapist's authority and result in a zero sum gain for the patient and family. Most useful is for the primary physician and the therapist to discuss the territory of the treatment and agree that certain issues will be dealt with in therapy (e.g., a recent affair), certain issues will be dealt with in primary care (e.g., the medical aspects of the wife's sexual dysfunction), and certain issues will be handled by both (e.g., both professionals will support the couple's strong parenting skills in the face of their current marital stress). Being explicit about the treatment plan allows the medical provider to redirect, for example, the wife who is looking for support after her husband's affair. ("That sounds painful. I think you need to discuss these issues further in your therapy.") It also allows the therapist to appropriately return medical issues to the physician. ("You have many concerns about your poor lubrication and your lack of interest in sex. You need to make an appointment with your physician and discuss with him your thoughts about these having a physiological basis. Then we can continue to work on other factors that may be inhibiting your desire for your husband.")

While the primary care physician has many responsibilities in making a successful referral, a good mental health specialist should also be responsible, responsive, and useful to you in many ways. If he or she is not, and you have other options, do not continue to use that person. Specifically, a good therapist should:

- provide timely feedback in the form that has been agreed upon,
- support your relationship with your patients,
- if a problem in this area arises, be direct and helpful in trying to get it resolved,
- give a practical and understandable evaluation of a patient and family,
- welcome contact and communication from you, and
- inform you regarding the ending and outcome of treatment so you can plan follow-up.

Working together under these circumstances results in effective collaboration that can yield both high quality patient care and education, support, and stimulation for the professionals involved. Consultation or referral to a mental health specialist is a powerful primary care intervention in and of itself for a patient. Even if the patient refuses the referral, such a discussion often helps the patient or family to view their problem differently and may motivate them to make changes that have been difficult until then. When the referral is successful, the patient, the family, and the relationship with the primary care provider may benefit.

References

1. Engel G: The need for a new medical model: A challenge for biomedicine. *Science* 1977;**196**:4286:129–136.
2. Bloch D: Family systems medicine: The field and the journal. *Fam Syst Med* 1983;**1**(1):3–11.
3. Bloch D: The partnership of Dr. Biomedicine and Dr. Psychosocial. *Fam Syst Med* 1988;**6**(1):2–4.
4. Glenn M: *Collaborative Health Care: A Family-Oriented Model.* New York, Praeger, 1987.
5. Wynne L, McDaniel SH, Weber T: *Systems Consultation: A New Perspective for Family Therapy.* New York, Guilford Press, 1986.
6. McDaniel SH, Campbell T, Wynne L, Weber T: Family systems consultation: Opportunities for teaching in family medicine. *Fam Syst Med* 1988;**6**(4):391–403.
7. Cummings NA, VandenBos GR: The twenty-year Kaiser-Permanente experience with psychotherapy and medical utilization: Implications for national health policy and national health insurance. *Health Policy Quarterly* 1981;**1**:159–175.
8. Mumford E, Schlesinger HJ, Glass GV, et al.: A new look at evidence about the reduced cost of medical utilization following mental health treatment. *Am J Psychiatry* 1984;**141**:1145–1158.
9. Gurman A, Kniskern D: Family therapy outcome research: knowns and unknowns, in Gurman A (ed.): *Handbook of Family Therapy.* New York, Brunner-Mazel, 1981.
10. Huygen FJA: *Family Medicine: The Medical Life History of Families.* New York, Brunner-Mazel, 1982.
11. Doherty WJ, Baird MA: *Family Therapy and Family Medicine.* New York, Guilford Press, 1983.
12. McDaniel SH, Campbell T: Physicians and family therapists: The risks of collaboration. *Fam Syst Med* 1985;**4**(1):4–8.
13. Bishop DS: Family therapy and family medicine. *Am J Fam Ther* 1981;**9**(2):68–70.
14. Simon R. Issues in the referral for family therapy. *Fam Syst Med* 1983;**1**(1):56–61.

PROTOCOL

When and How to Refer Primary-Care Patients to Mental Health Specialists

When to Treat and When to Refer Problems Seen in Primary Care

Problems commonly seen in primary care counseling	Problems commonly referred on to a mental health specialist
Adjustment to the diagnosis of a new illness	Suicidal or homicidal ideation, intent, or behavior
Other adjustment or situational disorders	Psychotic behavior
Crises of limited severity or duration	Sexual or physical abuse
Behavior problems	Substance abuse
Mild depressive reactions	Somatic fixation
Mild anxiety reactions	Moderate-severe marital and sexual problems
Uncomplicated grief reactions	Multi-problem family situations
	Problems resistant to change in primary care counseling

The Do's and Don'ts of Referral to Mental Health Specialists

A. The Do's

  1. Clarify the consultation or referral question.
  2. Refer to someone you know and trust whenever possible.
  3. Consult with the intended therapist as early as possible.
  4. Work to maximize the patient's motivation to use the referral in a productive way:
     a. Use the patient's language.
     b. Refer for "evaluation", "consultation", or "counseling."
     c. Refer to the specialist as a "counselor" or an "expert on help ing people with problems such as yours."
  5. Elicit family support for the referral.
  6. Have the patient call the therapist for an appointment before he or she leaves your office.
  7. Join the therapist for the first session, for those patients who are difficult and need your support to accept the referral.

8. Make explicit the frequency and kind of communication you want from the therapist.
9. Negotiate and clarify what you will work on with the patient, what the therapist will work on, and how you will work together.
10. When a patient strongly resists a referral:
    a. Take a longer view of the problem. Some difficult referrals take 1–2 years to accomplish.
    b. Wait for a crisis to occur, when referral is typically easier.
11. Support treatment with the mental health specialist.
    a. Communicate regularly with the therapist.
    b. Let the patient know you and the therapist are a team.
12. Follow-up with the patient after making the referral.
    a. Set up an appointment soon after the counseling begins to support treatment and reassure the patient of your interest.
    b. Set up an appointment with the patient soon after counseling ends to debrief and provide continuity.

B. The Don'ts

1. Don't assume the mental health specialist has a similar working style to that of a primary care physician. Work to get to know the differences between yourself and a therapist you respect. By recognizing differences, the ground for efficient collaboration will be established.
2. Don't wait until the last minute to refer a difficult patient or family. Therapists refer to this as a "dump" and feel it takes a very long time to bring the patient back to a place where treatment can be successful. Contact the therapist fairly early in the process, even for an informal consultation.
3. Don't use medical or psychiatric diagnoses with patients when making the referral. While patients may benefit from knowing their diagnoses, the language of the patient and the family is much more descriptive and understandable to them.
4. Don't refer to a "family therapist" for "family therapy". Unfortunately, most patients hear these labels as conferring blame or inadequacy on their family. Exceptions to this principle are those problems patients themselves label "marital" or "family" problems.
5. When patients strongly resist a referral, don't battle with them. Maintain your recommendation, monitor their functioning for deterioration, and just wait.
6. Don't allow the patient to pit you against the therapist.
    a. Encourage the patient to talk directly to the therapist about any complaints he or she has about the treatment.

   b. Encourage the patient to attend several sessions and "give it a fair try."
   c. Tell the therapist the patient is reporting difficulty.
   d. When treatment is stuck or ineffective, ask the therapist for his or her assessment. Consider consultation, termination, or referral to another mental health specialist.
7. Don't continue using a therapist who generally does not provide adequate feedback or effective treatment.

CHAPTER 23

Managing Personal and Professional Boundaries

How to Make the Physician's Own Issues a Resource in Patient Care

Empathy and sensitivity are resources in family-oriented primary care that are largely developed in the providers' own personal and family life. A physician's appreciation of the richness of emotional life, the complexity of human problems, and the humility inherent in human suffering forms the foundation for such empathy and fuels a successful doctor-patient relationship. A physician may be drawn to primary care in the first place because his or her upbringing has resulted in a highly developed sense of responsibility and altruism. Many primary care physicians played a caretaking role that was highly valued in their original families, and has led to a commitment to serving others and a sensitivity to illness and loss.

All this early family training is useful to the physician interested in the art of medicine. These caretaking dynamics contribute to making individuals into excellent, caring physicians. These same dynamics make it very important for providers to establish clear boundaries between work and family life to offset a tendency to get overinvolved with patients, patients' families, and work issues in general. Personal anxiety and/or a desire to maintain power or control over people can result in such overinvolvement (1). A clear sense of boundaries prevents this problem and supports the healthy dynamics that lead an individual to choose a career in primary care medicine. In this chapter, we will discuss several different aspects of managing personal and professional boundaries, including recognizing when one's own family of origin or one's own current family issues are impacting a patient encounter in a positive way and when to refer a patient to a colleague because of the potential negative effects of personal issues. We will also discuss the importance of role clarity in shifting from being a physician to being a spouse or family member, and vice versa, and provide some warning signals for problems in this area.

Physicians' Family of Origin Issues

A physician's past and current personal issues can be either a major resource or a profound hindrance in the doctor-patient relationship. Styles of caretaking and authority as well as tolerance for affect are all learned in our families of origin. Many physicians are able to use their past experiences to enhance their empathy and their credibility with patients. However, current problems or unresolved struggles from the past can cloud or distort our perceptions of patients and their families. Utilizing personal issues as a resource depends on being able to recognize these issues when they occur in our work. When the physician recognizes that a patient or family is stimulating an important personal issue, the physician then has the opportunity to decide whether to treat, collaborate with a colleague, or refer.

> Dr. Bayer came from a family of high achievers and heavy drinkers. When her parents divorced during her adolescence, she began attending Ala-Teen while her mother attended Al-Anon. After his second marriage, her father finally entered alcohol treatment and began attending AA regularly. Alcoholism had caused her much pain in the past and became an area of interest to her as a physician. She read articles and sought supervision during residency for patient problems that involved alcoholism. Drawing on her experience with her own family, supervision helped her recognize that alcoholic patients and their families were the only people who could decide to change the problem. Dr. Bayer saw her role as assessing the problem and providing advice and support. By using her personal experience and professional training to great advantage, she became known for her skill in evaluating alcoholic families and eventually getting them into treatment. She felt great pride and satisfaction in helping these patients and became a referral source for colleagues who recognized they did not have the same skills.
>
> Dr. Lane, by contrast, always had difficulty with her alcoholic patients. Her father was also a drinker. She suspected that his drinking contributed to the loud arguments and occasional physical fighting that still characterized her parents' marriage. Her father denied he was a "problem drinker" because he said he drank half as much as his own father who "did have a problem." Dr. Lane drank very little herself as did her husband, but her husband smoked marijuana on a daily basis because "it helps me relax." Dr. Lane found herself very interested in getting her alcoholic patients into treatment but felt she was never successful. She told her colleagues: "Alcoholics never change. There's no point in wasting your breath trying to convince them."

In this first example, Dr. Bayer was able to recognize and understand alcoholism clearly. She knew what she could contribute as a physician and what the patient and family would have to go through themselves.

She also had respect for the difficulty of the process. All these factors helped to make her comfortable working with alcoholic patients whether they were actively drinking or working to stay sober. Dr. Lane, on the other hand, was not clear how substance abuse had affected her own life. This same confusion occurred when trying to evaluate patients and whether or not they had a problem with drinking. Eventually, she became pessimistic about the potential for change, just as her own personal experience remained unchanged. For personal issues to be a resource, it is vital that the physician be able to recognize when an issue can be used to enhance professional skills (as with Dr. Bayer) and when it is unresolved (as with Dr. Lane). We all have issues in the latter category, and when patient problems overlap with them it is important to either refer, collaborate, or seek consultation. We do not do ourselves or our patients a service by treating them in isolation when our own unresolved personal experiences are a factor in their care.

A physician may be able to understand a particular problem in depth because of being personally familiar with it; on the other hand, the physician may not perceive a patient accurately because that patient reminds him or her of the physician's own family member. Recognizing when a patient or family triggers a personal issue for the provider is not always easy and requires sensitivity and experience. Each individual provider will have a set of idiosyncratic signals that alert him or her to a personally relevant dynamic occurring during an interview. The following are generic **signals that a patient or family may be activating a personal issue for the physician:**

1. **Becoming overinvolved** with a particular patient or family.
   - routinely having longer than usual sessions with this patient
   - allowing this patient or family easier access than is typical for you – e.g., allowing them to call you at home or interrupt you with another patient
   - your own family members complaining about this patient's behavior because it is pervading your own family life
2. **Being underinvolved** with a particular patient or family.
   - expanding the time between patient sessions because you would rather not see a patient
   - not returning a patient or family member's phone call
   - routinely asking your secretary or nurse practitioner to "take care of the problem"
3. **Undue pessimism** that people can change a particular problem behavior.
4. A strong **feeling that a patient must change** a particular problem behavior.
5. **Prescribing the same treatment or "educating" a patient over and over again** in spite of the fact that it is not working.

6. Feeling reluctant to see a particular patient when you see his or her name on the schedule sheet.

7. Confusion about why your treatment is not working with this particular patient when it typically works with others.

8. Over-medicalizing or intellectualizing when discussing a patient's illness or problem.

9. Boredom, anger, or sadness with a patient or family out of proportion to the patient's problem.

In the next examples, the first physician, Dr. Holmes, is able to recognize and utilize the signals that he is overreacting to the family while the second physician, Dr. Smith, does not attend to these signals and loses her patient.

> Dr. Holmes felt particularly badly about having to tell a long-time patient that he had terminal cancer. Just after finishing with this patient and his family, he noticed that Mrs. Gerber was next on his schedule. His stomach twitched, and he wondered if he was getting a headache. Mrs. Gerber was a demanding patient who made Dr. Holmes feel as if he never gave her enough. "I wonder what her complaint will be today," he thought. Sure enough, Mrs. Gerber looked irritated when he walked in the room. "What took you so long?" she asked. Dr. Holmes found himself wanting to say, "I had someone with a *real* illness to deal with." Instead, he said, "I'm sorry. We get backed up here from time to time. What can I do for you today?" After the session, while reflecting on his day, Dr. Holmes wondered why Mrs. Gerber got to him so much. While discussing it with his partner, he realized Mrs. Gerber made him feel the way he used to with his mother: no matter what he did, he couldn't please her. And perhaps for the same reason: as an adult Dr. Holmes had come to realize that his mother had a longstanding underlying depression. Now he began to wonder about Mrs. Gerber's psychosocial situation, how much support she had, and whether she might have a clinical depression. He decided to do a more in-depth evaluation of her mental status and her affect and try to involve her family and friends in the evaluation to test her support network. After the conversation with his colleague, Dr. Holmes realized he was actually looking forward to the next session with Mrs. Gerber because he was curious to find out what was driving her unhappiness.
>
> Dr. Smith had the reputation of being a caring, effective physician. She was responsible and responsive, though she did not have many friends. Dr. Smith did a lot of counseling in her practice. Though she did not enjoy it much, she felt it was part of her job as a doctor and she also was convinced that few patients would accept a referral to a mental health specialist. Today she had to see a patient in the ICU who had come very close to overdosing on the antidepressant Dr. Smith had prescribed for her. The overdose surprised Dr. Smith. She had been doing individual counseling with this young housewife for four months and had described the patient in her chart as "bright and sensible." At the hospital, the patient told her that she had had another argument with her husband, become frustrated, and "wanted a way out." Dr. Smith decided this woman was more impulsive than she had realized, and

bluntly told her in the hospital that she needed to see a psychiatrist. The patient was offended by Dr. Smith's abruptness. She decided Dr. Smith did not truly understand how miserable she felt, and she switched to another primary care physician.

Without realizing it, Dr. Smith was repeating a pattern established in her own family of origin. When she was 10, her own mother had committed suicide after several counseling sessions with her internist. The family had handled this death by trying to "move on." Dr. Smith's father remarried quickly and her mother was rarely discussed in family gatherings. Dr. Smith worked hard to take care of her brother and sister. She felt she had adapted to this tragedy as well as possible, but in fact she had little support and had spoken to virtually no one about the loneliness and confusion that plagued her memories of her mother. Instead, Dr. Smith poured herself into her work and was vulnerable to taking on too much counseling, too much responsibility with patients, and not recognizing patients at high risk for major depression or suicide.

Most providers find that utilizing personal issues as a resource requires trusted colleagues with whom to discuss challenging cases. Balint groups (2), and their latter-day offshoots that utilize a family perspective (3,4) offer a vehicle to physicians to explore their own personal issues vis-a-vis clinical cases. Some of these groups use both the patient's and the physician's genogram as tools to discover any similarities that may be meaningful in the doctor-patient relationship. Several family-oriented primary care physicians have recommended that physicians use a Bowenian approach (5) to work on their own family of origin issues as a method of becoming more effective professionally (6–8).

The Physician's Current Family Issues

Issues in the physician's current family life can also be either a resource or a problem for patient care.

Dr. Orion's parents visited her for the first time in her new home soon after the arrival of her first child. Because Dr. Orion practiced obstetrics, she was prepared for the joy, the physical pain, and the fatigue that accompanied having a child. She was not, however, prepared for what happened when her parents visited. Her parents were clearly delighted at the arrival of their first grandchild, however her mother could not stop telling her what to do with the baby. No matter what Dr. Orion did with her baby, her mother had a better way to do it. After breathing a sigh of relief at her parents' departure, Dr. Orion returned to patient care and found herself interested in how new parents negotiated the change in their relationship with their own parents. She collaborated with a family therapist on a study of the relationship between new parents, grandparents, and infant morbidity. She also developed clinical guidelines for patients to obtain support and guidance from their own parents, either before or soon after the delivery of their first child. Dr. Orion tested the guidelines by applying them to her relationship with her own parents and recognizing them in their new role as grandparents.

While Dr. Orion was able to use her own experience to be helpful to her patients, Dr. Waters found himself discontent and overwhelmed with patients whose problems resembled his own.

Dr. Waters felt drained and tired at the end of each workday. He realized that ever since he and his wife had been discussing separation, his tolerance for hearing about patients' marital problems was very low. One female patient that he had previously enjoyed working with now seemed demanding and needy. She complained her husband did not listen to her and cared more about work than he did about her, complaints amazingly close to those of Dr. Waters' own wife. Dr. Waters continued to see this patient, though he spaced her appointments out as much as she would tolerate.

All personal experiences have the potential of enriching our professional lives. However, private stresses and struggles that are occurring in the moment, and so by definition are unresolved, run the biggest risk of leading to difficulties in the doctor–patient relationship. A trusted colleague or a Balint-like group can be very helpful in sorting out these issues. It is important to us and to our patients that we give ourselves permission to collaborate or refer when patients' problems hit "too close to home."

Studies have shown physicians to have particular difficulty with depression and substance abuse (9–11). Additionally, they are susceptible to having problems in their own marriages related to workaholism, or what Gerber calls being "married to their careers" (12). Several **strategies** are important **to help the physician deal with current family problems:**

- develop a willingness to seek help oneself when it is needed,
- develop a lifestyle that provides a balance between work and personal life,
- establish appropriate boundaries between work and home life, so that some time is protected for personal and family needs to be met without the intrusion of patients, and
- develop clarity about when one is in a professional role, with the challenges and rewards of being a professional, and when one is in a family role, with the challenges and rewards of being a family member.

Role Clarity:
To Be or Not to Be Your Own Family's Physician

A natural facet of being a family member is caring about the health and well-being of loved ones. This function is somewhat complicated when one or more family members is a professional health provider. When and how much to use one's professional expertise with family members can be a challenging issue. Many families consciously or unconsciously train their children to be caretakers of some kind. It is quite natural then, when one does become a health care provider, to feel some conflict about how much to take care of one's own family's medical concerns. In any given situation if a provider decides to be his or her own family's physician, that role allows the physician to express concern and caring through using medical skills and it allows the patient/family member to feel cared about . . . until there is a bad outcome. Then, the physician and the family will question the medical decision-making process and an undue amount of guilt and responsibility may become part of the already complex relationships between the physician and his or her family. If the physician refuses to use his or her special expertise with family members, the patient/family member may feel uncared for or abandoned and the physician may feel badly about not being "helpful" in an area where he or she does have some special skill.

Being clear about whether one is functioning as a professional or as a family member is essential to resolving this dilemma. It is difficult to develop the neutrality and distance necessary to make clear diagnoses and implement potentially difficult treatment plans if one is a family member of the patient, and it is difficult to allow oneself to advocate for and care deeply about a family member if one is responsible for his or her medical care. One solution is to develop a relationship with a respected primary care physician who is outside the family. Turning to this person frees the physician to enjoy the family member role, yet have confidence that the patient is receiving quality medical care.

Without a clear distinction between the roles of health care provider and family member, it is easy for the physician to become either overinvolved or underinvolved in the family member's medical care. Some physicians may characteristically overfunction in their professional role, so that they tend to become overinvolved in the medical care of family members. In this situation, it is easy to avoid important emotional issues by intellectualizing or medicalizing about a loved one's condition. Others may underfunction and not provide concern or support unless a family member has a "truly serious" illness. Either problem is dangerous because it results in the physician underfunctioning as a family member. Every physician needs to examine his or her style, philosophy, and practice setting and consciously set boundaries with regard to dealing with family medical issues. The specifics of these boundaries will vary from individual to individual. Some practice settings with few physicians, such as those in rural settings, make setting boundaries more challenging though all the more important. The following are general **warning signs of overinvolvement with your own family's medical concerns,** signs of slipping into the difficult role of being your own family's physician:

1. When you counsel or advise family members about some health issue more than one time.

- when you give frequent advice about some family member's significant health concern and find that the relative is not going to his or her physician about the problem.
- when you repeatedly try to get a family member to adopt a more healthy lifestyle and change behaviors such as diet, smoking, and exercise.

2. **When you, and only you, take care of family health matters.**

   - when you are the only person who speaks to your ill family member's physician.
   - when you are the person who coordinates the care of the family member among the specialists.

3. **When you, instead of an independent physician, evaluates a family member's illness.**

   - when you do a physical exam on a family member.
   - when you order tests on a family member.
   - when you write a referral letter to have a family member evaluated further.

4. **When you treat a family member for an illness for which most people see a physician.**

   - when you write a prescription for medication for a family member.
   - when you assist in the surgery of a family member (deliver a baby, run a code, etc.).

The following is an example of a physician who became overinvolved in her grandmother's medical care.

> Dr. Rudder was raised by her grandmother after her mother died at a very early age. Her grandmother was very proud of "her granddaughter, the doctor." Soon after Dr. Rudder set up a practice as a primary care physician in a distant urban setting, her grandmother had a stroke in her rural hometown.
>
> Dr. Rudder rushed to the hometown hospital to see her grandmother and found her in the care of an older physician who she was unsure was "up to date" medically. Dr. Rudder was quite upset about her grandmother's illness and the thought that she might die, but she had difficulty focusing on these feelings. Instead, she found herself making demands of the floor nurses as if she were the attending, and strongly suggesting alternative treatment plans to her grandmother's physician. Dr. Rudder knew there was much she wanted to say to her grandmother: how she appreciated all her sacrifice in raising her, how she admired her stubborn strong will, how she loved her. But, instead, she found herself obsessed with her grandmother's medical care. Frustrated that perhaps it was not the best, Dr. Rudder suggested to her grandmother that she change physicians to one of her colleagues in residency who had opened a practice not too far away. To Dr. Rudder's disappointment and irrita-

tion, her grandmother made it clear that she had a long-term relationship with her physician, that she had complete confidence in him, and that she had no desire to change physicians at this point in time.

During the hospitalization, Dr. Rudder functioned as the primary family link to her grandmother's physician. Other family members pumped her for information and relied on her to relay any questions to her grandmother's doctor. Dr. Rudder felt trapped, unsatisfied with her role, worried about her grandmother and exhausted. Her grandmother died one week after being hospitalized.

Unfortunately, Dr. Rudder confused her role as physician with her role as family member. Her medical knowledge interfered with her being able to successfully deal with the important emotional issues that confronted her with the illness and impending death of her grandmother. Her lack of confidence in her grandmother's doctor made it that much more difficult for her to leave her medical care in his hands. As a result, she was unable to maintain a clear boundary around her most important role in this situation, that of granddaughter.

While some physicians tend to become overinvolved in family member's health issues, others respond to the same stress by becoming underinvolved. The following are **warning signs of underinvolvement with your own family's medical concerns,** signals that the rest of the family may read as a lack of caring:

1. **When you do not want to hear anything about a family member's symptoms.**
2. **When you never comment on or discuss the medical issues of a family member.**
3. **When you do not provide support or sympathy for the everyday symptoms or aches and pains of family members.**
4. **When you avoid contact or conversation with the ill family member.**

The following is an example of a physician who was underinvolved in his children's lives.

Dr. Christopher had a style his patients likened to Marcus Welby. He was always available to them, morning, noon, and night. They worshiped him, and even stopped his children on the street to tell them what a wonderful man he was. His family was organized around supporting Dr. Christopher's dedication to his job. His wife ran the household and raised the children. His children were used to the fact that he rarely came to their baseball games or school plays. They also knew that unless they had some dire illness or injury, their father was unlikely to show much concern. "He sees so much serious illness, he knows this is not a problem," their mother would tell them. Unfortunately, his children grew up not realizing their father's loneliness or the depth of feeling he had for them.

Under- or overinvolvement in family member's medical concerns can lead to personal pain and interpersonal difficulty. Conscious decisions about boundaries between work and family life make a balanced lifestyle more likely.

Conclusion

Family-oriented primary care begins at home. Physicians' unresolved past or current personal problems play a role in their diagnosis and management of patients, either wittingly or unwittingly. Stephens, in an essay that called for physicians to examine their personal and societal stands regarding the family, said: "Let us boldly become more 'pro family', perhaps attending first to ourselves in our own family roles" (13). The secret to successful caretaking may be the recognition that we cannot change another's behavior, rather we can only change our own. While we are responsible for professional medical care (the diagnosis and treatment), the patient remains in charge of his or her own health (reporting symptoms, collaborating in the history and exam, and final decision making regarding treatment). Patient care can benefit from physicians establishing these boundaries and focusing on changing our own behavior when needed. The dictum, "Physician, heal thyself," may be one of the most powerful therapeutic agents for any physician's patients.

References

1. Guggenbuhl-Craig A: *Power in the Helping Professions.* Irving, TX, Spring Publications, 1979.
2. Balint M: The Doctor, *His Patient, and the Illness.* New York, International Press, 1957.
3. McDaniel S, Bank J, Campbell T, Mancini J, Shore B: Using a group as a consultant, in Wynne L, McDaniel S, Weber T (eds.): *Systems Consultation: A New Perspective for Family Therapy.* New York, Guilford Publications, 1986. 4. Botelho R, McDaniel S, Jones JE: A family systems approach to a Balint-style group: An innovative CME demonstration project for primary care physicians. Submitted for publication, 1988.
5. Bowen M: Toward the differentiation of self in one's family of origin, in *Family Therapy in Clinical Practice.* New York, Jason Aronson, 1978.
6. Christie-Seely J, Fernandez R, Pardis G, Talbot Y, Turcotte R: The physician's family, in Christie-Seely J (ed.): *Working with the Family in Primary Care.* New York, Praeger, 1983.
7. Crouch M: Working with one's own family issues: A path for professional development, in Crouch M, Roberts L (eds.): *The Family in Medical Practice.* New York, Springer-Verlag, 1986.
8. Mengel M: Physician ineffectiveness due to family-of-origin issues. *Fam Syst Med* 1987;5(2):176–190.

9. Juntunen J, Asp S, Olkinuora N, Aarimaa N, Strid L, Kauttu K: Doctors' drinking habits and consumption of alcohol. *Br Med J* 1988;**297**:951–954.
10. McCue JD: The effects of stress on physicians and their medical practice. *N Engl J Med* 1982;**306**:458–463.
11. Vaillant GF, Sobowale AB, McArthur C: Some psychological vulnerabilities of physicians. *New Engl J Med* 1972;**272**:372–375.
12. Gerber L: *Married to Their Careers*. New York, Tavistock Publications, 1983.
13. Stephens G: On being "pro family" in family practice. *J Am Board Fam Prac* 1988;**1**(1):66–68.

PROTOCOL

How to Manage Personal and Professional Boundaries As a Health Care Provider

Patient care: signals that a patient or family may be activating a personal issue for the physician.

1. Becoming overinvolved with a particular patient or family.
2. Being underinvolved with a particular patient or family.
3. Undue pessimism that people can change a particular problem behavior.
4. A strong feeling that a patient must change a particular problem behavior.
5. Prescribing the same treatment or "educating" a patient over and over again in spite of the fact that it is not working.
6. Feeling reluctant to see a particular patient when you see his or her name on the schedule sheet.
7. Confusion about why your treatment is not working with this particular patient when it typically works with others.
8. Over-medicalizing or intellectualizing when discussing a patient's illness or problem.
9. Boredom, anger, or sadness with a patient or family out of proportion to the patient's problem.

Family life:
A. Warning signs of **overinvolvement** with your own family's medical concerns.

    1. When you counsel or advise family members about some health issue more than one time.
       a. when you give frequent advice about some family member's significant health concern and find that the relative is not going to his or her physician about the problem.
       b. when you repeatedly try to get a family member to adopt a more healthy lifestyle and change behaviors such as diet, smoking, and exercise.
    2. When you, and only you, take care of family health matters.
       a. when you are the only person who speaks to your family member's physician.
       b. when you are the person who coordinates the care of the family member among the specialists.
    3. When you, instead of an independent physician, evaluates a family member's illness.
       a. when you do a physical exam on a family member.

    b. when you order tests on a family member.

    c. when you write a referral letter to have a family member evaluated further.

4. When you treat a family member for an illness for which most people see a physician.

    a. when you write a prescription for medication for a family member.

    b. when you assist in the surgery of a family member (deliver a baby, run a code, etc.).

B. Warning signs of **underinvolvement** with your own family's medical concerns.

1. When you do not want to hear anything about a family member's symptoms.

2. When you never comment on or discuss the medical issues of a family member.

3. When you do not provide support or sympathy for the everyday symptoms or aches and pains of family members.

4. When you avoid contact or conversation with the ill family member.

Author Index

Subject Index

About the Authors

Susan H. McDaniel received her Ph.D. in clinical psychology from the University of North Carolina at Chapel Hill (1979). She then completed a postdoctoral fellowship in family therapy at the Texas Research Institute for the Mental Sciences in Houston, TX. Since 1980, she has been at the University of Rochester School of Medicine and Dentistry where she is now Associate Professor of Psychiatry and Family Medicine. With Dr. Campbell, she is in charge of Psychosocial Education at Family Medicine. Dr. McDaniel is also Director of the Family Therapy Training Program in Psychiatry. She is co-author of *Systems Consultation* with Lyman Wynne and Timothy Weber. She is also Book Review Editor for *Family Systems Medicine* and has published widely in this area.

Thomas L. Campbell received his undergraduate degree from Harvard College and his M.D. (1979) from Harvard Medical School. He completed his family practice residency and his fellowship in psychosomatic medicine at the University of Rochester School of Medicine and Dentistry. Since 1983, he has been Assistant Professor of Family Medicine and Psychiatry at the University of Rochester. With Dr. McDaniel, he is in charge of Psychosocial Education at Family Medicine. His interests include the role of the family in medical practice and research on the influence of the family on physical and mental health. His National Institute of Mental Health monograph, *Family's Impact on Health*, has been an influential review of the current research in this area. He is board certified in family practice and a member of the Society of Teachers of Family Medicine. Dr. Campbell has also written many articles in the area of family systems medicine.

David B. Seaburn has received masters' degrees from Boston University, School of Theology and the State University of New York at Brockport. He is currently a family therapist and faculty member in the Departments of Psychiatry and Family Medicine at the University of Rochester School of Medicine and Dentistry. Mr. Seaburn's primary interests include working with families experiencing chronic illness and teaching family medicine residents how to utilize a family systems orientation in primary care. Mr. Seaburn has published a variety of articles in the family therapy and family medicine fields.